NURSING RESEARCH USING ETHNOGRAPHY

Mary de Chesnay, PhD, RN, PMHCNS-BC, FAAN, is professor and immediate past-director of WellStar School of Nursing, Kennesaw State University, Georgia, as well as a licensed psychotherapist and a nurse–anthropologist researcher. In her private psychotherapy practice (active practice since 1973), Dr. de Chesnay has specialized in treating sexually abused and trafficked children, has developed culturally based interventions, and has taught content about vulnerable populations for many years. The third edition of Dr. de Chesnay's book, *Caring for the Vulnerable,* was published in 2012. She has also authored six book chapters and 19 journal articles. She is principal investigator (PI) or co-PI on numerous grants and has served as a consultant on research, academic, continuing education, and law enforcement projects. Recently, Dr. de Chesnay was invited to serve on the Georgia State Governor's Task Force called CSEC (Commercial Sexual Exploitation of Children). She has presented nationally and internationally in nursing and anthropology, and has published on incest and sex tourism and about applying various qualitative approaches to clinical research. She has been invited as a keynote speaker at numerous conferences including Sigma Theta Tau and the International Society of Psychiatric Nurses.

Nursing Research Using Ethnography

Qualitative Designs and Methods in Nursing

Mary de Chesnay, PhD, RN, PMHCNS-BC, FAAN

Editor

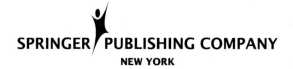

SPRINGER PUBLISHING COMPANY

NEW YORK

Springer Publishing Company, LLC
11 West 42nd Street
New York, NY 10036
www.springerpub.com

Acquisitions Editor: Joseph Morita
Production Editor: Brian Black
Composition: Exeter Premedia Services Private Ltd.

ISBN: 978-0-8261-3465-3
e-book ISBN: 978-0-8261-3466-0

14 15 16 17/ 5 4 3 2 1

The author and the publisher of this Work have made every effort to use sources believed to be reliable to provide information that is accurate and compatible with the standards generally accepted at the time of publication. The author and publisher shall not be liable for any special, consequential, or exemplary damages resulting, in whole or in part, from the readers' use of, or reliance on, the information contained in this book. The publisher has no responsibility for the persistence or accuracy of URLs for external or third-party Internet websites referred to in this publication and does not guarantee that any content on such websites is, or will remain, accurate or appropriate.

Library of Congress Cataloging-in-Publication Data
Nursing research using ethnography : qualitative designs and methods in nursing / Mary de Chesnay, editor.
   p. ; cm.
   Includes bibliographical references and index.
   ISBN 978-0-8261-3465-3—ISBN 978-0-8261-3466-0 (e-book)
   I. De Chesnay, Mary, editor.
   [DNLM: 1. Nursing Research—methods. 2. Anthropology, Cultural—methods. 3. Qualitative Research. 4. Research Design. WY 20.5]
   RT81.5
   610.73072—dc23

                                                                    2014007301

Printed in the United States of America by Gasch Printing.

QUALITATIVE DESIGNS AND METHODS IN NURSING

Mary de Chesnay, PhD, RN, PMHCNS-BC, FAAN, Series Editor

For Kathleen Logan Martin, first a teacher and always a friend.
—MdC

CONTENTS

Contributors

Mary E. Abrums, RN, MN, MA, PhD, is a sociocultural anthropologist and an associate professor in the Nursing and Health Studies Program at the University of Washington, Bothell. Her ethnographic and life history narrative research with poor and working-class African American women is published in a book titled *Moving the Rock: Poverty and Faith in a Black Storefront Church*. Her teaching and research focuses on culture, diversity, and disparity in health and health care.

Mary Applegate, MN, The chapter in this text represents the master's research of Mary Applegate under the direction of Dr. Janice Morse. Financial support was provided by the Alberta Foundation for Nursing Research, the Alberta Association of Registered Nurses, and by an NHRDP/MRC Research Scholar Award to Dr. Morse.

Nana Yaa Boadu, MPH, is a PhD candidate at the School of Public Health, University of Alberta, Edmonton, Canada. She has a master of public health degree from Emory University in Atlanta, Georgia, and a bachelor of science (BSc, biochemistry) from the University of Ghana. Her PhD program was funded through Alberta Innovates-Health Solutions (AIHS), formerly Alberta Heritage Foundation for Medical Research (AHFMR). Nana's doctoral research involves a focused ethnography to investigate guideline compliance for malaria management in Ghana. She is a 2011 doctoral research awardee of the International Development Research Center (IDRC) in Ottawa, Ontario, Canada. Nana is jointly supervised by Dr. Stephanie Yanow and Dr. Gina Higginbottom. Her research interests include health system strengthening, policy development, and primary care delivery in limited-resource settings.

Joan L. Bottorff, PhD, RN, FCAHS, FAAN, is professor of nursing at the University of British Columbia, Okanagan campus, faculty of Health and Social Development. She is the director of the Institute for Healthy Living and Chronic Disease Prevention at the University of British Columbia.

Pamela J. Brink, RN, PhD (Anthropology), FAAN, is professor emeritus (nursing and anthropology) at the University of Alberta. A founding member and past president of the Council of Nursing and Anthropology, she is the founder, and has been editor for 25 years, of the *Western Journal of Nursing Research.* Author of an early text in nursing and anthropology (*Nursing and Anthropology: A Book of Readings*) and two texts in nursing research, her anthropology research was conducted on a Native American reservation, in a mountain county in southeastern Kentucky, and in Eastern Nigeria. Her other research projects have been on inpatient heroin addicts and successful dieters.

Mary de Chesnay, PhD, RN, PMHCNS-BC, FAAN, is professor of nursing at Kennesaw State University and secretary of the Council on Nursing and Anthropology (CONAA) of the Society for Applied Anthropology (SFAA). She has conducted ethnographic fieldwork and participatory action research in Latin America and the Caribbean. She has taught qualitative research at all levels in the United States and abroad in the roles of faculty, head of a department of research, dean, and endowed chair.

Gina Marie Awoko Higginbottom, PhD, RN, RM, RHV, is professor and Canada Research Chair in Ethnicity and Health and professor in the Faculty of Nursing at the University of Alberta. Gina's research portfolio focuses on ethnic minority populations and immigrant health using participatory models of research and ethnography. Her particular focus is on the broad issue of social exclusion and equity in health care and lay understanding of health and illness. A second theme in her research portfolio has focused on maternal health and well-being including parenting issues, early parenthood, and postnatal depression in different ethnic minority groups. Gina has concluded as principal investigator in 22 nationally and internationally funded qualitative research studies, and currently holds three Canadian Institute for Health grants. Gina is assistant editor of the *Ethnicity and Health* journal and co-chair of the International Institute for Qualitative Methodology (IIQM)'s 2013 Thinking Qualitatively Conference and an Affiliate Scholar of IIQM as well as an advisory board member of IIQM. Gina is an experienced educator with a professional teaching qualification who has facilitated many undergraduate, graduate, and doctoral programs in the United Kingdom and Canada. Her forthcoming text, *Using Participatory Research Methods in Qualitative Health Research,* is scheduled for publication in 2014.

Carol Holtz, PhD, RN, is a professor of nursing, teaching at Kennesaw State University for the past 32 years. She is the editor and author of Jones and Bartlett's first and second editions of *Global Health Care*, past member and vice chair of the Cobb County, Georgia, Board of Health and the Cobb County Community Services Board for 14 years. She teaches undergraduate and doctoral nursing students at her institution, and is a member of the Scholar's Group of the International Transcultural Nursing Society. Her recently published research projects use both qualitative and quantitative methodologies addressing HIV/AIDS in indigenous women in rural Oaxaca, Mexico.

Diane Keen, MSN, RN, CNE, is a lecturer at Kennesaw State University (KSU) and a student in the doctorate of nursing science program at KSU. She teaches in community health, and her field of research is intergenerational relationships between older adults and young adults with developmental disabilities.

Ditsapelo M. McFarland, PhD, RN, RM, is an associate professor at the Adelphi University College of Nursing and Public Health, Garden City, New York. The focus of her research is screening of the cervix for cancer in women in Botswana, Africa. She has conducted both qualitative and quantitative research in this area. She has also taught a research course at both the University of Botswana and Adelphi University. She has received two grants to support her research on cancer of the cervix, one from the University of Botswana and the other from Adelphi University. She is currently a chairperson of the research council at the Adelphi University College of Nursing. She has reviewed doctoral and master's theses for foreign as well as local universities.

Mikki Meadows-Oliver, PhD, RN, is an associate professor of nursing at Yale University in New Haven, Connecticut. She has conducted qualitative research with a variety of women such as adolescent mothers, foster mothers, and homeless mothers. She has conducted meta-ethnographies of qualitative research on homeless adult mothers and homeless adolescent mothers.

Jeri A. Milstead, PhD, RN, NEA-BC, FAAN, is dean and professor emerita, University of Toledo College of Nursing. She has worked in the public policy arena as advisor to a U.S. senator, teaches policy to doctoral and master's students of nursing, and serves actively on boards, task forces, and committees in the public and private sectors. She has conducted research and consultation in The Netherlands, China, Jordan, Nicaragua, and Cuba. She is editor and senior author of *Health Policy and Politics: A Nurse's Guide*, Fifth ed. (in process).

Janice M. Morse, PhD, FAAN, is professor and the Barnes Presidential Chair, in the College of Nursing, University of Utah, and professor emerita, University of Alberta. She was the founding director and scientific director of the International Institute for Qualitative Methodology, University of Alberta, and founding editor for the *International Journal of Qualitative Methods.* She is the founding editor for *Qualitative Health Research.* From 1998 to 2007 she served as editor for the Qual Press, and is currently editor for the series Developing Qualitative Inquiry and the Basics of Qualitative Inquiry. She is a recipient of the Lifetime Achievement in Qualitative Inquiry from the International Congress for Qualitative Inquiry (2011), was awarded the International Nurse Researcher Hall of Fame, Episteme Award (Sigma Theta Tau), and was awarded honorary doctorates from the University of Newcastle (Australia) and Athabasca University (Canada). She is the author of 370 articles and 23 books on qualitative research methods, suffering, comforting, and patient falls.

Tommie Nelms, PhD, RN, is professor of nursing at Kennesaw State University. She is director of the WellStar School of Nursing and coordinator of the Doctor of Nursing Science program. She has a long history of conducting and directing phenomenological research and has been a student of Heideggerian philosophy and research for many years. Her research is mainly focused on practices of mothering, caring, and family.

Leslie K. Robbins, PhD, RN, PMHNP-BC, PMHCNS-BC, is an associate professor and the assistant dean of graduate education and director of the doctor of nursing practice program in the School of Nursing at the University of Texas at El Paso. She holds the J. Edward and Helen M. C. Stern Endowed Professorship in Nursing. She also has an adjunct faculty position in the Interdisciplinary Health Sciences PhD program in which she teaches qualitative research courses. Dr. Robbins has chaired many PhD students' qualitative research dissertations. She has conducted qualitative research with women in recovery from alcohol abuse, women who are homeless, and women affected by mental health issues. She is both a psychiatric mental health nurse practitioner and a clinical nurse specialist and maintains a part-time practice that focuses on women's issues.

Carl Ross, PhD, FNP-BC, CNE, is a university professor of nursing and coordinator of international programs at Robert Morris University School of Nursing and Health Sciences. He has conducted qualitative research utilizing ethnographic fieldwork and participatory action research in Nicaragua, where he has made over 80 trips. Dr. Ross is a practicing family nurse practitioner and currently runs a men's health clinic in Nicaragua. He has directed many doctor of nursing practice students' capstones utilizing qualitative methods.

Joanne K. Singleton, PhD, RN, APRN, FNP-BC, FNAP, FNYAM, is a professor of nursing at Pace University, College of Health Professions, Lienhard School of Nursing, chairperson for the department of graduate studies, and doctor of nursing practice program director. She has conducted ethnographic fieldwork in the culture of nursing practice, and qualitative inquiry in nursing and health care. She is a past director of an International Institute of Qualitative Methods Cooperating site and has taught and advised on qualitative research at the master's and doctoral levels.

FOREWORD

What can ethnography, developed as a field method from anthropology, offer nursing? Ethnography emerged as a method to determine cultural perspectives, cultural differences, and to document cultural patterns of beliefs and behaviors. Many of the theories of culture underlie ethnography, only a slice of which—albeit a large slice—is pertinent to nursing.

Medical anthropologists carved their domain, examining cultural perspectives of illness causation, traditional healing practices, and traditional medicine. Recognizing its potential for nursing, Madeleine Leininger (1985) developed ethnonursing, moving the cultural gaze from cultures in the broadest sense to caring practices within cultures, including our own. And in the past 40 years, we have seen the basic strategies inherent in ethnography adapted and immersed into other qualitative methods such as grounded theory.

But what can ethnography, as a method, offer nursing? Must it be adapted and its techniques and strategies moved away from its anthropological origins? Once ethnography was the most commonly used qualitative method in nursing. Why not now?

The most obvious use for ethnography in nursing is associated with community health. The anthropological perspective of cultural groups as a comprehensive unit of analysis is very pertinent and significant as we think about healthy communities. From the time of Margaret Mead (1935/1963), ethnographic methods have been mixed method designs, enriching qualitative data with quantitative, and producing ethnographic results that permitted comparison between communities and over time. Nurses first used ethnographic methods within communities in different cultures (see Brink, this volume), but later focused on cultural phenomena that were of interest to nursing. We have seen Kay's (1982) studies of childbirth as well as Morse's ethnographies on pain and privacy (Chapter 15, this volume).

Gradually nursing (and education) moved ethnography away from the geographical community, considering the hospital (or school), or even the hospital unit (or classroom) as the unit of analysis. Germain's (1979) cancer unit quickly became such a model. For nursing, this was an important way to see the patients' perspectives of illness, and interactions with caregivers and families. About this time, culture became important, and nursing branched into transcultural care and ethnonursing (Leininger, 1985).

The next change in ethnographic methods in nursing was when people with a particular illness were considered as a cultural group for focused ethnography (Muecke, 1994). Although we treat persons with diabetes, schizophrenia, or spinal cord injuries *as if* they were defined by the common experiences that result from their diseases, this does not violate ethnographic methods. But the fact that usually a diabetic does not have interactions with other diabetics, and the isolation of each person in the study, does somewhat stretch the assumptions of ethnography. But they learn how to "act like a diabetic" from their physicians, and obtain clues from others (even their support group) about what is expected from them. Nevertheless, the ethnographic method does "work" with these studies, which has been labeled *focus ethnography* (Muecke, 1994).

Ethnographic methods are now being weakened: They have been reduced to, for instance, telephone interviews as studies that exclude the observational components. We read that researchers are using "ethnographic interviews" alone, and considering that a method. Traditional anthropologists are fighting back for richer and deeper studies, for larger samples, for observational components, for comparison, and for the inclusion of quantitative measures (Pelto, 2013).

This book goes a long way to assist in this effort of bringing ethnography back to its proper place—Mary de Chesnay is to be congratulated. Ethnography has much to offer nursing; and nursing has much to gain from ethnography.

Janice M. Morse, PhD (Nursing), PhD (Anthropology), FAAN
Professor and Presidential Research Chair
College of Nursing, University of Utah

REFERENCES

Germain, C. (1979). *The cancer unit: An ethnography*. Wakefield, MA: Nursing Resources.
Kay, M. A. (1982). *The anthropology of human birth*. Philadelphia, PA: F.A. Davis.
Leininger, M. (Ed). (1985). *Qualitative research methods in nursing*. New York, NY: Grune Stratton.

Mead, M. (1935/1963). *Sex and temperament in three primitive societies* (pp. 175–185). New York, NY: Morrow.

Muecke, M. (1994). On the evaluation of ethnographies. In J. M. Morse (Ed.), *Critical issues in qualitative research methods* (pp. 187–209). Thousand Oaks, CA: Sage.

Pelto, P. (2013). *Applied ethnography: Guidelines for field research.* Walnut Creek, CA: Left Coast Press.

SERIES FOREWORD

In this section, which is published in all volumes of the series, we discuss some key aspects of any qualitative design. This is basic information that might be helpful to novice researchers or those new to the designs and methods described in each chapter. The material is not meant to be rigid and prescribed because qualitative research by its nature is fluid and flexible; the reader should use any ideas that are relevant and discard any ideas that are not relevant to the specific project in mind.

Before beginning a project, it is helpful to commit to publishing it. Of course, it will be publishable because you will use every resource at hand to make sure it is of high quality and contributes to knowledge. Theses and dissertations are meaningless exercises if only the student and committee know what was learned. It is rather heart-breaking to think of all the effort that senior faculty have exerted to complete a degree and yet not to have anyone else benefit by the work. Therefore, some additional resources are included here. Appendix A for each book is a list of journals that publish qualitative research. References to the current nursing qualitative research textbooks are included so that readers may find additional material from sources cited in those chapters.

FOCUS

In qualitative research the focus is emic—what we commonly think of as "from the participant's point of view." The researcher's point of view, called "the etic view," is secondary and does not take precedence over what the participant wants to convey, because in qualitative research, the focus is on the person and his or her story. In contrast, quantitative researchers take pains to learn as much as they can about a topic and focus the research data collection on what they want to know. Cases or subjects that do not provide information about the researcher's agenda are considered outliers and are discarded or treated as aberrant data. Qualitative researchers embrace outliers and actively seek diverse points of view from participants to enrich the data. They sample for diversity within groups and welcome different perceptions even if they seek fairly homogenous samples. For example, in Leenerts and Magilvy's (2000) grounded theory study to examine self-care practices among women, they narrowed the study to low-income, White, HIV-positive women but included both lesbian and heterosexual women.

PROPOSALS

There are many excellent sources in the literature on how to write a research proposal. A couple are cited here (Annersten, 2006; Mareno, 2012; Martin, 2010; Schmelzer, 2006), and examples are found in Appendices B, C, and D. Proposals for any type of research should include basic elements about the purpose, significance, theoretical support, and methods. What is often lacking is a thorough discussion about the rationale. The rationale is needed for the overall design as well as each step in the process. Why qualitative research? Why ethnography and not phenomenology? Why go to a certain setting? Why select the participants through word of mouth? Why use one particular type of software over another to analyze data?

Other common mistakes are not doing justice to significance and failure to provide sufficient theoretical support for the approach. In qualitative research, which tends to be theory generating instead of theory testing, the author still needs to explain why the study is conducted from a particular frame of reference. For example, in some ethnographic work, there are hypotheses that are tested based on the work of prior ethnographers who studied that culture, but there is still a need to generate new theory about current phenomena within that culture from the point of view of the specific informants for the subsequent study.

Significance is underappreciated as an important component of research. Without justifying the importance of the study or the potential impact of the study, there is no case for why the study should be conducted. If a study cannot be justified, why should sponsors fund it? Why should participants agree to participate? Why should the principal investigator bother to conduct it?

COMMONALITIES IN METHODS

Interviewing Basics

One of the best resources for learning how to interview for qualitative research is by Patton (2002), and readers are referred to his book for a detailed guide to interviewing. He describes the process, issues, and challenges in a way that readers can focus their interview in a wide variety of directions that are flexible, yet rigorous. For example, in ethnography, a mix of interview methods is appropriate, ranging from unstructured interviews or informal conversation to highly structured interviews. Unless nurses are conducting mixed-design studies, most of their interviews will be semi-structured. Semi-structured interviews include a few general questions, but the interviewer is free to allow the interviewee to digress along any lines he or she wishes. It is up to the interviewer to bring the interview back to the focus of the research. This requires skill and sensitivity.

Some general guidelines apply to semi-structured interviews:

- Establish rapport.
- Ask open-ended questions. For example, the second question is much more likely to generate a meaningful response than the first in a grounded theory study of coping with cervical cancer.

  Interviewer: Were you afraid when you first heard your diagnosis of cervical cancer?

  Participant: Yes.

  Contrast the above with the following:

  Interviewer: What was your first thought when you heard your diagnosis of cervical cancer?

  Participant: I thought of my young children and how they were going to lose their mother and that they would grow up not knowing how much I loved them.

- Continuously "read" the person's reactions and adapt the approach based on response to questions. For example, in the interview about coping with the diagnosis, the participant began tearing so the interviewer appropriately gave her some time to collect herself. Maintaining silence is one of the most difficult things to learn for researchers who have been classically trained in quantitative methods. In structured interviewing, we are trained to continue despite distractions and to eliminate bias, which may involve eliminating emotion and emotional reactions to what we hear in the interview. Yet the quality of outcomes in qualitative designs may depend on the researcher–participant relationship. It is critical to be authentic and to allow the participant to be authentic.

Ethical Issues

The principles of the Belmont Commission apply to all types of research: respect, justice, beneficence. Perhaps these are even more important when interviewing people about their culture or life experiences. These are highly personal and may be painful for the person to relate, though I have found that there is a cathartic effect to participating in naturalistic research with an empathic interviewer (de Chesnay, 1991, 1993).

Rigor

Readers are referred to the classic paper on rigor in qualitative research (Sandelowski, 1986). Rather than speak of validity and reliability we use other terms, such as accuracy (Do the data represent truth as the participant sees it?) and replicability (Can the reader follow the decision trail to see why the researcher concluded as he or she did?).

DATA ANALYSIS

Analyzing data requires many decisions about how to collect data and whether to use high-tech measures such as qualitative software or old-school measures such as colored index cards. The contributors to this series provide examples of both.

Mixed designs require a balance between the assumptions of quantitative research while conducting that part and qualitative research during that phase. It can be difficult for novice researchers to keep things straight. Researchers are encouraged to learn each paradigm well and to be clear about why they use certain methods for their purposes. Each type of design can stand alone, and one should never think that qualitative research is *less than* quantitative; it is just different.

Mary de Chesnay

REFERENCES

Annersten, M. (2006). How to write a research proposal. *European Diabetes Nursing*, 3(2), 102–105.

de Chesnay, M. (1991, March 13–17). *Catharsis: Outcome of naturalistic research*. Presented to Society for Applied Anthropology, Charleston, SC.

de Chesnay, M. (1993). Workshop with Dr. Patricia Marshall of Symposium on Research Ethics in Fieldwork. Sponsored by Society for Applied Anthropology, Committee on Ethics. Memphis, March 25–29, 1992; San Antonio, Texas, March 11–14, 1993.

Leenerts, M. H., & Magilvy, K. (2000). Investing in self-care: A midrange theory of self-care grounded in the lived experience of low-income HIV-positive white women. *Advances in Nursing Science*, 22(3), 58–75.

Mareno, N. (2012). Sample qualitative research proposal: Childhood obesity in Latino families. In M. de Chesnay & B. Anderson (Eds.), *Caring for the vulnerable* (pp. 203–218). Sudbury, MA: Jones and Bartlett.

Martin, C. H. (2010). A 15-step model for writing a research proposal. *British Journal of Midwifery*, 18(12), 791–798.

Patton, M. Q. (2002). *Qualitative research and evaluation methods* (3rd ed.). Thousand Oaks, CA: Sage.

Sandelowski, M. (1986). The problem of rigor in qualitative research. *Advances in Nursing Science*, 4(3), 27–37.

Schmelzer, M. (2006). How to start a research proposal. *Gastroenterology Nursing*, 29(2), 186–188.

PREFACE

Qualitative research has evolved from a slightly disreputable beginning to wide acceptance in nursing research. Approaches that focus on the stories and perceptions of people, instead of what scientists think the world is about, have been a tradition in anthropology for a long time and have created a body of knowledge that cannot be replicated in the lab. The richness of human experience is what qualitative research is all about. Respect for this tradition was long in coming among the scientific community. Nurses seem to have been in the forefront, though, and though many of my generation (children of the 1950s and 1960s) were classically trained in quantitative techniques, we found something lacking. Perhaps because I am a psychiatric nurse, I have been trained to listen to people tell me their stories, whether the stories are problems that nearly destroy the spirit, or uplifting accounts of how they live within their cultures, or how they cope with terrible traumas and chronic diseases. It seems logical to me that a critical part of developing new knowledge that nurses can use to help patients is to find out first what the patients themselves have to say.

In the first volume of this series, the focus is on ethnography, in many ways the grandparent of qualitative research. Subsequent volumes address grounded theory, life history, phenomenology, historical research, participatory action research, and data analysis. The volume on data analysis also includes material on focus groups and case studies, and two types of research that can be used with a variety of designs, including quantitative research and mixed designs. Efforts have been made to recruit contributors from several countries to demonstrate global applicability of qualitative research.

There are many fine textbooks on nursing research that provide an overview of all the methods, but our aim here is to provide specific information to guide graduate students or experienced nurses who are novices in the designs represented in this series in conducting studies from the point of view of our constituents—patients and their families. The studies conducted by contributors provide much practical advice for beginners as well as new ideas for experienced researchers. Some authors take a formal approach, but others speak quite personally in the first person. We hope you catch their enthusiasm and have fun conducting your own studies.

Mary de Chesnay

ACKNOWLEDGMENTS

In any publishing venture, there are many people who work together to produce the final draft. The contributors kindly shared their expertise to offer advice and counsel to novices, and the reviewers ensured the quality of submissions. All of them have come up through the ranks as qualitative researchers and their participation is critical to helping novices learn the process.

No publication is successful without great people who not only know how to do their own jobs but also how to guide authors. At Springer Publishing Company, we are indebted to Margaret Zuccarini for the idea for the series, her ongoing support and her excellent problem-solving skills. The person who guided the editorial process and was available for numerous questions, which he patiently answered as if he had not heard them a hundred times, was Joseph Morita. Also critical to the project were the people who proofed the work, marketed the series, and transformed it into hard copies, among them Chris Teja.

At Kennesaw State University, Dr. Tommie Nelms, director of the WellStar School of Nursing, was a constant source of emotional and practical support in addition to her chapter contribution to the phenomenology volume. Her administrative assistant, Mrs. Cynthia Elery, kindly assigned student assistants to complete several chores, which enabled the author to focus on the scholarship. Bradley Garner, Chadwick Brown, and Chino Duke are our student assistants and unsung heroes of the university.

Finally, I am grateful to my cousin, Amy Dagit, whose expertise in proofreading saved many hours for some of the chapters. Any mistakes left are mine alone.

> I want to understand the world from your point of view. I want to know what you know in the way you know it. I want to understand the meaning of your experience, to walk in your shoes, to feel things as you feel them, to explain things as you explain them. Will you become my teacher and help me understand?
>
> —James P. Spradley in *You Owe Yourself a Drunk: An Ethnography of Urban Nomads*

CHAPTER ONE

OVERVIEW OF ETHNOGRAPHY

Mary de Chesnay

*I*n the first volume of this series, we examine ethnography as a research design of particular relevance to nursing. To many scholars, nothing is more fascinating than the study of culture, the life-ways of a people. In particular, practicing nurses might find this field of inquiry a rich source of ways to help us make patients more comfortable as they experience a variety of illnesses and injuries for which they seek treatment. Developing an understanding of some of the differences among cultures in terms of social rules, values, and interaction styles can help nurses work more effectively with people from cultures different from their own. In the days of cultural competence for applied fields such as ours, this is even more important than knowledge for its own sake.

Working effectively with people who are different from ourselves is the essence of cultural competence. For example, knowing that the Navajo may consider it rude to look people directly in the eye when conversing, we would not interpret their behavior as avoidance or resistance (Charlene, personal communication, 1975; Chiang, 1993).

Knowing that Chinese women consider pregnancy to be a "hot" condition, helps us understand why they may prefer cold foods during pregnancy; and knowing they consider childbirth a "cold" condition, we understand why they prefer to eat hot foods during the postpartum period (Brathwaite & Williams, 2004; Liang, personal communication, 2000). However, there is a danger in considering these tidbits of cultural knowledge to be sufficient when working with patients or clients of different cultures. People are members of cultures, but they are also individuals and may or may not subscribe or adhere to the rules and norms of their own culture. In this sense, the patient is the best guide to what is appropriate for that person or family.

To be culturally competent is to work effectively with people of different lifestyles, whether these lifestyles are derived from ethnicity (African American, Anglo-Caribbean), country of origin (Brazil, Taiwan, Somalia), job (truck driving, factory worker), profession (medicine, law, nursing), or other life condition (prostituted children, alcoholic, victim of violent crime, gang member). It is not practical for most nurses to become knowledgeable about all the diverse cultures represented in the world or even in our own countries, but it is feasible to learn a few things about the major cultures represented in the communities in which we practice.

The work of ethnographers, who study cultures intensively over time, is disseminated in many forms such as books, articles, and the Internet. Ethnographic material is readily available to all who can access the Internet or who work with people who represent those cultures. Two resources that are particularly valuable are the Human Relations Area Files (HRAF) archived at Yale University (www.yale.edu/hraf) and the website organized by the University of Washington–Seattle called Ethnomed (www.ethnomed.org). HRAF is a compilation of ethnographic reports collected over many years by traditional ethnographers who lived in the cultures described. Ethnomed was a project of the University of Washington to describe the health needs and beliefs of the people from those cultures represented in the Seattle area.

Some nurses want more depth and breadth of knowledge about diverse cultures whether to increase knowledge for its own sake or to become better practitioners. Some believe that, to be a good practitioner, one must understand culture if only to move beyond our own ethnocentric biases when working with people who do not share our biases. To *do* ethnography as one's research methodology choice is the focus of this book. From the background and history of the methodology to the state of art in nursing, the contributors to this volume present a thorough picture of how to conduct an ethnographic study in nursing. The book is designed to help both novice researchers and those experienced in other designs use the techniques of ethnography to expand their skills in conducting significant research that benefits patients.

OVERVIEW OF ETHNOGRAPHY

Philosophical Derivation

Ethnography is the research design of anthropology, though adopted by sociologists, educators, nurses, and others interested in the culture and social interactions of groups. The primary method is fieldwork, which consists of intense periods of living with the people being studied. The ethnographer observes, participates in varying degrees depending on purpose and context, interviews key cultural informants who can teach about their culture, and reviews any other material that seems relevant to the purpose of the study. Other material might include the arts, news reports, written records, or, in more primitive societies without written language, stories told by the elders. For example, during my doctoral fieldwork in Jamaica, I had trouble initially with being on time everywhere and having to wait for others to arrive. I mentioned this (actually I complained about it) to a Jamaican friend with whom I had lunch, and she immediately laughed and invited me to a local play in Kingston, called *8 o'clock Jamaica Time*. The joke was that the curtain rose at 8:30. This simple experience taught me the different priorities of the people I would later meet and the need to meet them where they were figuratively and not where I thought they should be according to my own ethnocentric bias.

One of the first things that many ethnographers do when visiting for the first time is to map the community of interest. Simple mapping involves drawing a picture of the community with key buildings, homes of participants, schools, offices, shops, parks, and so on. Orienting the placement of key structures in the community is useful when conducting participatory action research or community-based action research such as the project described by Aronson, Wallis, O'Campo, Whitehead, and Schafer (2007) in the evaluation of the Baltimore City Healthy Start Program. This federally funded program provides services designed to prevent infant mortality, and the research team was interested in documenting its effectiveness in three low-income neighborhoods. Mapping allowed them to see relationships within and among the three neighborhoods.

A more sophisticated example of the use of mapping involved using geographic information systems (GIS) to map the structures and streets of Darwin, Australia (Brennan-Horley, Luckman, Gibson, & Willoughby-Smith, 2010). In addition to the high-tech GIS, the team also included maps handwritten by participants that showed perceptions of interviewees about the relationships among people and places. The results of the study showed that the creative people themselves preferred the natural environment of the city over the creative spaces designed for that purpose. Nurses, who have had to live with architectural designs for hospitals that did not involve nurses in the planning stages, can identify with how important it is to obtain stakeholder input.

Participant observation as a qualitative method is dominant in cultural anthropology, whereas surveys and other quantitative methods are particularly useful to medical sociologists (Dougherty & Tripp-Reimer, 1985). Participant observation can be viewed as a continuum in which a researcher progresses from *observer* to *participant observer* to varying degrees to *participant*. Combined with interviews, participant observation of a variety of cultural aspects, practices, and rituals distinguishes ethnography from other qualitative methods although it can be used in other designs.

Traditional ethnographies are reports of the observation of the community as it is (Brink, 2013). No experiments are done to change the nature or amount of interactions among members. By being a participant observer, the ethnographer has an influence on the community and cannot know the community as an insider would but can gain the trust of the community to the extent that cultural informants or members of the community will teach the researcher about their culture. In contrast, critical ethnography is designed for political action and change.

Traditionally the term *cultural informant* was used to name the person who is interviewed by the ethnographer and is still widely used by anthropologists. The meaning is simply that the person informs or teaches the ethnographer about the culture. A key informant is one who has more information to offer or is more open to talking with the ethnographer and helping to guide the process. However, the term *informant* is objectionable to many because it conjures images of spies and snitches and can place the members of the culture who choose to talk with the ethnographer at risk of retaliation for revealing the secrets of the community. Modern alternatives to *cultural* or *key informant* are *participant, respondent, teacher, or coach*.

The term *subject* is inappropriate, because there are no experiments being performed on the person being interviewed. In addition, and this term may lead novices to become confused and think of ethnography as a quantitative method. Confusion about philosophical orientation may lead to awkward decisions about methods and, subsequently, errors in data analysis by creating threats to accuracy. For example, viewing ethnography as primarily a quantitative undertaking might put into place too much structure in data collection and cause the researcher to miss opportunities for learning as much as possible from the people.

Ethnographic techniques have developed over the years into highly adaptable methods for diverse purposes. Wolf (2012) presents several types of ethnographies among which are traditional, focused, mini-, micro- and maxi-ethnographies, visual, auto-ethnography, cognitive, critical, deconstructed, disrupted, performance, practitioner, reflexive, and specialist ethnographies. Because this series on qualitative research is designed for doctoral students and experienced researchers who want to use new designs, the chapter will focus on only a few main types and leave the others to investigators who want to delve more deeply into the nuances of ethnographic research.

TRADITIONAL ETHNOGRAPHY

Early Ethnographers in Anthropology

Early explorers recorded observations of the exotic places and people they met on their travels in diaries, letters home, and official reports. These might be considered ethnographic accounts because they made note of the strange customs and other cultural material discovered although field observations were not the purpose of the trips. Later, scholars went into the field for the purpose of studying cultures. Although many early ethnographers influenced modern methods and the development of anthropology as a science, this volume is not long enough to do justice to all their work. A few had a profound influence on the field and are mentioned here.

One of the earliest scholarly ethnographies was published by Malinowski (1913) after his fieldwork with the aboriginal Australians. He documented kinship patterns, family relationships, sexual relationships, and ways of obtaining a wife. Malinowski also addressed family violence in the tribes he studied. Violence of men against their wives was perceived by all, including the wife, as justice if punishment for an offense committed by the wife (e.g., adultery) or as brutality (from bad temper of the husband). Much of Malinowski's book is a discussion of his findings in comparison to those of other writers who had published their observations of the aborigines.

A physicist by training, Franz Boas is viewed as the Father of American Anthropology (Stocking, 1960). His early book on race and civilization (Boas, 1911) tackled the problem of why some civilizations were able to advance and assimilate more than others. In so doing, he maintained that race was not a matter of superiority of one race over another but rather of the development of civilizations in different ways. He later wrote books that became classic texts in modern anthropology (Boas, 1928, 1940).

Margaret Mead, a student of Boas, conducted her initial graduate fieldwork in Samoa, and the resulting publication about the sexual mores of Samoan adolescent girls caused a public stir (Mead, 1928). She later published an account of her fieldwork in New Guinea (Mead, 1930). Mead chose to study adolescent girls both for practical reasons (she was a young woman and could more easily develop rapport with them) and because there was a lack of ethnographic material on women (parallel to the lack of women ethnographers). The following passage captures the essence of fieldwork and why it is necessary to immerse oneself in the community in order to understand it.

I did something very different from what I would do if I concentrated upon a study of the adolescent girl in Kokomo, Indiana. In such a study, I would go right to the crux of the problem. I would not have to linger long over the Indiana language, the table manners or sleeping habits of my subjects, or make an exhaustive study of how they learned to dress themselves, to use the telephone, or what the concept of conscience meant in Kokomo. (Mead, 1928, p. 9)

One of the most heated controversies in anthropology was the failed attempt to debunk Mead's work by another anthropologist who criticized her methods as flawed. He claimed to have repeated field interviews with two of Mead's informants who claimed they were joking with her and exaggerated their sexual activity (Freeman, 1983). However, his interviews took place almost 20 years later, and he was a man talking to women, whereas Mead was a young woman talking with young women. Although he continued to refute Mead's work until his death, his views are not generally accepted by anthropologists as proof of Mead's fallacy.

Ruth Benedict, a student of Boas and contemporary of Mead, was one of the first professional women to hold a place in the academy of the early 20th century. Mentored by Boas, she was appointed as faculty under his leadership in the anthropology department at Columbia ("Ruth Benedict," Columbia University, n.d.) She worked with the Zuni tribe of the American Southwest and the Canadian Blackfoot tribe as apart from writing a manuscript for the War Department on Japanese culture (Benedict, 1946). Her view of culture was that of the personality of cultures; that is, we must understand the individual within his or her culture and the culture as a collection of individuals expressing their culture. Her work contributed to the argument for racial equality (Benedict, 1934).

Early Ethnographies by Nurses

The first doctoral degree in anthropology awarded to a nurse was to Madeleine Leininger, who earned a PhD from the University of Washington in the mid-1960s (Boyle & Hinrichs, 2013). While teaching at the University of Cincinnati, she met with visiting professor Margaret Mead about her concern that cultural knowledge was lacking in her discipline of psychiatric nursing. Leininger subsequently decided to study anthropology at the University of Washington, Seattle and earned the first doctoral degree in anthropology in 1965 (The Madeleine M. Leininger Collection Papers, 1953–1995). She later published a landmark book linking nursing and anthropology (Leininger, 1970) and developed her ideas about the two disciplines into a new way of looking at culture within nursing that she called transcultural nursing (Leininger, 1978). Later, as dean of nursing at the University of Colorado, she helped establish the nurse–scientist programs of the 1960s. However, Leininger departed from traditional anthropology by creating a new focus she called *ethnonursing* that linked her culture care theory with anthropological research methods (Leininger, 1997).

Traditional ethnographies that require a year or more immersed in the field (usually in remote geographic areas) are rare in nursing. The early nurse–anthropologists conducted traditional fieldwork but did not necessarily publish whole volumes of their studies as was common among anthropologists An exception was Jody Glittenberg (1994). In the discipline of anthropology, students tend to progress seamlessly from the baccalaureate to the doctoral degree. However, in nursing, students are usually required or at least strongly encouraged to practice for a year or more before entering a master's degree program. Then due to the financial burden of education, added to the fact that many nurses are the breadwinners as single parents or have children if theirs is a two-career family, they cannot take a year to go abroad for traditional fieldwork. Consequently, after the first generation of anthropologists who were first nurses, nurse–researchers tend to choose focused ethnographies. Dr. Pam Brink is one of the early nurse–anthropologists, and her reflections on a long and varied career are presented in this volume. Others in the first generation of nurse–anthropologists were Margarita Kay, Eleanor Bauwens, and Agnes Aamodt (1976), all of whom conducted traditional fieldwork. Subsequently, many other nurses have earned doctoral degrees in anthropology or used their cognate courses to "minor" in anthropology, and their work is highlighted in Chapter 2 as well as subsequent chapters by ethnographers.

CRITICAL ETHNOGRAPHY

Whereas traditional ethnography describes a culture as it is, critical ethnography is designed for change. Critical ethnography represents an evolution of ethnography with a political or activist mission (Breda, 2013). In critical ethnography, the researcher engages with the participants to bring to awareness the imbalance of power that disenfranchises marginalized people and to change the culture so the oppressed are set free (Soyini, 2005; Thomas, 1993; Thompson, 1987). This approach is appealing to nurses, whose work usually involves caring for vulnerable populations. Activism to address health disparities and reverse injustices in the system can be an important role of the nurse.

Manias and Street (2000) studied power relationships among nurses and between nurses and physicians in a critical care unit. In their analysis of their ethnographic study as an example of critical ethnography, they identified three methodological issues: researcher/participant subjectivity, the movement from empowerment to reflexivity, and the construction of one form of ethnographic "truth" (Manias & Street, 2001). To address subjectivity, they advise an ongoing evaluation by researchers and participants of the effect of the researcher on the process. The concept of empowerment implies dominant and subordinate roles with the researcher as dominant and the participants as subordinate. Language that addresses this inequity is the term *reflexivity* with the researcher as a co-participant. In this sense, reflexivity involves much sharing of material, information, and ideas between researcher and participant, not simply validation by participants of the researcher's interpretation. Finally, the concept of truth is challenged. Unlike traditional ethnography, no attempt is made to produce ethnographic reports that are "messy" and never final.

VISUAL ETHNOGRAPHY

A subspecialty in ethnography that has been developing since Mead's early work (Mead, 1995) is visual ethnography in which photos and films are used to study culture. The use of visual techniques has long been used in anthropology to help understand how people see themselves. Now in the age of digital photography, it is easy to incorporate photos and film into research as demonstrated in the chapter by Moreno in the forthcoming *Participatory Action Research* volume of this series, in which she discusses photovoice as a technique for working with communities to produce health outcomes.

There are several excellent sources on visual anthropology, and the American Anthropological Association has a subgroup on the specialty. Readers are referred to classic works by Pink (2001), Ruby (2000), and Powdermaker (1950). Pink (2008) expanded the techniques of visual ethnography to describe how visual ethnography can be used to understand how people move in their environments.

Garcia and Saewye (2007) conducted a focused ethnography with 14 Latino adolescent immigrants to elicit health perceptions and experiences in the United States. Each was given a disposable camera to take pictures that represented their lives in the United States, and a follow-up interview was conducted to discuss their impressions. Their study was the only one found in the visual ethnography literature that was conducted by nurses.

Nine Korean children living with an autistic sibling were asked to produce home movies about life with their siblings. They provided commentary in the films that was of their own choosing. A key component of the method was that the Korean children, rather than the researcher, owned their data. The investigators also used various forms of play such as finger puppets to make the data collection fun for the children. Finally their parents were interviewed about the process. Children's activities are often taken for granted and are somewhat invisible to adults; so the use of videos made by children seems a particularly interesting method when the focus is on their perceptions (Hwang & Charnley, 2010).

The tourism industry might be viewed as applied anthropology in which visual ethnography plays an important role to portray images of contemporary life in the settings of interest (Rakic & Chambers, 2009). Whereas the marketing people might want to use visual techniques to present the best of the place for attracting revenue, local governments might be more concerned with the social and political climate to attract economic development. Furthermore, using visual techniques can increase involvement in the research and yield better data (Brace-Govan, 2007).

FOCUSED ETHNOGRAPHY

Focused ethnographies are much more commonly conducted by nurses or other professionals whose major field is not anthropology or by those applied anthropologists who do contract work. Focused ethnographies are characterized by fieldwork during intense but not necessarily continuous periods of participant observation, interviews with key members of the culture who are willing to be interviewed in depth, and collection of specific data that relate to a narrower research question than in a traditional ethnography.

In a focused ethnography, the researcher looks at cultural factors within a narrower scope of inquiry rather than trying to understand the culture of a people as a whole in all its dimensions. For example, the author, as a nurse–psychotherapist, conducted a focused ethnography of Jamaican family structure (de Chesnay, 1986) to satisfy doctoral fieldwork requirements; but as a family therapist, she also wanted to understand cultural differences when treating Jamaican families in her practice in the United States. Over about 2 years, she conducted many interviews, spent hours progressing from just "hanging out" to participant observation to participating fully in activities of the family with whom she lived, but remained focused on family structure and processes.

An excellent example of a focused ethnography that took place over a long period of time (15 years with shorter periods of funding) was focused on childhood obesity, a timely topic that is receiving much attention as a result of Michelle Obama's adoption of it as her cause as First Lady. For example, Clark, Johnson, O'Connor, and Lassetter (2013) studied Latino parents' and grandparents' approaches to the childcare issues surrounding feeding and nutrition—the cultural constructions and how they acted upon these.

Wilkinson and Callister (2010) conducted a focused ethnography of Ghanian women who gave birth. The researchers, a physician and a nurse, recognized the impact on health care of the immigrants from Ghana in the United States and the need to provide culturally competent care. During a volunteer medical activity in Ghana, they interviewed 24 women who presented at the Salvation Army clinic for delivery after a period of intense participant observation at the clinic. Their findings were invaluable in helping the clinic to develop safe motherhood practices, to increase knowledge about family planning, and to implement better data-collection practices at the clinic.

Focused ethnographies are useful methods in understanding organizational culture. In a study of a pediatric critical care unit, Scott and Pollack (2008) were concerned about nurses using research to improve practice. After a period of participant observation over 7 months, they conducted interviews with 29 unit members. Four aspects of the organizational culture contributed to the lack of nursing research utilization: hierarchical structure, technology-driven bedside care, lack of appreciation for innovation, and emphasis on clinical experience.

Examples of other focused ethnographies conducted by nurses are easily found in the literature (Bland, 2007; Bull & Fitzgerald, 2006; Clabo, 2008; Cricco-Lizza, 2006; Field, 1983; Lesser, Koniak-Griffin, & Anderson, 1999; Shepherd, 2011). Many more examples can be found, and Chapter 2 includes a more thorough review of the nursing literature using ethnography.

Focused ethnographies are useful to practice disciplines other than nursing. For example, in business, anthropological approaches can clarify organizational structure and culture (Moore, 2011; Oliveiro, 2010). Qirko (2007) argues for a mixed-design approach that captures the richness of qualitative research with the generalizability of quantitative research. Marketing researchers can target specific aspects of consumer behavior.

Social work researchers have found ethnographic approaches beneficial in studying the structures and cultures of institutions, such as the paradoxical nature of residential childcare institutions, for which they are accountable (Palomares & Poveda, 2010). They can then apply their results to interventions with their client populations.

Characteristics of focused ethnographies are that they are time limited, usually do not involve extensive periods of living in the field, and have research questions that are narrower in scope than traditional ethnographies (Knoblauch, 2005). Although the duration of data collection periods is shorter, the overall data collection might involve several trips over a longer time. Focused ethnographies might focus on social interactions among people of the same cultural group as the investigator in contrast to immersion in the remote settings of traditional ethnographies, or they might involve shorter trips to remote settings. Whereas some are skeptical that focused ethnographies qualify as ethnography, it can be argued that as long as the focus is on cultural material or the context is cultural, then it is legitimate to focus the research to answer specific questions.

SUMMARY

This chapter presents an overview of ethnography as a design and offers examples of how ethnography can help nurse researchers identify cultural factors that can improve care. Whereas knowledge for its own sake is necessary and admirable, applied knowledge is needed in nursing to promote culturally relevant ways of caring for patients. As long as cultural competence is a cornerstone of practice, ethnography is a major tool for understanding culture and interacting with patients.

REFERENCES

Aamodt, A. (1976). Observations of a health and healing system in a Papago community. In M. Leininger (Ed.), *Transcultural health care: Issues and conditions* (pp. 23–36). Philadelphia, PA: F.A. Davis.

Aronson, R., Wallis, A., O'Campo, P., Whitehead, T., & Schafer, P. (2007). Ethnographically informed community evaluation: A framework and approach for evaluating community based initiatives. *Maternal and Child Health Journal, 11,* 97–109.

Benedict, R. (1934). *Patterns of culture.* New York, NY: Houghton Mifflin.

Benedict, R. (1946). *The chrysanthemum and the sword: Patterns of Japanese culture.* Rutland, VT and Tokyo, Japan: Charles E. Tuttle.

Bland, M. (2007). Betwixt and between: A critical ethnography of comfort in New Zealand residential aged care. *Journal of Clinical Nursing, 16,* 937–944.

Boas, F. (1911). *The mind of primitive man.* New York, NY: MacMillan.

Boas, F. (1928). *Anthropology and modern life.* New York, NY: W.W. Norton.

Boas, F. (1940). *Race, language, and culture.* New York, NY: MacMillan.

Boyle, J., & Hinrichs, J. G. (2013). Madeleine Leininger, PhD, LHD, RN, FRCA, FAAN: A remembrance. *Journal of Transcultural Nursing, 24*(1), 5.

Brace-Govan, J. (2007). Participant photography in visual ethnography. *International Journal of Market Research, 49*(6), 735–750.

Brathwaite, A. C., & Williams, C. C. (2004). Childbirth experiences of professional Chinese Canadian women. *Journal of Obstetric, Gynecologic, and Neonatal Nursing, 33*(6), 748–755.

Breda, K. (2013). Critical ethnography. In C. Beck (Ed.), *Routledge International handbook of qualitative nursing research* (pp. 230–241). New York, NY: Routledge.

Brennan-Horley, C., Luckman, S., Gibson, C., & Willoughby-Smith, J. (2010). GIS, ethnography, and cultural research: Putting maps back into ethnographic mapping. *The Information Society, 26,* 92–103.

Brink, P. (2013). Traditional ethnography. In C. Beck (Ed.), *Routledge handbook of qualitative research* (pp. 203–212). New York, NY: Routledge.

Bull, R., & Fitzgerald, M. (2006). Nursing in a technological environment: Nursing care in the operating room. *International Journal of Nursing Practice, 12,* 3–7.

Chiang, L. (1993). *Beyond the language: Native Americans' nonverbal communication.* Paper presented at the annual meeting of the Midwest Association of Teachers of Educational Psychology, October 1–2. Anderson, IN.

Clabo, L. (2008). An ethnography of pain assessment and the role of social context on two postoperative units. *Journal of Advanced Nursing, 61*(5), 531–539.

Clark, L., Johnson, S. L., O'Connor, M. E., & Lassetter, J. (2013). Cultural aspects of Latino early childhood obesity. In C. T. Beck (Ed.), *Routledge international handbook of qualitative nursing research* (pp. 103–118). New York, NY: Routledge.

Cricco-Lizza, R. (2006). Black non-Hispanic mothers' perceptions about the promotion of infant-feeding methods by nurses and physicians. *Journal of Obstetric, Gynecologic, and Neonatal Nursing, 35*(2), 173–180.

de Chesnay, M. (1986). Jamaican family structure: The paradox of normalcy. *Family Process, 25,* 293–300.

Dougherty, M., & Tripp-Reimer, T. (1985). The interface of nursing and anthropology. *Annual Review of Anthropology, 14,* 214–291.

Ethnomed. Retrieved August, 1, 2013, from http://ethnomed.org

Field, P. (1983). An ethnography: Four public health nurses' perspectives of nursing. *Journal of Advanced Nursing, 8,* 3–12.

Freeman, D. (1983). *Margaret Mead and Samoa: The making and unmaking of an anthropological myth.* Cambridge, MA: Harvard University Press.

Garcia, C. M., & Saewye, E. M. (2007). Perceptions of mental health among recently immigrated Mexican adolescents. *Issues in Mental Health Nursing, 28,* 37–54.

Glittenberg, J. (1994). *To the mountain and back: The mysteries of Guatemalan family life.* Long Grove, IL: Waveland Press.

Human Relations Area Files. Retrieved September 1, 2013, from http://www.yale.edu/hraf

Hwang, S. K., & Charnley, H. (2010). Honourable sacrifice: A visual ethnography of the family lives of Korean children with autistic siblings. *Children and Society, 24,* 437–448.

Knoblauch, H. (2005). Focused ethnography [30 paragraphs]. *Forum: Qualitative Social Research, 6*(3), Art. 44, http://nbn-resolving.de/urn:nbn:de:0114-fqs0503440

Lesser, J., Koniak-Griffin, D., & Anderson, N. (1999). Depressed adolescent mothers' perceptions of their own maternal role. *Issues in Mental Health Nursing, 20,* 131–149.

Leininger, M. (1970). *Nursing and anthropology: Two worlds to blend.* New York, NY: John Wiley & Sons.

Leininger, M. (1978). *Transcultural nursing: Concepts, theories, and practices.* New York, NY: John Wiley & Sons.

Leininger, M. (1997). Overview of the theory of culture care with the ethnonursing research method. *Journal of Transcultural Nursing, 8*(2), 32–52.

Madeleine M. Leininger Collection Papers, 1953–1995. Retrieved February 21, 2013, from https://www.reuther.wayne.edu/files/WSP000725.pdf

Malinowski, B. (1913). The family among the aboriginal Australians: A sociological study. London, UK: University of London Press.

Manias E., & Street, A. (2000). Possibilities for critical social theory and Foucault's work: A tool box approach. *Nursing Inquiry, 7,* 50–60.

Manias, E., & Street, A. (2001). The interplay of knowledge and decision making between doctors and nurses in critical care. *International Journal of Nursing Studies, 38,* 173–184.

Mead. M. (1928). *Coming of age in Samoa.* New York, NY: William Morrow.

Mead, M. (1930). *Growing up in New Guinea.* New York, NY: William Morrow.

Mead, M. (1995). Visual anthropology in a discipline of words. In P. Hockings (Ed.), *Principles of visual anthropology* (pp. 3–10). New York, NY: Mouton de Gruyter.

Moore, F. (2011). Ambivalence, anthropology and business: A review of ethnographic researchin international organisations. *Social Anthropology/Anthropologie Sociale, 19*(4), 506–519.

Oliveiro, P. (2010). Focused ethnography through thematic networks: Defining validity in business anthropology research. *International Journal of Business Anthropology, 1*(2), 14–31.

Palomares, M., & Povada, D. (2010). Linguistic ethnography and the study of welfare institutions as a flow of social practices: The case of residential child care institutions as paradoxical institutions. *Text & Talk, 30*(2), 193–212.

Pink, S. (2001). *Doing visual ethnography images, media and representation in research.* London, UK: Sage.

Pink, S. (2008). Mobilising visual ethnography: Making routes, making place and making images. *Forum Qualitative Social Research, 9*(3), 1–18.

Qirko, H. (2007). Diversity and cultural assessments in business organizations. *The International Journal of Diversity in Organizations, Communities, and Nations, 7*(3), 151–158.

Powdermaker, H. (1950). *Hollywood: The dream factory.* Boston, MA: Little, Brown.

Rakic, T., & Chamber, D. (2009). Researcher with a movie camera: Visual ethnography in the field. *Current Issues in Tourism, 12*(3), 255–270.

Ruby, J. (2000). *Picturing culture: Explorations of film and anthropology.* Chicago, IL: University of Chicago Press.

"Ruth Benedict" Department of Anthropology. (n.d.). Retrieved February 21, 2013, from Columbia University website http://anthropology.columbia.edu/ruth -fulton

Scott, S., & Pollack, C. (2008). The role of nursing unit culture in shaping research utilization behaviors. *Research in Nursing & Health, 31*, 298–309.

Shepherd, M. L. (2011). Behind the scales: Child and family health nurses taking care of women's emotional wellbeing. *Contemporary Nurse, 37*(2), 137–148.

Soyini, M. D. (2005). *Critical ethnography: Methods, ethics and performance*. Thousand Oaks, CA: Sage.

Stocking, G. W. (1960). Franz Boas and the founding of the American Anthropological Association. *American Anthropologist, 62*, 1–17.

Thomas, J. (1993). *Doing critical ethnography*. Newbury Park, CA: Sage.

Thompson, J. (1987). Critical scholarship: The critique of domination in nursing. *Advances in Nursing Science, 10*(1), 27–28.

Wilkinson, S., & Callister, L. (2010). Giving birth: The voices of Ghanaian women. *Health Care for Women International, 31*, 201–220.

Wolf, Z. R. (2012). Ethnography: The method. In P. Munhall (Ed.), *Nursing research: A qualitative perspective* (pp. 285–338). Sudbury, MA: Jones and Bartlett.

Chapter Two

State of the Art in Nursing Research Using Ethnography

Diane Keen and Mary de Chesnay

This chapter on ethnographic literature in nursing captures the widest array of studies published to date. Many of the early doctoral dissertations were conducted as traditional ethnographies, but were not always published (Boyle, 1982; Brink, 1969, 2013; Osborne, 1968; Reid, 1969). However, there is an emerging tradition of newer focused ethnographies in which the ethnographer studies specific aspects of the culture of interest. Some were published as books (Dougherty, 1978) and some as journal articles (Germain, 1979).

Early nurse–anthropologists earned degrees in nursing at the baccalaureate and master's degree levels, but because there were no doctoral programs in nursing, they earned doctoral degrees in related fields. Many were employed in academic institutions and so earned the EdD or PhD in Education majoring in higher education or academic administration. Many others earned a PhD in the sciences or social sciences such as anthropology in what were called the nurse–scientist programs.

Nurses who studied anthropology conducted traditional fieldwork in which they lived in a community for an extended period of time. Madeleine Leininger, the first nurse to earn a PhD in anthropology, conducted her early fieldwork in New Guinea (Leininger, 1966). She later published her first book blending nursing and anthropology. Nurses who conduct ethnographic research beyond their doctoral programs tend to conduct focused or limited ethnographies in which they study a specific health problem within the context of a cultural group.

In this chapter, we present an overview of the state of the art ethnographies conducted by nurses. A 10-year search was conducted but special attention is given to the published work of early nurse–anthropologists. An important source for the perceptions of the pioneers is a special issue of the *Western Journal of Nursing Research* (2001) edited by Dr. Pam Brink who gathered the so-called "grandparents papers" into a special issue that includes essays by the early nurse–anthropologists. Edited by Dr. Nancy Anderson, the issue includes reflections by Aamodt, Brink, Leininger, Osborne, Barbee, Byerly, Kay, and Chrisman. These names are highly recognizable to all those of us who came after. The next section highlights a few works by the early generation.

TRADITIONAL ETHNOGRAPHIES AND EARLY NURSE–ANTHROPOLOGISTS

Because the first generation of nurses with doctoral degrees in anthropology was required to fit into the existing education model for nonnurse–anthropologists, they tended to conduct traditional fieldwork. However, they did not always publish (Brink, 2013). Madeleine Leininger was the first nurse to earn a PhD in anthropology. She was followed by the following nurses who can be viewed as the first generation of nurse–anthropologists (with apologies to any we have missed):

Pamela J. Brink: My clinical area of expertise is psychiatric nursing. My research and publications have focused on transcultural nursing, women's health, ethical issues, qualitative research methods, obesity, and successful dieters. I have completed ethnographies on a small community in southeastern Kentucky, one reservation of the Northern Paiute Indians of Nevada, and one clan of the Annang speaking peoples of southeastern Nigeria. With the Annang peoples, I examined their health care decision making; the role of traditional birth attendants; women's secret societies and value orientations; and the fattening room. (http://www.nursing.ualberta.ca/en/Staff/Emeritae/PBrink.aspx)

Elizabeth Lee Byerly (1969, 1970, and 1981) conducted fieldwork in the hospital and analyzed relationships according to general system theory. She later conducted funded fieldwork on agricultural migrants in central Washington. She made a case for using participant observation in nursing settings at a time when nursing curricula did not include such techniques.

Agnes Aamodt (1971, 1992) conducted research with the Tohono O'odham children in southern Arizona, to learn how they structure health knowledge, and with Norwegian American women living in the Midwest. She taught for many years at the University of Arizona and wrote a history of the school of nursing.

Margarita A. Kay (1977, 1982, 1996, 2001) conducted research on health and illness in a Mexican American barrio. She later wrote about natural remedies and created a medical dictionary and reference book on healing with plants.

Eleanor Bauwens (1978) published a book from her dissertation in which she applied anthropological theory to patient care. She conducted ethnographic research in prenatal clinics, hospital deliveries, and studied the healing practices of five ethnic groups in Miami. Her edited volume includes work by other early nurse–anthropologists who focused on the interface between culture and health.

Oliver H. Osborne conducted research in Africa and was named a chief of the tribe with which he worked. He used anthropological skills to develop social programs in the United States and taught at the University of Washington for many years.

Antoinette Ragucci (1972) published on how to employ anthropological methods in nursing research. She was probably one of the first to make the case for qualitative research in general.

Afterward came the following who can be viewed as the second generation of nurse–anthropologists: Nancy Anderson, Toni Tripp-Reimer, Molly C. Dougherty (1978), Jody Glittenberg, Lydia De Santis, Lauren Clark, Evelyn Barbee, and Carol Germain (1979), whose dissertation was an ethnographic study on an oncology unit.

FOCUSED ETHNOGRAPHIES

An extensive search of the literature was conducted to identify ethnographies completed by nurses. Ethnographies were reviewed for authorship; only studies conducted by nurses, or multidisciplinary studies with nurses on the team, were considered for review. Over 40 studies were reviewed and are summarized in the following paragraphs. In the literature review it was apparent that qualitative research in general has become more acceptable in the past 10 years, with ethnography being much more common in recent years.

Studies were reviewed globally. Eleven articles reviewed were on research conducted in Canada. The United States followed with 10 studies, the United Kingdom 9, and Australia 5. One study was identified as having been conducted in each of the following countries: Bangladesh, Iceland, Brazil, Ghana, Sri Lanka, India, New Zealand, Nicaragua, and Taiwan. The clinical focus of the studies varied. The majority of the studies were conducted in inpatient and community settings, but there were also studies conducted in educational settings, long-term care facilities, and a prison. As was mentioned previously, a common thread in the ethnographies reviewed was an attempt to understand a group of people or culture better. The studies will be discussed by clinical focus.

STATE OF THE ART OF NURSING LITERATURE
USING ETHNOGRAPHY

Inpatient Settings

Lin, Chaboyer, Wallis, and Miller (2012) conducted an ethnographic study using activity theory as the theoretical framework for the study. Activity theory provided a methodological manner for the researchers to perform interviews, observation, and examination of existing documents. The stated purpose of the study was "to explore the factors that influence intensive care patient discharge" (Lin et al., 2012, p. 1054). An inpatient adult intensive care unit (ICU) in Australia was the setting for the study. Researchers gathered information through ethnographic methods described earlier by observing 28 ICU patient discharges and conducting 56 interviews. Researchers identified several major problems such as discharge, which was often delayed because of limited availability of beds and after-hours discharge, which also presented problems, and the fact that patients had little input in the discharge decision. Researchers made recommendations for improved discharge processes, which included availability of tools and procedures to facilitate discharge. In addition, in a patient-centered environment researchers advocated that patients should have input into decision making.

Paiva, Rossi, Costa, and Dantas (2010) also conducted an ethnography in an ICU setting; the location for this study was Brazil. The purpose of the study was to understand the trauma experience of patients in the ICU, with the ultimate goal being to provide resources for health professionals to identify aspects of trauma. The ethnographic method chosen was informed by medical anthropology and included direct observation, semi-structured interviews, and field notes. Patients and their relatives were interviewed post-discharge. Paiva and colleagues (2010) concluded that living through a trauma experience shapes those involved in the experience, and contributes to the well-being of the patient. The researchers suggested that incorporation of the perspective of individuals, who have been impacted by trauma, is important in planning and would be beneficial in meeting the needs of other patients.

Elmir, Schmied, Wilkes, and Jackson (2010) conducted a meta-ethnography on traumatic birth in Australia. The purpose of the study was to report "women's perceptions and experiences of traumatic birth" (Elmir et al., 2010). Ten qualitative studies were evaluated and common themes identified. Women reported "feeling invisible and out of control," discussed the need to be treated humanely, felt trapped, and described emotions as being on a roller-coaster. A traumatic birth experience has a significantly negative impact on the life of those women who experience it. Researchers concluded that health care workers could have a positive impact on the patient by recognizing the women's need to be informed and involved in making decisions about the birth. In addition, researchers pointed out the need for debriefing after a traumatic birth. Nursing can assist women by allowing them the opportunity to talk about their experience, this could be added to the postnatal assessment for psychological distress.

Continuing with ethnographies that focus on trauma, Cole (2006) conducted a study to "explore the culture of a trauma team in relation to human factors" in an emergency department in a teaching hospital in the United Kingdom. Using interviews and observational methods, researchers identified five categories that impacted the competence of the trauma team. They included leadership, role competence, conflict, communication, and environment. Recommendations for clinical practice included developing formal roles for team leaders and professional development.

Griffiths (2010) conducted an ethnography to "explore the nurses' role on a medical assessment unit." The nurses were triaging emergency room patients in a hospital in Wales, United Kingdom. By using participant observation, semi-structured interviews, and document reviews, Griffiths identified three concepts: first, organization of clinical space; second, professional knowledge; and finally, ability to work under pressure. Nurses developed strategies that incorporated these concepts into their practice to meet the demands of working autonomously. Griffith cautioned that the medical assessment unit may actually hinder holistic nursing care in favor of organization and efficiency.

De Silva and Rolls (2010) conducted an ethnographic study and reported on the health care system and nursing in Sri Lanka. The methods used by the researchers included observation, semi-structured interviews, and field notes. Two major categories that emerged during a larger study on nurses' cancer pain management were nursing and the health care system. The health care system was found to be wanting because of the lack of staff, poor infrastructure, and lack of resources. This, in combination with the number of patients and inadequate management, created a poor health care situation in Sri Lanka. Nursing roles included not only patient care and medication administration, but other duties such as janitorial duties. Nurses reported feeling powerless. Authors identified knowledge deficit, attitudes, beliefs, and medication direction as contributors to powerlessness. Increasing workloads, minimal career opportunities, and task-oriented nursing contributed to the nurses feeling trapped. Currently nursing is undervalued in the medically dominated health care system. DeSilva and Rolls (2010) suggested that for nursing to progress in Sri Lanka, separation from medicine and improved nursing education is needed.

Patient satisfaction related to response to call bells was the topic of an ethnography conducted by Deitrick, Bokovoy, Stern, and Panik (2006). The purpose of the study was collecting "call bell data in addition to information about the broader topic of the components of patient satisfaction" (Deitrick et al., 2006, p. 316). Ethnographers used mapping, photography, observations, and interview methods to understand patient satisfaction better. Patients indicated that the response to call bells was slow and ineffective in that they did not receive what they needed or it took a long time to meet their needs. One problem identified was that staff disagreed on who should respond to the call bells and therefore no one responded. Researchers recommended that leadership should develop standards for responding to call bells. This study provided insight into a problem in the hospital with potential recommendations for a solution.

Bull and FitzGerald (2006) investigated the ways operating room (OR) nurses provided care for patients in the midst of the technological environment of the OR in an Australian hospital. Researchers used intense observation and interviews to study the contribution of nurses in the OR. Nurses blended technology and caring in their ways of providing care for the patient. Technology is important in the OR and often skills seemed to be the primary concern of nurses. However, through observation and interviews, the researchers discovered that the act of the nurse caring for the patient made the nurse more competent in his or her skills.

Children's interpretation of being in the hospital was the focus of a critical ethnography conducted by Livesley and Long (2013) in England. The stated purpose of the study was "to develop insight into children's subjective interpretations and knowledge of being hospital inpatients" (Livesley & Long, 2013, p. 1292). Researchers engaged children by using age-appropriate strategies such as storytelling and drawing. Although the study was conducted to understand the children's hospital inpatient stay better, interviews were conducted in the home of children who had been in the nephro-urology hospital ward of the hospital. In addition to interviews the researchers conducted over 100 hours of fieldwork in the hospital setting over a period of 6 months, again using age-appropriate methods to interact with the children. Constant comparative methods were used to analyze the data. Researchers determined that there was an urgent need for nursing to employ an inclusive participatory model to enhance interaction with the children. Livesley and Long (2013) referred to the children's expression of their feelings and needs as "children's voices," and they indicated that the children's voices were not being heard as a result of outdated ineffective methods being used by nurses.

Angus, Hodnett, and O'Brien-Pallas (2003) described the method used to implement an evidence-based practice study in Canada. Bringing Research to Intrapartum Nursing Care (BRINC) was a study that evaluated evidence-based intrapartum nursing practice. This follow-up ethnographic study reviewed the effectiveness of intrapartum practices. The BRINC trial provided proof of the effectiveness of the evidence-based practices that were implemented in intrapartum nursing. This ethnographic study illustrated the benefits and struggles encountered while implementing evidence-based practices in the two nursing units in Canada.

Mitchell and Steeves (2012) conducted an ethnography to "explore the cultural acceptability of clean delivery kits (CDKs) on the Atlantic Coast of Nicaragua." International efforts to provide adequate supplies for delivery led to improved outcomes during birth. CDKs provided midwives the supplies necessary to assist in a delivery. Health care is provided primarily through the governmental agency in Nicaragua and they prefer that births occur in institutions. However, as a result of the difficulty in traversing the terrain and other transportation issues, there are problems in getting to facilities. Because inpatient births are desired it is likely that the CDKs will not be provided for home births. The CDKs were assessed for their content, their need, their usefulness, and their political acceptability. Cultural competence was addressed by meeting with stakeholders to discuss cultural issues. The researchers concluded that the kits were acceptable and also needed to help improve birth outcomes.

Two ethnographic studies that focused on mental health were reviewed, one conducted in Australia, and the second in the United Kingdom. First, Grigg, Endacott, Herrman, and Harvey (2004) conducted an ethnographic study in an effort to enhance mental health nurses' understanding of participant observation in Australia. The researchers reviewed the effectiveness of triage programs to identify the factors that influence speed of treatment of patients. Researchers commented on the benefits of a native participant observer. In addition, the ethnographic approach was found to be an effective method to gain a deeper understanding of the phenomenon being studied, namely, mental health triage.

An ethnographic document analysis was conducted by Deacon and Fairhurst (2008) at an inpatient mental health facility in the United Kingdom. Researchers completed a document analysis on a previous ethnographic study. This work focused on identifying the work that nurses do in an acute care setting. Deacon and Fairhurst (2008) reviewed those documents in an effort to determine if the mental health nursing role correlated to the nursing role in general. The researchers concluded that seven of the eight bundles of work were the same in mental health nursing, and the eighth was similar. These bundles described what nurses actually do. Bundles that were comparable to both mental health and acute care nursing roles included managing multiple agendas, circulating patients, bringing the individual into the organization, managing the work of others, mediating occupational boundaries, maintaining records, and prioritizing care. Communicating information was similar; however, because of the nature of mental health nursing and the lack of hard diagnostic testing, the communication patterns of a mental health nurse with the physician involve interpretation of the patient's behavior. Interestingly though, the researchers found many similarities between the different nursing roles using an ethnographic document analysis and concluded that the work of the nurse is summed up as a health care intermediary.

Community Settings

Nineteen ethnographic studies that were conducted by nurses in the community setting were reviewed. The settings for these studies included the United States, United Kingdom, Canada, and a few other smaller countries. Similar to the studies that were conducted in the inpatient setting, the ethnographies in the community focused on understanding a phenomenon better to enhance nursing practice. In the first study, Kelly and Kelly (2013) had families of children with cancer from a minority ethnic group, whose parents were working during treatment, as participants. They found that the workload and the nature of cancer treatment put tremendous pressure on parents. Through participant observation in homes and community clinical settings, the researchers observed eight families of children who were undergoing treatment. Kelly and Kelly (2013) concluded that nursing could have a positive impact on the lives of cancer patients and their families by acknowledging the amount of work parents do on behalf of their children. Further research to understand additional challenges that parents of minority children may experience was recommended.

Drew (2011) pointed out the lack of research in general in community nursing. In addition, she stated that community nurses expertise is not well known. The stated purpose of the article was "to present some of the processes and findings of a qualitative, ethnographic study into the culture of community nurses through the vehicle of the handover nurse" (Drew, 2011, p. 161). The study was conducted in West Midlands, England, in a primary care trust. The ethnography was conducted using participant observation, field notes, and semi-structured interviews over a 6-month period. Key issues identified included teamwork with colleagues, working across teams, morale and use of humor, referral of patients, and rituals and routines of handover reports. The authors found two important issues: first, adequate time for handover report is essential and second, group identity was important to manage stress. Community nurses often feel isolated, and the support of the group was helpful.

Remote villages in Ladakh, India, were the settings for the next community ethnography to be discussed. The investigators used focused ethnography to study disability cross-culturally (McElroy et al., 2011). Information was gathered from interviews and participant observation. There were 30 participants, 3 individuals with a disability, 13 caregivers, and 14 village leaders. The questions addressed were on how ready the Ladakhi communities are to work with individuals with disabilities and what the individuals with disabilities would say are the factors or barriers. Because of the participatory nature of ethnography, the study allowed a deeper understanding of community readiness to work for those persons with disabilities that the study was aimed at. Use of research methods such as ethnography helps communities to plan programs that are significant to the community and that address the concerns of the community.

In response to the need for cultural competence in caring for women in childbirth in Ghana, Wilkinson and Callister (2010) conducted a focused ethnography aimed at understanding Ghanian women's perceptions on childbearing. The purpose of this study was to "describe the perceptions of childbirth among Ghanaian women" (Wilkinson & Callister, 2010, p. 201). Once again, ethnography is used as a method of understanding a phenomenon in an effort to improve care. The study was conducted in villages in Ghana, primarily in the Salvation Army clinic. Authors obtained culturally relevant information on women in Ghana that could be used by other health care workers. A common point that emerged during the interviews was that all the pregnancies were unintended. Authors suggested education on family planning might be of benefit while respecting the religious views of the community. This was the first study to explore childbirth in Ghana.

Nurses from Canada conducted a meta-ethnography searching for qualitative studies on telephone triage and advice from 1980 to 2008. Sixteen studies were identified. Five major themes were identified; they were "gaining and maintaining skills, autonomy, new work environment, holistic assessment, and stress and pressure" (Purc-Stephenson & Thrasher, 2010, p. 482). Common concerns found in telenursing included the lack of visual cues and the autonomous role of the nurse. The review included the psychosocial aspects of telehealth, which was a void in the literature. Authors found that isolation, heavy workload, independent decision making, and stress all had an impact on on-the-job satisfaction of telehealth nurses (Purc-Stephenson & Thrasher, 2010). As previously stated, this review included ethnographic studies conducted by nurses. Nurses are concerned with the individual as a whole, and consequently some of their studies are not focused on direct patient care but rather on holistic caring for individuals and communities.

The next study was an ethnography that explored Latino immigration to a Midwest city in the United States and the consequent impact on their cultural practices and community connectedness. Bathum and Baumann (2007) found that the immigrants had experienced a loss of community and that working to build the community could help eliminate some of the health problems this vulnerable population experiences. As holistic caregivers, nurses, in community settings particularly, seek solutions to problems that people experience beyond acute medical problems. By identifying solutions that may impact the community by reducing health issues, the nurse is caring for the whole person.

Ethnography was combined with participatory research to explore the perceptions and expressions of young African American men between the ages of 18 and 25 years. Participant observations and interviews were used along with participatory research methods. Young men in the study were happy to have the opportunity to share their story. They admitted they did not always disclose their true feelings. As a whole they saw depression as a weakness. Although the participants were not poor, they did identify social stress. Some of the problems identified in the interview included stress, which appeared to be used sometimes to mean depression; coping with stress; a feeling of being treated differently by individuals of other races as well as by the police; and depression, which they saw as simply a fact of life. Kendrick, Anderson, and Moore (2007) concluded that psychological interventions were needed.

Cricco-Lizza (2006) used ethnography to describe how infant breastfeeding was promoted by health care workers. The population studied included low-income Black non-Hispanic women in the New York metropolitan area. In particular, Black mothers who were enrolled in a special supplemental nutrition program were interviewed and the interviews recorded. The author found that trusting relationships are essential between health care provider and patient. Participants in this study identified trust/mistrust issues with health care providers. Cricco-Lizza (2006) recommended focusing efforts on developing trusting relationships between the patient and health care provider in an effort to improve breastfeeding education and care and to decrease disparities related to breastfeeding.

The nature of knowledge was studied by Kennedy (2003) as a part of a larger study. District nurses (DNs) in the United Kingdom require a vast amount of knowledge, and theoretical knowledge is needed in practice. This study examined the role of the DN, specifically with reference to the knowledge used during assessment visits. Kennedy (2003) found that the DNs were required to combine their theoretical knowledge with their practice knowledge. This is an interesting finding in an ethnographic study as the relevance gap is discussed throughout the nursing literature (Risjord, 2010). This study details the need for both knowledge bases to effectively assess patients and adds to the evidence supporting the closure of the relevance gap by uniting theory and practice knowledge.

Gates, Lackey, and Brown (2001) conducted a focused ethnography using photography evaluating caring behaviors as they relate to African American women and breast cancer diagnosis. Three themes were identified. First, caring behaviors for self and others were meaningful in diagnosis and continued treatment for breast cancer. Next, professionals displaying caring behaviors supported continued treatment. And, finally, noncaring behaviors were barriers to early diagnosis and treatment. The authors concluded that the act of caring encouraged African American women to seek treatment. Gates and colleagues (2001) called on nurses to work as advocates for African American women in encouraging them to seek screening and treatment as well as challenge the "wait and see" attitude taken by some providers.

Thirty years ago, Field (1983) found that ethnography was a good way of developing understanding of participants in a study, specifically nurses in this case. The author noted several other areas in which ethnography might be useful, including families and their understanding of health and illness, and understanding families' choices in health care better. The purpose of this study was "to describe four nurses' perspectives of nursing" (Field, 1983, p. 3). Four nurses were interviewed while the researcher immersed herself in the nurses' environment for observation. The criteria examined to identify the nurses' framework of beliefs included the goal of public health, the goal of nursing, the role of the nurse, the source of the client's actual or potential problems, focus and modes of intervention, and expected results of nursing activity. All four nurses reported health promotion or disease prevention as the goal of public health. Another similarity was in their perception of the role of the nurse, all four nurses reported that helping the client and problem solving were part of the role of the nurse. This article contributed to nursing knowledge in two ways. It provided knowledge on nurses' perspectives on nursing and also provided a detailed explanation of how ethnographic studies could be used to enhance nursing knowledge at a time when the research method of ethnography was beginning to be used more frequently in nursing.

Critical ethnography was used as a method to study satellite hemodialysis (Bennett, 2010). Nurses identified three areas of quality that they were focused on: what is, what is not, and what influences quality. Quality was determined to be primarily technical skills on the part of the nurse. Other issues such as blood pressure management were not considered to be quality care. The authors concluded that quality improvement was needed in outpatient dialysis and that improvement will require nursing to not only recognize the need for improvement but also integrate improved practices.

Lipson (1994) conducted interviews with 32 Afghan refugee women as a part of a larger ethnographic work. Lipson's findings were divided into three age groups: Elderly Afghan women who were refugees in the United States experienced isolation, women from the middle generation reported bearing the burden of caring for the family, and young and single women experienced cultural issues, especially in finding a spouse. Nurses needed this knowledge so that their interventions could be aimed at addressing the isolation, burdens, and cultural conflict that these women were experiencing to improve the overall well-being of these refugees.

McInnes, Seers, and Tutton (2011) conducted a literature review and identified themes and concepts through a meta-ethnographic approach related to older individuals' perception of their risk for falls and of appropriate interventions. Researchers found that older individuals acknowledged their increased risk for falls and wanted to be involved in developing a plan for fall prevention. This study reinforces the nurse's responsibility in acknowledging the patient's autonomy. The authors concluded that by respecting the patient's autonomy and involving the patient in developing interventions to prevent falls, the patient may be more likely to follow the fall prevention protocol.

O'Mahony, Este, and Bouchal (2012) explored postpartum depression in immigrant women. Use of critical ethnography in a pragmatic way allowed the participants to interact and share experiences. This interaction gave the researchers an opportunity to understand their experiences better. The aim to empower women was accomplished by including the women themselves in the sharing of their stories. By identifying the needs of this vulnerable group, it was recommended that mental health support be developed for this population.

Kennedy (2011) identified a gap in research related to family-centered care (FCC). Because FCC grew out of adult patient care, research on how FCC enhances care for the pediatric population was required. The purpose of the study was to give children, ages 7 to 11, a voice in expressing their role in FCC and to recommend possible ways to enhance FCC for this population. The children included in the study had a bleeding disorder for which they were being treated. Ethnographic methods were used, including unstructured interviews, document reviews, and validation interviews. Use of a treasure map and online games were interesting methods used to confirm the domains identified in interviews that support the children's role in their care. Kennedy (2011) found that children do want to be involved in FCC as part of the health care team. Exploration to include youth in such care was recommended.

In an effort to understand adolescent mothers' experience with depression and their maternal role Lesser, Koniak-Griffin, and Anderson (1999) conducted an ethnography to learn more about young mothers' personal experiences. The authors reported that previous quantitative methods had not been adequate to evaluate the maternal role in young mothers. Using interviews and data from the literature, the researchers found that motherhood may improve previous negative activities such as drug use and other risky behaviors. In addition, the interviews revealed further need for research to develop and expand nursing interventions to assist these young mothers. In particular, school nurses were identified as a group that had access to these young mothers and hence, the ability to have a positive impact on the young mothers by assessment of their depression and education.

In a focused ethnography, Higgins and Learn (1999) interviewed Hispanic women who were between 20 and 40 to evaluate their health practices. Each woman was interviewed multiple times. The results included information on their positive view of health, health promotion knowledge, use of safety measures, lack of cultural practices for disease prevention, and the importance of integrating spirituality in health practices. The authors concluded that adult Hispanic women are knowledgeable about health and that health care workers should be aware of their knowledge.

Chang, Hayter, and Wu (2010) performed a systematic review of the literature to assess women's experience with menarche. A meta-ethnography was conducted with the information gained through the review of the literature. Five key concepts emerged from the 14 studies reviewed. The concepts included "menarche preparation, significant others' response to menarche, physical experience of menarche, psychological experience of menarche and social-cultural perspective of menarche" (Chang et al., 2010, p. 447). Authors concluded that menarche has a major impact on women and that this information would be useful, in particular, to school nurses who work with young women as they begin menarche.

Educational Settings

Four ethnographic studies related to nursing education were evaluated. Three of those four were related to high-fidelity simulation and all were conducted in Canada. Harder, Ross, and Paul (2013a) conducted a focused ethnography aimed at understanding the culture of learning related to high-fidelity simulation and student learning. Methods included participant observation, interviews, and document analysis. The authors found that a clear role assignment is essential to student learning. Students learn more in roles that are familiar; being assigned to the role of the medical doctor was problematic for the students as they were trying to learn the role of the nurse. Structured and active role assignments enhanced participation and learning.

The same authors, Harder, Ross, and Paul (2013b), described the instructors' role in simulation in a second article. The research included 20 instructors, 2 interviews, participant observations, and field notes. Data were coded and themes identified. Harder and colleagues (2013b) found that the comfort level of the instructor makes an impact on student learning. They recommended ongoing support for faculty involved in high-fidelity simulation to increase faculty comfort level, thereby increasing student learning.

Limoges (2010) used institutional ethnography to explore high-fidelity simulation in nursing education. In particular, the author was looking at the organization and regulation of the simulation laboratory in nursing education. The author conducted nine student interviews exploring how learning was organized. Organization and knowledge processes identified included the social context of the simulation laboratory, discussion of biomedicine dominance in the hospital, the simulation laboratory being representative of nurses' actual work environment, and feeling accountable for their own knowledge.

In another institutional ethnography reviewing the literature, Dyjur, Rankin, and Lane (2011) explored nurses' math skills and medication safety. The authors challenge the standard that math examination proves medication competency. They suggest that the focus on math competency can detract from other risks that are not seen by the instructor when a student passes the math exam. Overall, the literature review showed a lack of math competence among nurses. Dyjur and colleagues (2011) recommended improving education as the solution.

Long-Term Care Settings

Kirshbaum, Olson, Pongthavornkamol, and Graffigna (2013) conducted an ethnography in hospice settings. The stated purpose of the study was "to examine the perception and experiences of fatigue held by patients attending a hospice in England; identify the behavioral patterns that distinguish fatigue from tiredness and exhaustion; provide conceptual definitions of tiredness, fatigue and exhaustion" (Kirshbaum et al., 2013, p. 146). The focus of the study was to assess clinical fatigue at the end of life in hospice care. Nine individuals were interviewed using a semi-structured method. The authors identified three markers of progressive decline; they were tiredness, exhaustion, and fatigue. Mental and physical challenges both resulted in fatigue. The authors concluded that the conceptual meanings of the three markers are socially constructed. Further, the authors suggested that the meanings could be used in constructing interventions that are socially appropriate for different social contexts.

In an effort to understand care for elderly individuals who are dying, Emilsdóttir and Gústafsdóttr (2011) conducted an ethnographic study with a clinical focus on end of life care in a nursing home in Iceland. Participant observation, semi-structured group interviews with registered nurses (RNs), and review of official records were all methods that were used. Themes that emerged included the importance of palliative care in the home, the central nature of the RN's caring in the home, importance of including families in early decisions in hospice care, the value of the RN's work toward a peaceful death for the patient, the knowledge of the RN as a contributor to good care, and the need to increase awareness of palliative care. Implementing changes that incorporated these themes would improve care for elderly individuals in hospices.

In a critical ethnographic study conducted in a long-term residential facility in British Columbia, Canada, Baumbusch (2010) discovered that building trusting relationships between the researcher and the participant was essential. Use of critical ethnography was a good method of inquiry that allowed the development of trust, possibly because of the close relationships that are developed. Implications for practice include the validation that nurse–researchers are in a position to affect change using critical ethnography by implementing findings from research into their practice.

Using critical ethnography Bland (2007) explored comfort in three nursing homes in New Zealand. In addition, the researcher examined how nursing impacts comfort. Bland (2007) found that ensuring residents' comfort should be a key nursing priority in nursing homes. Nurses and other health care workers need to empower residents in nursing homes and provide individualized care, which is fundamental to patient comfort.

Ethnography was used as a method to understand the strengths and learning needs of nurses in rural Canadian nursing homes. Cruttenden (2006) identified many strengths of the health care team. The team included directors of care, RNs, licensed practical nurses, and resident assistants. Four areas were reviewed, and each area had its strengths identified. Those strengths included leadership abilities, caring, openness to learning, and critical thinking. Cruttenden (2006) then identified the learning needs of the team. One common need among RNs and directors was gerontological nursing education. The study concluded that focusing on the strengths of the team and increasing knowledge related to gerontology will enhance care for individuals living in nursing homes.

Heinze and Nolan (2012) conducted a meta-ethnography using a systematic review of the literature to better understand parents' viewpoints on end of life care. The authors reviewed 35 articles and chose appropriate articles to be included in the study. Using data from parent surveys, focus groups, participant observations, and interviews, the researchers synthesized the data and determined three common themes related to parental decision making during end-of-life care for children; they were "communication, extending time, and understanding prognosis" (Heinze & Nolan, 2012). The knowledge developed in this study could be used by pediatric nurses to improve family care by recognizing the needs of the parents in decision making and providing the support the parents need.

The purpose of the ethnography conducted by Chuang and Abbey (2009) was to provide improved care for residents of a Taiwanese nursing home. The researchers stated that the aim of the study was to "explore and understand the culture of nursing home life for older residents in Taiwan" (Chuang & Abbey, 2009, p. 1640). Three themes were identified; they were collective life, care rituals, and embedded beliefs. These themes or concepts summarize the common statements residents made about their experiences in the nursing home. Life in the nursing home was described as tedious and monotonous, and residents expressed loneliness. Residents considered themselves more like patients in a hospital than residents living in a home. This better understanding of the culture of a Taiwanese nursing home provided the knowledge necessary to initiate positive changes to improve care for older individuals living in a nursing home.

Prison Settings

One ethnography aimed at nurses' experiences in prison health care was reviewed. Twelve prisons in England were included in the study. Interviews with managers and focus groups with key informants were conducted. Nurses identified their work as meeting the needs and maintaining the health of the individuals in prison. In addition, health care workers discussed nurses delivering primary care. Authors concluded that nurse-led primary care in prisons has been beneficial to the individual's health in prison. Powell, Harris, Condon, and Kemple (2010) recommended that nurse-led health care in the prison achieve an equivalent level of care as that given in the community.

SUMMARY

Areas of Commonality

Nursing knowledge was a common thread throughout the literature reviewed. Kennedy (2003) specifically addressed the importance of using theoretical knowledge in practice. Risjord (2010) defined the lack of a theory and practice relationship as the relevance gap. The literature review revealed the progress nursing is making in recognizing this gap and attempting to close it. Nursing knowledge is essential in patient care. Using the ethnographic method of inquiry, nurses have been able to identify areas of need both in knowledge and practice and make recommendations for enhanced practice.

Caring and patient advocacy were other common themes in the literature. Nurses studied a variety of research questions, but all had caring for the patient as the motivation. Caring is the essence of nursing (Watson, 2008) and consequently should be incorporated in nursing research. RNs were described as "pillars of caring for the dying elderly in the nursing home" (Emilsdóttir & Gústafsdóttir, 2011). OR nurses blended technology and caring (Bull & FitzGerald, 2006). Caring for patients in a culturally competent way was studied in Ghana (Wilkinson & Callister, 2010) as was caring for African American women with breast cancer (Gates, Lackey, & Brown, 2001). Nurses care for patients in multiple settings; those discussed in this review include inpatient settings, community settings, long-term care facilities, and prisons. As a result of caring for patients, the nurses are called to respond as advocates (Gates, Lackey, & Brown, 2001).

The common purpose of the ethnographic studies reviewed was to explain or understand a phenomenon to increase nursing knowledge. As mentioned above, nursing knowledge impacts practice. Using ethnographic methods to better understand the role of the nurse in caring for patients affords the ability to investigate a research question and determine the essence of the concept being studied. Application of this knowledge has the potential to improve nursing practice in caring for patients.

Areas of Difference

The literature reviewed covered literature from over 40 years and 13 different countries. The literature was sparse in the early years with a plethora of studies being conducted in recent years. Developed countries were well represented in the research; Canada, the United Kingdom, and the United States accounted for the majority of the studies reviewed. Smaller countries were either completely unrepresented in ethnographic studies, or only have one focused study, such as Ghana. Nurses have focused on diverse research questions that were identified in practice. Nursing education; prison nursing; and inpatient, community, and long-term care were all studied. Finally, although all studies reviewed were ethnographic, the researchers used a variety of methods and theories to support their studies.

In summary, the evolution of ethnographic research in nursing has expanded beyond nurses who obtain doctoral degrees in anthropology to anyone with a broad focus on culture or an intense interest in the delivery of so-called culturally competent care. Nurses conduct ethnographic research in a variety of settings, and most of these are focused ethnographies or traditional ethnographies in the home countries of the researchers. Wherever the studies are conducted, their publication enriches the practice of our discipline.

ACKNOWLEDGMENT

The authors are indebted to Dr. Nancy Anderson and Dr. Pam Brink for their assistance.

REFERENCES

Aamodt, A. M. (1971). *Enculturation process and the Papago child an inquiry into the acquisition of perspectives on health and healing.* Unpublished dissertation. Seattle: University of Washington.

Aamodt, A. M. (1992). Toward conceptualizations in nursing: Harbingers from the sciences and humanities. *Journal of Professional Nursing, 8*(3), 184–194.

Angus, J., Hodnett, E., & O'Brien-Pallas, L. (2003). Implementing evidence-based nursing practice: A tale of two intrapartum nursing units. *Nursing Inquiry, 10*(4), 218–228. doi:10.1046/j.1440-1800.2003.00193.x

Bathum, M. E., & Bauman, L. C. (2007). A sense of community among immigrant Latinas. *Family & Community Health, 30*(3), 167–177. doi:10.1097/01.FCH.0000 277760.24290.de

Baumbusch, J. L. (2010). Conducting critical ethnography in long-term residential care: Experiences of a novice researcher in the field. *Journal of Advanced Nursing, 67*(1), 184–192. doi:10.1111/j.1365-2648.2010.05413.x

Bauwens, E. (1978). *The anthropology of health.* St. Louis: C.V. Mosby.

Bennett, P. N. (2010). Satellite dialysis nursing: Technology, caring and power. *Journal of Advanced Nursing, 67*(1), 149–157. doi:10.1111/j.1365-2648.2010.05474.x

Bland, M. (2007). Betwixt and between: A critical ethnography of comfort in New Zealand residential aged care. *Journal of Clinical Nursing, 16,* 937–944. doi:10.1111/j.1365-2702.2006.0756.x

Boyle, J. (1982). *Dimensions of illness behavior among urban Maya.* Unpublished dissertation. Salt Lake City, UT: University of Utah.

Brink, P. J. (1969). *The Pyramid Lake Paiute of Nevada.* Unpublished doctoral dissertation. Boston, MA: Boston University.

Brink, P. (2013). Traditional ethnography. In C. T. Beck (Ed.), *Routledge International handbook of qualitative research* (pp. 203–212). New York, NY: Routledge.

Bull, R., & FitzGerald, M. (2006). Nursing in a technological environment: Nursing care in the operating room. *International Journal of Nursing Practice, 12,* 3–7. doi:10.1111/j.1440-172X.2006.00542.x

Byerly, E. L. (1969). The nurse researcher as participant observer in a nursing setting. *Nursing Research, 18*(3), 230–236.

Byerly, E. L. (1970). *Registered nurse role behavior in the hospital sociocultural system: A systems approach.* Dissertation Abstracts. Ann Arbor, MI: University Microfilms.

Byerly, E. L. (1981). *Health care alternatives of multiethnic migrants.* (Report of the ICNE Rural Health Research Project to the Division of Nursing, USPHS) [Microfilm]. National Technical Information System (NTIS No. HJRP-0903462).

Chang, Y., Hayter, M., & Wu, S. (2010). A systematic review and meta-ethnography of the qualitative literature: Experiences of the menarche. *Journal of Clinical Nursing, 19,* 447–460. doi:10.1111/j.1365-2702.2009.01019.x

Chuang, Y., & Abbey, J. (2009). The culture of a Taiwanese nursing home. *Journal of Clinical Nursing, 18,* 1640–1648. doi:10.1111/j.1365-2702.2008.02698.x

Cole, E. (2006). The culture of a trauma team in relation to human factors. *Journal of Clinical Nursing, 15,* 1257–1266. doi:10.1111/j.1365-2702.2006.01566.x

Cricco-Lizza, R. (2006). Black non-Hispanic mothers' perceptions about the promotion of infant-feeding methods by nurses and physicians. *Journal of Obstetric, Gynecologic, & Neonatal Nursing, 35,* 173–180. doi:10.1111/J.1552-6909 ,206.00033.x

Cruttenden, K. E. (2006). Long-term care planning study: Strengths and learning needs of nursing staff. *Canadian Journal on Aging, 25*(4), 347–361. doi:10.1353 /cja.2007.0016

De Silva, B. S., & Rolls, C. (2010). Health-care system and nursing in Sri Lanka: An ethnography study. *Nursing and Health Sciences, 12,* 33–38. doi:10.111/j.1442-2018 .2009.00482.x

Deacon, M., & Fairhurst, E. (2008). The real-life practice of acute inpatient mental health nurses: An analysis of 'eight interrelated bundles of activity.' *Nursing Inquiry, 15*(4), 330–340. doi:10.1111/j.1440-1800.2008.00426.x

Deitrick, L., Bokovoy, J., Stern, G., & Panik, A. (2006). Dance of the call bells: Using ethnography to evaluate patient satisfaction with quality of care. *Journal of Nursing Care Quality, 21*(4), 316–324. Retrieved from www.journals.lww.com /jncqjournal

Dougherty, M. (1978). *Becoming a woman in rural Black culture.* New York, NY: Holt, Rinehart & Winston.

Drew, D. (2011). Professional identity and the culture of community nursing. *British Journal of Community Nursing, 16*(3), 126–131.

Dyjur, L., Rankin, J., & Lane, A. (2011). Maths for medications: An analytical exemplar of the social organization of nurses' knowledge. *Nursing Philosophy, 12*(3), 200–213. doi:10.1111/j.1466-769X.2011.00493.x

Elmir, R., Schmied, V., Wilkes, L, & Jackson, D. (2010). Women's perceptions and experiences of a traumatic birth: A meta-ethnography. *Journal of Advanced Nursing, 66*(10), 2142–2153. doi:10.1111/j.1365-2648.2010.05391.x

Emilsdóttir, A., & Gústafsdóttir, M. (2011). End of life in an Icelandic nursing home: An ethnographic study. *International Journal of Palliative Nursing, 17*(8), 405–411. Retrieved from www.ijpn.co.uk

Field, P. A. (1983). An ethnography: Four public health nurses' perspectives of nursing. *Journal of Advanced Nursing, 8*(1), 3–12. doi:10.1111/j.1365-2648.1983.tb00284.x

Gates, M. F., Lackey, N. R., & Brown, G. (2001). Caring demands and delay in seeking care in African American women newly diagnosed with breast cancer: An ethnographic, photographic study. *Oncology Nursing Forum, 28*(3), 529–537. Retrieved from www.ons.org

Germain, C. (1979). *The cancer unit: An ethnography.* Wakefield, MA: Nursing Resources.

Griffiths, P. (2010). A community of practice: The nurses' role on a medical assessment unit. *Journal of Clinical Nursing, 20,* 247–254. doi:10.1111/j.1365-2702.2009.03135.x

Grigg, M., Endacott, R., Herrman, H., & Harvey, C. (2004). An ethnographic study of three mental health triage programs. *International Journal of Mental Health Nursing, 13*(3), 146–151. doi:10.1111/j.1440-0979.2004.0326.x

Harder, B. N., Ross, C. J. M., & Paul, P. (2013a). Student perspective of roles assignment in high-fidelity simulation: An ethnographic study. *Clinical Simulation in Nursing, 9*(9), e329. doi:10.1016/j.ecns.2012.09.003

Harder, B. N., Ross, C. J. M., & Paul, P. (2013b). Instructor comfort level in high-fidelity simulation. *Nurse Education Today, 33*(10), 1242. doi:10.1016/j.nedt.2012 .09.003

Heinze, K. E., & Nolan, M. T. (2012). Parental decision making for children with cancer at the end of life: A meta-ethnography. *Journal of Pediatric Oncology Nursing, 29*(6), 337–345. doi:10.1177/1043454212456905

Higgins, P. G., & Learn, C. D. (1999). Health practices of adult Hispanic women. *Journal of Advanced Nursing, 29*(5), 1105–1112.

Kay, M. (1977). Health and illness in a Mexican American barrio. In E. Spicer (Ed.), *Ethnic medicine in the Southwest*. Tucson, AZ: University of Arizona Press.

Kay, M. (1982). *The anthropology of human birth*. Philadelphia, PA: F.S. Davis.

Kay, M. (1996). *Healing with plants in the American and Mexican West*. Tucson: University of Arizona Press.

Kay, M. (2001). *Southwestern medical dictionary*. Spanish/English, English/Spanish (2nd ed.). Tucson: University of Arizona Press.

Kelly, P., & Kelly, D. (2013). Childhood cancer-parenting work for British Bangladeshi families during treatment: An ethnographic study. *International Journal of Nursing Studies, 50*(7), 933–944. doi:10.1016/j.ijnurstu.2012.11.004

Kendrick, L., Anderson, N. L. R., & Moore, B. (2007). Perceptions of depression among young African American men. *Family & Community Health, 30*(1), 63–73. Retrieved from www.journals.lww.com/familyandcommunityhealth/Abstract /2007/01000/Perceptions_of_Depression_Among_Young_African.8.aspx

Kennedy, A. P. (2011). Systematic ethnography of school-age children with bleeding disorders and other chronic illnesses: Exploring children's perceptions of partnership roles in family-centered care of their chronic illness. *Child: Care, Health, and Development, 38*(6), 863–869.

Kennedy, C. M. (2003). A typology of knowledge for district nursing assessment practice. *Journal of Advanced Nursing, 45*(4), 401–409. doi:10.1111/j.1440-0979 .2004.0326.x

Kirshbaum, M., Olson, K., Pongthavornkamol, K., & Graffigna, G. (2013). Understanding the meaning of fatigue at the end of life: An ethnoscience approach. *European Journal of Oncology Nursing, 17*(2), 146–153.

Leininger, M. (1966). *Convergence and divergence of human behavior: An ethnopsychological comparative study of two Gadsup villages in the eastern highlands of New Guinea*. Unpublished dissertation. Seattle, WA: University of Washington.

Lesser, J., Koniak-Griffin, D., & Anderson, N. L. R. (1999). Depressed adolescent mothers' perceptions of their own role. *Issues in Mental Health Nursing, 20*, 131–149.

Limoges, J. (2010). An exploration of ruling relations and how they organize and regulate nursing education in the high-fidelity patient simulation laboratory. *Nursing Inquiry, 17*(1), 57–63. doi:10.1111/j.1440-1800.2009.00484.x

Lin, F., Chaboyer, W., Wallis, M., & Miller, A. (2012). Factors contributing to the process of intensive care patient discharge: An ethnographic study informed by activity theory. *International Journal of Nursing Studies, 50*, 1054–1066. doi:10.1016 /j.ijnurstu.2012.11.024

Lipson, J. G. (1994). Changing roles of afghan refugee women in the United States. *Health Care for Women International, 15*, 171–184.

Livesley, J., & Long, T. (2013). Children's experiences as hospital in-patients: Voice, competence and work. Messages for nursing from a critical ethnographic study. *International Journal of Nursing Studies, 50*(10), 1292–1303. doi:10.1016/j.ijnurstu .2012.12.005

McElroy, T. A., Davis, A., Hunt, C., Dadul, J., Stanba, T., & Larson, C. (2011). Navigating a way forward: Using focused ethnography and community readiness to study disability issues in Ladakh, India. *Disability and Rehabilitation, 33*(1), 17–27. doi:10.3109/09638288.2010.485670

McInnes, E., Seers, K., & Tutton, L. (2011). Older people's views in relation to risk of falling and need for intervention: A meta-ethnography. *Journal of Advanced Nursing, 67*(12), 2525–2536. doi:10.1111/j.1365-2648.2011.05707.x

Mitchell, E. M., & Steeves, R. (2012). The acceptability of clean delivery kits on the Atlantic coast of Nicaragua: A focused ethnography. *Hispanic Health Care International, 10*(1), 36–41. doi:10.1891/1540-4153.10.1.36

O'Mahony, J. M., Este, D., & Bouchal, S. R. (2012). Using critical ethnography to explore issues among immigrant and refugee women seeking help for postpartum depression. *Issues in Mental Health Nursing, 33*, 735–742. doi:10.3109/01612 840.2012.701707

Osborne, O. H. (1968). *The Egbado of Egbaland* (PhD thesis). Michigan State University, Deptartment of Anthropology: Ann Arbor.

Paiva, L., Rossi, L. A., Costa, M. C. S., & Dantas, R. A. S. (2010). The experiences and consequences of a multiple trauma event from the perspective of the patient. *Latino-Am Enfermagem, 18*(6), 1221–1228. Retrieved from www.eerp.usp.br/rlae

Powell, J., Harris, F., Condon, L., & Kemple, T. (2010). Nursing care of prisoners: Staff views and experiences. *Journal of Advanced Nursing, 66*(6), 1257–1265. doi:10.111 /j.1365-2648.2010.05296.x

Purc-Stephenson, R. J., & Thrasher, C. (2010). Nurses' experience with telephone triage and advice: A meta-ethnography. *Journal of Advanced Nursing, 66*(3), 482–494. doi:10.1111/j.1365-2648.2010.05275.x

Ragucci, A. (1972). The ethnographic approach and nursing research. *Nursing Research, 21*(6), 485–490.

Reid, M. B. (1969). *Persistence and change in the health concepts and practices of the Sukuma of Tanzania, East Africa*. Unpublished Doctoral dissertation. Washington, DC: The Catholic University of America.

Risjord, M. (2010). *Nursing knowledge: Science, practice, and philosophy*. West Sussex: UK: Wiley-Blackwell.

Watson, J. (2008). *Nursing: The philosophy and science of caring*. Boulder: University Press of Colorado.

Western Journal of Nursing Research. (2001). Special issue: The anthropology of nurse anthropologists, 23(8), 767–847.

Wilkinson, S. E., & Callister, L. C. (2010). Giving birth: The voices of Ghanaian women. *Health Care for Women International, 21*, 201–220. doi:10.1080/0739933090334858

CHAPTER THREE

ETHNOGRAPHIC METHODS

Mary de Chesnay

*T*o many scholars, nothing is more fascinating than the study of culture, the lifeways of a people. The opportunity to live within another culture, observe the scene, and participate in the rituals and festivals is priceless. Yet, it can be frightening to immerse oneself in another culture and to spend extended periods of time away from family and friends. In this chapter, the process of conducting ethnographic research is described in a step-by-step format from the idea for the study through the methods one uses to explore the research question to the dissemination of results. Ethnography is fluid, though, and readers should feel free to adapt these ideas for their own settings and purposes. There are many ways to the same end and part of the beauty of ethnography is taking different paths to discover the richness of culture.

CONCEPTUALIZATION PHASE

Deciding What to Study

Identifying the research question can be the hardest part of conducting research, whether quantitative or qualitative. One usually has an "itch" or a question that drives the person to a specific area of study. For example, in the author's ethnographic work in Jamaica, the impetus was to find out more about family structure in order to work more effectively with Jamaican clients in a private psychotherapy practice (de Chesnay, 1986). It was necessary to suffer some teasing by family and colleagues about working on a tan, but the clinical application of the research results was well worth the expense and effort.

Asking the Question

The way the research question is framed dictates the methodology. In some cases ethnographers might be interested in specific patterns and use a mixed-design approach to gather both emic and etic data. Emic data refers to data from the point of view of the participant, and etic is from the point of view of the researcher. Some ethnographers use a blended approach in which they set out to test a hypothesis about the culture they plan to study. Others lay the groundwork for a hypothesis-testing study by first conducting ethnographic research. For example, a group of emergency department staff nurses wants to improve response times to the most serious patients who present in the emergency department. They all have different ideas about why response times are slow and it rapidly becomes clear that they need help understanding this aspect of their own culture before they can make effective changes to their procedures.

First, they need to understand the barriers to fast response, so with the guidance of the hospital's director of research, they design a two-phase study. The first is a focused ethnography in which the participant observer plays the role of the potted plant and records response times to all new patients. To reduce bias, they recruit Dr. Jones, a faculty member from the affiliated school of nursing, to be the principal investigator and participant observer. Dr. Jones writes the proposal, coordinates the human subjects' approval process, interviews the staff, sets up times for a graduate student to observe, and trains the student on data collection. Once data are collected and analyzed, Dr. Jones meets with the staff to discuss the results. The results indicate that there is no consistent procedure for triaging patients by a nurse; rather, the triaging is usually done by the administrative secretary who has not been trained and by any nurse who happens to be at the front desk and happens to observe the patients who are waiting. The second phase of the project is to design an experimental study to test the hypothesis that triaging by a registered nurse in a consistent manner will decrease response times. The experiment is conducted and the null hypothesis rejected. The staff redesigns the policy and procedure manual to mandate that intakes are completed under the guidance of a registered nurse.

Others are focused on finding out, discovering as many aspects of the culture as possible. Traditional ethnographies were designed to describe fully the culture of a specific people in a specific place. There might be research questions about a specific topic such as Mead's work with adolescent girls in New Guinea as described in Chapter 1 or the study by Glittenberg (1994) reported in her book.

In contrast to the hypothesis-testing model, the traditional ethnography is the more common approach to ethnographies conducted by nurses, social workers, teachers, and counselors. The approach is to ask questions around a specific topic but to be open to exploring any aspects of the culture under study. The danger here lies in the distractions that will entice the ethnographer into many interesting but different directions and slow the study to the point where the original questions do not get answered. This format involves focusing on one aspect of the culture where the aim is to identify cultural factors that contribute to problems affecting the people they serve.

An example of this type of focused ethnography might be the following. A rural community health agency director realizes that the geographic area the agency serves has an influx of Mayan immigrants. Many of these people speak neither English nor Spanish. While some are able to get by in Spanish, many speak only Mayan. The federal government, Office of Minority Health has developed a blueprint for improving health care by implementing culturally and linguistically appropriate services (CLAS) referred to as the CLAS standards (Office of Minority Health, 2001). In order to comply with CLAS mandates, the director realizes that she needs more information about Mayan culture. She designs a focused ethnography in which she identifies a bilingual research assistant, trains the person in participant observation and interviewing, and sends the person into the community to collect data. The nurses then use the data to develop assessment and intervention protocols for their Mayan patients.

Purpose Statement

Federal grant proposals often require a purpose statement that captures succinctly the research questions and objectives of the study. An example of how to frame a purpose statement for an ethnographic study of a convenience store backroom clinic in urban Florida that caters to Central Americans might be the following.

> The purpose of the study is to describe the culture of a backroom clinic serving a Latin American population in an urban Florida community. The short-term specific aim is to identify the practitioners, types of illnesses and injuries, methods of treatment, and follow-up care of the residents who use the clinic. The long-term specific aim is to improve the funding base of such clinics that can relieve the burden on local emergency departments and thereby save health care costs in the community.

Reviewing the Literature

A controversial question in conducting qualitative research is how much literature review should be performed before the study. In quantitative research, a thorough literature review is conducted because it is necessary to account for as many sources of bias as possible, to develop sound theoretical support for the study, and to write a tight hypothesis. However, in qualitative research, there is a danger of biasing oneself by reviewing too much of the literature before the study because the investigator knows what other researchers have said and may not hear what the participants say. A useful approach is to review enough literature before the study to determine whether the study needs to be done and to obtain a background on the problem that will direct fieldwork. The follow-up literature review then matches the study findings to the literature on the concepts and themes that emerge from the data. However, some ethnographic studies are designed to look for evidence to support existing theory. In these cases, a thorough literature review would be done before the study is conducted. For example, many of the ethnonursing studies examine phenomena in light of Madeleine Leininger's sunrise model, so it would be appropriate to test aspects of her model. To determine whether and how certain aspects should be tested, a full literature would have to be done.

Significance of the Study

One of the most important aspects of conducting research is to justify the study. The investigator's time and effort, and possibly a sponsor's money, need to be spent to generate knowledge to preserve the culture of isolated peoples or to lay the groundwork for interventions that will help people. Knowledge development alone is a worthy goal of any research, but in nursing, we are concerned ultimately with helping people in a culturally appropriate way that will promote health and healing. Therefore, we emphasize significance.

Over the years of working with doctoral students and reviewing grant proposals, I have noticed two major issues in discussing significance. The first is that investigators often simply state that the study is significant without specifying how it is significant. For example, consider the following vague statement "a" about a study mentioned previously in which emergency department nurses want to improve response times versus the next statement "b" that clearly says how the investigator thinks the study will improve nursing.

a. "The significance of this study is that the results will be used to improve nursing care in the emergency department."

b. "This study will be significant in identifying the causes of slow response times in triaging in the emergency department so that new protocols can be put in place that eliminate the barriers identified in order to achieve the goal of improving response times for the most critically ill or injured patients."

Consider the following statement about significance from the published literature. This statement is an effective argument for the need to conduct studies from the emic point of view because not all members of a cultural group subscribe to the same beliefs.

> Clearly, not all Hispanic women have exactly the same cultural health practices. Beliefs in traditional medicine are changing. It is important to understand what cultural practices adult Hispanic women use to keep themselves and their families healthy. This information is critical as we begin to identify specific aspects of Hispanic women's health. (Higgins & Learn, 1999, p. 1107)

By studying the variability in cultural beliefs of Hispanic women, nurses can avoid stereotyping yet make their interventions relevant for the women they serve.

In the next section, we discuss methodology in detail with specific recommendations for conducting ethnographic research in the field. The discussion centers around traditional ethnography and readers who plan to conduct focused ethnographies are invited to ignore any techniques that are not relevant to their design. For example, issues of language and living arrangements may not apply because many nurses who conduct focused ethnographies do so in their own communities.

METHODOLOGICAL PHASE

Design

Once the research question is developed, the first step is to consider the design choices. It is tempting to decide on the design first and to make the question fit the design, but that is not the best approach. If a nurse researcher wants to conduct a traditional ethnography and has the time to immerse herself or himself in that culture, then the following information will be useful.

I conducted doctoral fieldwork in another culture, although I conducted a focused ethnography on family structure in Jamaica (de Chesnay, 1986) rather than a traditional ethnography. I made several trips over the course of 2 years, and will use this study to illustrate the steps I took to prepare for fieldwork and to enter the field. The research question involved identifying types of family structure and how they function as families. Other examples are given from the literature as well.

Setting and Sample

Deciding on the culture in which fieldwork will be conducted and the people one will interview is largely a function of practical access. Where does one go to answer the research question, what language requirements are there, and how much money can one spend on the project with or without funding? Answering these questions is a useful beginning.

Once the setting is decided, review the literature to learn as much as possible about the setting, but be open to the inevitable surprises—both pleasant and unpleasant—that will occur once you arrive in the field. Ethnography is not for the faint of heart or for those who do not tolerate ambiguity. Knowing oneself is probably the most important skill one can develop as a researcher, particularly an ethnographer.

Sometimes the initial sample can be identified ahead of time, such as when I knew I would be living with the family of a Jamaican living in the United States. She contacted her mother and sister and got permission for me to stay with them and to interview them. She was extremely helpful in coaching me on the etiquette of living in that community, from what to wear and how to behave ("You are a nice person, just be yourself") to what gifts to bring the mother and sister. She stressed not to offer to pay them, but to bring gifts and take them to dinner. Once I was there and the family got to know me, they referred me to others in the community and were extremely helpful in smoothing the way.

Identifying gatekeepers and stakeholders is a major part of deciding on the sample. Formal meetings with people who can answer your questions and informal meetings with others in the setting are invaluable. Be honest about the purpose of the research and act in a professional way and you are more likely to gain trust. One of the women in my hostess's neighborhood was initially antagonistic to me as a white North American woman trying to study Jamaicans. She created many little tests to trap me and prove to everyone I was not to be trusted. Finally she demanded: "How can we trust anyone with White skin?" I responded with: "Well just pretend my skin is dark and I was dipped

in Clorox." This was a somewhat sarcastic response because of my inexperi-
ence and impatience, which I instantly regretted, until she started laughing
and that brought the whole group along with her. Later I took her aside to
apologize for being so flippant and to reassure her I meant no disrespect and
she said: "Don't ever apologize for being real—the reason I don't trust most
Whites is that they are not real—always got to be pretending to be so cool." We
then became friends and she was one of my best cultural informants. She was
a gatekeeper and referred me to several other women to interview.

Finding the right gatekeepers can be a challenge. Sometimes, the
obvious person in charge is not the gatekeeper for an agency or program.
For example, in an academic setting, the administrators are certainly formal
gatekeepers and usually need to give permission for any research conducted
in their institution, but the staff members are the ones who control much of
the information you might need.

Another setting in which gatekeepers might not be apparent is churches.
A doctoral student who wished to conduct an ethnographic study in a southern U.S. African American church obtained permission from the pastor, but
neither he nor the student thought to get permission from the deacons. The
student was prohibited from collecting data by the deacon and had to find
another church.

In traditional Muslim families, nurses might want to conduct research
with women, but must seek not only their permission but that of their husbands or adult sons. Failure to obtain permission from the right gatekeepers
can sabotage the study before it begins. However much we might balk at
the idea of obtaining anyone else's permission except the person we want to
interview, we must respect the cultural rules and values or risk being blocked.

Similarly, it is important to identify the right stakeholders in a setting
to capture a holistic view of the phenomenon under study. For example, to
examine breastfeeding practices and challenges of mothers in urban areas
of Guatemala, one would naturally interview breastfeeding mothers. However, it might also be important to interview mothers who are no longer
breastfeeding and mothers who unsuccessfully breastfed as well as nurses in
clinics that provide support to new mothers.

If the ethnographer does not have a contact in the field, then it is useful
to "hang out" to identify people to interview. On one field trip to Jamaica, I
stayed at a Kingston hotel that catered to professors and other professionals
who had business in the capital. One of the professors became a friend and
gave me insights into how other Caribbeans perceived Jamaicans.

The sample will depend on the research question, but it is customary
to sample for diversity—that is, find as many people within the range you
need and interview them one by one or in small groups. The sample consists

of any participants or key informants who can teach you what you want to know about the culture. Sometimes the sample is narrow (e.g., breastfeeding mothers and others who advise them) or broad (e.g., Jamaican families).

How many participants does one need? The answer is, as many as it takes to answer the research question. This is usually determined by saturation, which is simply redundancy or learning nothing new from subsequent interviews. More is provided on saturation under data analysis.

Human Subjects Issues

The institutional review board (IRB) of the investigator's school will review the proposal and provide approval before data collection can begin. In developing countries, similar human subject committees may or may not exist. In that case it is helpful to get permissions from government agencies such as the Ministry of Health or a local academic institution. One problem that sometimes arises with human subjects committees is that members tend to be appointed from the "hard sciences" and do not understand qualitative research. They review the proposal as if it is a quantitative study and object to anything not fitting the positivistic paradigm of traditional scientific study. In qualitative research, particularly ethnography, many decisions are made in the field and cannot be made ahead of time because life in the field is unpredictable. This concept is difficult for some quantitative researchers to grasp.

One problem lies in the confidentiality aspect. For example, we customarily choose pseudonyms for participants to protect their privacy. However, in many cultures, people are insulted by the idea that the researcher will publish their data under a name that is not their own. They see this as stealing their ideas and crediting another, even though the pseudonym is for their privacy. For the Jamaica study, I had reassured the IRB that I would not use real names, but one potential informant insisted I use his name and was adamant that if I would not, he would not participate. After a long discussion, we finally agreed I could use his real middle name, because he was known by his first name. The reason he was sensitive to this was that he had his father's full name and was proud not to be illegitimate.

Another problem is that the questions are not always known. A semi-structured interview guide is just that—a guide—not the same as a questionnaire that has been validated in a specific format. Sometimes the questions the participant wants to answer cannot be developed before entering the field because the ethnographer cannot know what the person wants to tell us about his or her culture.

Finally, the idea of signed consent forms is frightening to many people who view signing their name to any document as giving away too much autonomy. Primitive or illiterate people are not accustomed to doing business in writing, so the idea of signed consents is a barrier to establishing trust. The ways to get around this are to do an oral consent with a witness or on audiotape.

Incentives

Paying participants is both an ethical and practical matter. The IRB would frown on paying so much that the participant feels compelled to join the study. Practically, the researcher needs to have funds to cover all expenses of the travel, living arrangements, data collection, analysis, and any in-country expenses. Because the ethnographer is not likely to know before the data collection trip who and how many to interview, it is hard to predict how much by way of funds would be needed for cash payments. When living in the field, it might be more appropriate to provide services or gifts of food to participants. For example, the researcher might invite participants to accompany her to the market to shop for groceries and then offer to buy the staples or treats. Women participants may refuse anything for themselves but will readily and gratefully accept help for their children. I have bought clothing for children and food treats for the family, such as ingredients for local dishes that I wanted to learn how to prepare. In one case I asked a participant to teach me how to make peas and rice and brought enough supplies to make a meal for the whole family and some neighbors.

The researcher is the best instrument of ethnography and establishing rapport, and compensating people for their time can be done by using the ethnographer's own talents and skills. For example, as a nurse I had special skills that I could use to provide emergency first aid and to refer people to physicians on the island. One *quid pro quo* I used in Jamaica was swimming lessons for children. In the days of British rule, Jamaicans told me they were not taught how to swim because many beaches were limited to tourists and locals had no access. I had been a lifeguard and taught swimming in my high school and college years and readily agreed to teach the children.

Instrumentation

Ethnography consists of participant observation and interviewing and may include many other methods of data collection such as photovoice, statistical analysis, community mapping, surveys, and content analysis of news reports, films, the arts, and so on. In ethnography, the researcher is the primary instrument, and it is the skill of the interviewer that determines the quality of results. Establishing rapport is necessary to establish trust that generates accurate data. The ability to know one's own strengths and weaknesses and to be open to learning at all times helps establish credibility.

The ability to observe both as a participant and by blending into the scenery is critical. As discussed in the next section, one school of thought is that ethnography should be conducted by outsiders and the traditional ethnographies involved in conducting fieldwork far from home in societies different from one's own. The idea behind this is that outsiders can be more objective. A notable exception was Zora Neale Thurston, a Black female anthropologist who studied with Boas at Barnard College and was encouraged to collect her data in the South where she was a member of the community. She started her major data collection on Black folklore in her hometown of Eatonville, Florida, because she knew people she grew up with would talk to her (Thurston, 1935).

Participant Observation

Participant observation includes a blend of observing the scene and being a part of it. It is a fluid process and rarely is as clearly delineated as "Now I am just observing and now I am a participant." If trust is established, by immersion in the culture, the researcher becomes a temporary member and can be treated almost as any other member. Researchers who have not established rapport and trust can usually tell by the degree of warmth and degree of comfortableness they experience from members. In early traditional ethnography, the researcher was an outsider immersed in a culture foreign to that of the subject (Breda, 2013). The rationale for this was to eliminate or minimize bias. The fallacy in this point of view is that it is not possible to eliminate bias, but it is possible to control it; that is, acknowledge bias and set it aside while being immersed in the field. More recently, it has become common for insiders to conduct ethnographic research on aspects of their own culture.

Participant observation includes formal data collection such as going on rounds with physicians and participating in healing ceremonies in a study on nonadherence of tuberculosis patients in urban Bolivia (Greene, 2004). Driving around the neighborhood to obtain a sense of the street rhythms is informal. Attending staff meetings of a free clinic that serves the homeless and observing treatments would be formal and scheduled data collection. Hanging out at lunch with the staff is informal. Whether formal or informal, it is critical to write field notes as soon as possible while the observations are fresh. It is not always possible to take notes at or tape meetings.

Reflective Journals and Field Notes
Reflective journals are the scourge of undergraduate students who are often assigned to submit these after clinical experiences. However, they are excellent ways of integrating and making sense of the data, as well as expressing the feelings of loneliness, empathy, and anger that the fieldworker experiences when far from home and away from loved ones.

Semi-Structured Interviews

Interviews that begin with a general set of a few broad questions are customary in ethnographic research. For the Jamaican family study, I started with six broad questions about families, but these were rapidly tossed away as I learned to let participants start where they wanted to start. Eventually I was able to ask everything I wanted to ask, but had I stayed with my own format, I would have sacrificed the richness of data that comes from letting people tell their own stories their own way.

Other Interviews

Sometimes interviews are informal, such as when "hanging out" at a local café and just making conversation with people. Sometimes, interviews are structured such as when one wishes to identify all members of the family and what their roles are within the family and community. Ways of conducting interviews vary widely but a good source for detailed information on conducting interviews is Patton who provides detailed examples of issues (Patton, 2002).

Rigor

As in any qualitative research project, when we discuss the rigor or quality of the study, we cannot simply use quantitative terms of validity (does the instrument measure what it is supposed to measure) and reliability (does it measure consistently)? We speak instead of accuracy and replicability. Accuracy is whether we report what people were actually trying to tell us, and replicability refers to whether we clearly stated our decision trail so that readers of our research reports can understand how we arrived at our conclusions. There cannot be true reliability because the nature of interviews involves interaction between two people, interviewer and respondent, and both change over time. Therefore, the interpretation varies, even if the same questions are asked, because the person being interviewed processes his or her stories slightly differently as age brings wisdom. For a thorough discussion of rigor see Sandelowski's (1993) classic article.

One way of looking at science is the pursuit of truth. We like truth, we think truth is a good thing, and we search for truth when we conduct research. But what is truth? In quantitative research we move toward truth by eliminating as much bias as possible from our methodology, and we take measures to prevent bias from influencing our conclusions. In contrast, qualitative research acknowledges bias. Particularly relevant to ethnography is ethnocentric bias, the belief that our cultural values are the correct ones. Ethnocentric bias just is—it is neither good nor bad—except insofar as we try to force our views on others. Our interpretation of truth in qualitative research is dependent on our skills as interviewers. Did we establish enough rapport with the participants to trust that they told us the truth *as they see it*?

Data Analysis

Narrative analysis and content analysis of field notes and audiotapes or interview notes are the usual methods of data analysis in ethnography. The last volume of this series is devoted to data analysis, and authors of the chapters have described how they analyzed data. Some of us are "old school" using colored index cards to help in content analysis. We read and reread transcripts until we are confident we have captured the meaning and then organize bits of data onto cards that we can shuffle around. The outcome might be a typology or model of concepts and their subconcepts laid out in a pattern with arrows to show direction of relationships. Other models are generated that can look either simple or complex with few or many concepts and their relationships.

Depending on the research question, the ethnographer might develop a theory (set of propositions) that explains a phenomenon. This theory would be developed from the narrative of analysis of themes as well as concepts. Ethnographers might describe the theory as "grounded" in empirical data. Sources for further discussion of data analysis are Agar (1986, 1996) and Atkinson and colleagues (2001).

PROCEDURES

Preparation for the Field

A few things to consider while preparing for the field will help, but one must develop one's own lists. For example, my anthropology professor gave me the usual list, but one thing I had not thought about when I asked her for advice was when she reminded me I am a nurse and suggested I review emergency childbirth procedures. I did not deliver any babies, but I did help with postpartum care suggestions and talked with many mothers about their newborns. The following list is somewhat of a standard and should be adapted as needed:

- Language, predicting problems, and deciding how one will address people in the field (learning local language before leaving home with tutor or after arrival takes time)
- Talking with people who have been there—other anthropologists, professors, immigrants, and so on (I met with Jamaicans in the United States before I went—they actually arranged home stay for me)
- Funding—write full proposal, get IRB approval
- Health issues—vaccinations
- Host country permissions
- Take care of personal details—how will your bills be paid? Do you understand exchange rates? Pets, children, and their education?
- Packing—clothing, supplies, medical supplies
- Cameras—for example, digital-Polaroid, sensitivity to having photos taken—permissions
- Bags to carry equipment during fieldwork
- Money—how much and how to keep safe.

Entering the Field

- Living arrangements
- Language and dialects—clarify meanings
- Decide on activities of daily living: Where will you sleep? Floor, hammock, what to wear to sleep? How and where to brush teeth, bathe, and so on.
- Getting used to food
- Mapping the community to familiarize oneself with areas—safe and unsafe
- Hanging out—one of the most important activities—a wealth of information can be gained from observing the scene

Conducting the Research

- Setting up experiences for participant observation and interviews
- Conducting interviews

- Digital dictation, audiotapes, field notes
- Tension between respecting privacy and using information—there are variations among locals about who owns the data. The ethnographer might believe that he or she owns the data, but locals may see their own cultural material as belonging to themselves and may object to certain things being made known outside the community. On one hand it can be argued that if everyone knows the ethnographer is an outsider, then anything said is fair game, but on the other hand, sometimes friendships develop and people say things in what they believe is in confidence. When in doubt, ask.

Sampling

- Obtaining IRB approval before the trip and getting permission from locals
- Establishing rapport to identify the right stakeholders, cultural informants, and so on
- Equipment—low-tech versus high-tech:
  o Old school—pens, pencils, colored index cards; easy to carry, can duplicate, harder to protect data, can get lost, flooded, destroyed accidentally
  o High-tech: computers, software (The Ethnograph, Nudist, etc.)—easier to back up and store data, risks with taking high-tech equipment to the field—theft (poor and desperate people do bad things)
- Holistic understanding—for example, reading newspapers, watching TV, radio, informal conversations with people on buses, in restaurants or coffee shops—while doing formal interviews
- Levels of observation—participant observation, participation with observation
- Dealing with loneliness—getting into sexual situations with locals—friendships with locals

Leaving the Field

The attachments and friendships developed in the field stay with one long after one leaves the field (Tamakoshi & Cross, 1996). It is important to prepare for termination even as one arrives. Be clear and truthful about intentions and limitations. Do not make promises you cannot keep. Fieldwork is fascinating, difficult, and time consuming. Presumably the ethnographer learns much from the study period, but that knowledge is useless if the ethnographer is the only one who benefits. The ethnographer needs to find the right balance between publishing data for the scientific community and respecting the people who gave of their time to welcome the researcher into their lives.

SUMMARY

Much of the material in this chapter is relevant to other qualitative research, but the ideas presented here represent only few perspectives of the author and those cited. There are many ways to achieve the same goal, and the authors in this volume have only scratched the surface of possibilities for conducting ethnographic research. Those of us who have been privileged to be welcomed into the lives of people from other cultures have been enriched ourselves beyond whatever insights we have provided to the scientific community through our work.

REFERENCES

Agar, M. (1986). *Speaking of ethnography*. Thousand Oaks, CA: Sage.

Agar, M. (1996). *The professional stranger: An informal introduction to ethnography* (2nd ed.). New York, NY: Academic Press.

Atkinson, P., Coffey, A., Delamont, S., Lofland, J., & Lofland, L. (Eds.). (2001). *Handbook of ethnography*. Thousand Oaks, CA: Sage.

Breda, K. (2013). Critical ethnography. In C. Beck (Ed.), *Routledge International handbook of qualitative nursing research* (pp. 230–241). New York, NY: Routledge.

de Chesnay, M. (1986). Jamaican family structure: The paradox of normalcy. *Family Process, 25*, 293–300.

Glittenberg, J. (1994). *To the mountain and back: Guatemalan family life*. Long Grove, IL: Waveland Press.

Greene, J. (2004). An ethnography of nonadherence: Culture, poverty and tuberculosis in urban Bolivia. *Culture, Medicine and Psychiatry, 28*, 401–425.

Higgins, P., & Learn, C. (1999). Health practices of adult Hispanic women. *Journal of Advanced Nursing, 29*(5), 1105–1112.

Office of Minority Health. (2001). *Final report: CLAS standards*. Retrieved July 12, 2013, from http://minorityhealth.hhs.gov/assets/pdf/checked/finalreport.pdf

Patton, M. Q. (2002). *Qualitative research and evaluation methods*. Thousand Oaks, CA: Sage.

Sandelowski, M. (1993). Rigor or rigor mortis: The problem of rigor in qualitative research revisited. *Advances in Nursing Science, 16*(2), 1–8.

Tamakoshi, L., & Cross, B. (1996). *Going home*. Retrieved July 10, 2013, from http://www.theanthropologistinthefield.com/goingho.htm

Thurston, Z. N. (1935). *Of mules and men*. Philadelphia, PA: J.B. Lippincott.

CHAPTER FOUR

CAMINANDO MAS CERCA CON DIOS (A CLOSER WALK WITH THEE): AN ETHNOGRAPHY OF HEALTH AND WELL-BEING OF RURAL NICARAGUAN MEN

Carl A. Ross

Nicaragua is located in the middle of the Central American isthmus and lies between Honduras and Costa Rica. The current population is approximately 4.3 million people with an annual increase of 3.1%. Nicaragua is divided topographically into three regions: Pacific, Atlantic, and Central. The population is unevenly distributed, with most of the population concentrated in the Pacific region. The Pacific region occupies 15.3% of the national territory, and has 61.5% of the total population. Nicaragua is cited by the Pan American Health Organization (PAHO, 1998) as one of the poorest third world countries. The people of Nicaragua are ethnically mixed, with 69% being a mix of Indian and Spanish known as mestizo, 9% Black, 17% Caucasians, and 5% Indians. The life expectancy for males is 66 and for females 71 years. In rural areas, life expectancy is almost 10 years lower than the urban areas. Females have a higher life expectancy than males in both urban and rural areas. The overall mortality rate estimated for Nicaragua from 1990 to 1995 was 10%, which is higher than the Latin American mortality average of 7% (PAHO, 1998).

The Ministry of Health is the governmental branch that controls the national health care system of Nicaragua. The mission of the Ministry of Health is to ensure that the population has access to health services. The newest statement in the mission emphasizes health care that is in response to the people's real and perceived needs and that focuses on health promotion and illness prevention. The current health care system does not address health promotion and is disease-oriented in practice. Nicaraguans only seek health care for illness, not for health promotion. According to Nicaragua's health care plan, health care priorities should be assigned to women and children with greater attention given to adolescents and the elderly. Men's health is not effectively addressed as part of the current national health plan. Work is under way to develop a new model that will approach health problems through a preventive and participatory strategy.

The purpose of this ethnographic dissertation is to understand and describe the meaning of health and well-being from the emic viewpoint of rural Nicaraguan men. Research in the United States, Nicaragua, or Central America has not revealed any studies that investigate the cultural meaning of health and well-being of Nicaraguan men. This vulnerable population can benefit from research studies that identify the meaning of health and well-being from the emic perspective. Once the emic perspective is understood, nurses and other health care practitioners will be better able to develop and implement health promotion programs, impact health policy, and meet the health care needs of rural Nicaraguan men. To date, the nursing literature provides minimal knowledge for nurses who care for men in rural areas. No studies were found that provided guidance to nurses caring for Nicaraguan men.

Men in Nicaragua have a 5-year shorter life expectancy than women and higher death rates for all the leading causes of death identified by the PAHO (1998). As a result of many trips to Nicaragua, this researcher observed that men are less likely than women to participate in health promotion activities provided by the local clinic. This seems to suggest that it would be helpful to investigate the effects of gender on the health of both men and women to understand the broader health perspective of these two groups.

Much of the literature that compares male and female issues attributes health differences to biological differences between the genders. Current research supports that the idea that differences in male-female health are a result of learned behaviors. It is described in the literature that men acquire masculinity from their culture (Artinian & Duggan, 1995). Understanding one's cultural orientation and the impact it has on health and well-being needs further exploration and direction in health care. Nurses must increase awareness and sensitivity to the cultural diversity of clients to provide culturally sensitive and culturally competent care. Learning that there are differences between cultures must become part of the nurses' knowledge base to develop cultural awareness when providing nursing care. It is essential that nurses develop cultural awareness. Cultural awareness is essential if nurses are to provide holistic individualized nursing care.

Globally there are many definitions of culture. One of the most well-known definitions is that of Madeleine Leininger, a leading nurse anthropologist. According to Leininger (1995), culture is:

The learned, shared, and transmitted knowledge of values, beliefs, norms, and lifeways of a particular group that guides an individual or group in their thinking, decisions, and actions in patterned ways. (p. 60)

Lustig and Koester (1993) share a definition of culture similar to that of Leininger (1995). According to them, culture is a learned set of shared perceptions about beliefs, values, and norms. These shared perceptions, in turn, affect the behavior of a relatively large group of people. Definitions of culture according to Leininger (1995) and Lustig and Koester emphasize individualized definitions of health and well-being, illness, and preferred treatments according to the individual's culture.

Nicaraguan men appear to be a vulnerable population. Nicaraguan men have limited access to and inadequate resources of health care. Health care professionals must establish a public health program that focuses on primary prevention for Nicaraguan men. Currently, the model of health care for Nicaraguan men falls under the traditional medical model of diagnosing and treating (Ministerio de Salud [MINSA], 1996). Understanding the emic view of this population will provide the starting point for the development of appropriate public health strategies and policies for this population.

Nicaraguans comprise a sizeable subgroup within the U.S. Hispanic population. It has been estimated that 300,000 Nicaraguans currently live in the United States. The majority of Nicaraguans in the United States currently reside in Florida (Nicaraguan Consulate, Miami, FL, personal communication, 2000). Based on these statistics, it is evident that health care personnel need to be aware of and sensitive to the Hispanic culture when providing nursing care to this population. What is learned from this study of rural Nicaraguan men's health care may be transferable to the United Sates and other Hispanic populations.

RESEARCH QUESTIONS

1. How do rural Nicaraguan men define health and well-being?
2. What variables influence health and well-being of rural Nicaraguan men?
3. What are the self-care behaviors of rural Nicaraguan men related to health and well-being?

DEFINITIONS

Rural Nicaraguan man—Any Nicaraguan male living in La Reforma and of 18 years of age and older

Emic view—Nicaraguan men's perspective of reality, "native's view"

THEORETICAL SUPPORT

Leininger (1991) developed the "Theory of Culture Care Diversity and Universality." Leininger's (1991) transcultural nursing theory was used as the theoretical support to operationalize the study. Her theory is derived from constructs of nursing and anthropology. Based on assumptions that culture influences one's definition of health and well-being, the purpose of the nursing theory is to examine culture care diversities and universalities to "discover ways to provide culturally congruent care to people of different or similar cultures to maintain or regain their well-being, health, or face death in a culturally appropriate way" (Leininger, 1991, p. 39).

Leininger's (1991) model is referred to as the sunrise model. This model serves as a cognitive map to orient and depict the influencing dimensions, components, facets, and major concepts of her theory, with an integrated total view of these dimensions. The seven rays of the sunrise conceptual model serves as the focus for the semi-structured interview guide. The top portion of the model focuses on the worldview, the social structure, and the cultural factors. The seven rays of the sunrise model are universalities that have been identified throughout all cultures. Through an inductive study of the sunrise model, the knowledge that becomes evident will serve to guide nurses in providing culturally congruent nursing care practices to Nicaraguan men.

The emic approach provides the researcher with rich data obtained directly from informants in their natural setting. This type of knowledge is essential to accurately assess, know, and understand the world of clients. This knowledge base then allows nurses and other health care providers to design and implement culturally congruent care that enhances health and well-being. Leininger (1991) asserted that only emic knowledge can "provide the truest knowledge base for culturally congruent care" (p. 36) and stressed the need for nurses to use the ethnographic design.

Culturally congruent care refers to those cognitively based assistive, supportive, facilitative, or enabling acts or decisions that are tailor made to fit with individual, group, or institutional cultural values, beliefs, and lifeways to provide or support meaningful, beneficial, and satisfying health care, or well-being services (Leininger, 1991). Leininger (1985) states that:

Ethnography, in the broadest and simplest sense, can be defined as the systematic process of observing, detailing, describing, documenting, and analyzing the lifeways or particular patterns of a culture or subculture in order to grasp the lifeways or patterns of the people in their familiar environment. (p. 35)

One's culture influences personal beliefs about health and well-being. All cultures and subcultures differ in various degrees. Noncongruent care can lead to dissatisfaction and frustration on the part of the recipient and the provider of care. The recipients and providers of health care will both benefit tremendously if health care providers adopt practices that are identified by specific cultures. Allowing this process to come alive will make health care highly personal, meaningful, and successful.

ASSUMPTIONS

1. There are different expressions, meanings, and experiences that influence how a person defines his or her health and well-being.
2. A person's behaviors, meanings, and life experiences are influenced by his or her culture.
3. The emic perspective is important in identifying cultural components of health and well-being.
4. Informants will respond to research questions honestly.

SIGNIFICANCE

The mission of the Ministry of Health is to ensure that the population has access to health services that respond to or meet real and perceived needs. The health system emphasizes health promotion and prevention through an integrated and humane approach (MINSA, 1996). Work is under way to develop a new health care model. In Nicaragua the new model will approach health problems through a preventive, integrated, inter-programmatic, and participatory strategy based on risk factors. Nicaragua's health care priority at present continues to be focused on women and children. However, the new model will give greater attention to adolescents and elderly individuals than the current model does. Men continue to be identified as a nonpriority group even in the new Nicaraguan health care model (MINSA, 1996).

The PAHO (1998) identified Nicaragua as one of the poorest countries in Latin America. Significant problems exist with obtaining everyday necessities of life such as adequate water and sanitation. Health care in Nicaragua might be called a luxury. The majority of the population cannot afford to pay for health care. Prior to the Sandinista government in the 1970s, there was little value placed on health care. According to White and Johnson (1998), by 1978 social aspects of life for the Nicaraguan people had deteriorated to a level of total failure. Only 28% of the population had access to any form of medical care, and 50% of the population was illiterate (White & Johnson, 1998). The Sandinista government created a unified health system making primary health care a basic right for all citizens. Unfortunately, due to many years of revolution, the initiative was abandoned and financial sanctions were imposed on existing health care systems. The government cut funding by 40% and the focus changed to curative and private health care, leaving little access for the majority of the population (Lane, 1995). Significant setbacks have since occurred as a result of the Contra war. Efforts have primarily focused on emergency care and containment of epidemics with little emphasis on aspects of prevention such as immunizations and sanitation (Lawton, 1988).

It is important for Nicaraguan nurses to understand the meaning of health and well-being of rural Nicaraguan men to provide comprehensive health care to this vulnerable population. It is also important from the perspective that nurses can help to empower Nicaraguan men to be better consumers of health care. American nurses can also benefit from the study results due to the large number of Nicaraguan immigrant population in the United States. Obtaining data from this vulnerable population of health care recipients will enable nurses to provide culturally congruent nursing care and ultimately influence health care policy.

The emic point of view emphasized in this study was sought because it is imperative to design programs that are relevant and congruent with the population they serve. Everyone has a system of beliefs to justify his or her level of health, be it good or bad, and unless health promotion programs match up with those beliefs, they are destined to fail. The results of this study will provide a database to assist nurses and other health care professionals in providing culturally congruent health care to Nicaraguan men in both Nicaragua and the United States. Nurses and other health care providers will be better prepared to assist these individuals in meeting their spiritual, social, physical, political, and emotional health care needs.

The results of this study can be influential in shaping health policy as well as the development of the new health care system in Nicaragua. As a result of the small percentage of monies made available for health care from the gross domestic product, Nicaragua's health care system continues to function with limited resources. In keeping with the mission of the Ministry of Health, initiatives for health care reform are moving from a "diagnose and treat" health care system to a system that responds to real and perceived needs of the Nicaraguan people.

It is anticipated that this new health care initiative will emphasize a "promote and prevent" approach to health care.

METHODOLOGY

Design

Ethnography is the best method for conducting cultural research. The use of the ethnographic approach allows for the researcher to explore the holistic nature of society and to ask questions relevant to nursing and health care. The naturalistic setting in which ethnographic research is conducted will allow the researcher the worldview of the informants being studied. Ethnography allows the researcher to understand people, what they do, what they say, how they relate to one another, what their customs and beliefs are, and how they derive meaning from their experiences (Goetz & LeCompte, 1984; Spradley, 1980). The researcher used ethnography because the cultural meaning of health and well-being has not been described by rural Nicaraguan men. Ethnography provides an opportunity to identify, learn, and understand predictable patterns of human thought and behavior. The investigator is the instrument of data gathering, and fieldwork is the heart of data collection. The researcher has been involved in Nicaraguan health care for the past 6 years and with this vulnerable rural male population for the past 3 years. The researcher has provided health care, health education, and screening programs to the rural Nicaraguan men of the community studied.

The planning and implementation of this ethnographic study took place in four phases. The first phase was preparation, which occurred from December 1994 through December 1999. During this phase, the researcher made preparations needed to conduct the study and formulated a systematic plan of investigation, searched the literature to find information on the people and concepts under investigation, and obtained Duquesne University's institutional review board (IRB) approval. Phase II involved fieldwork, working with the informants, and data collection.

Instrumentation

In qualitative research, the researcher is the primary instrument for it is the skill of the interviewer that enables the participant to be open in expressing his or her views. For the past 5 years the researcher was involved with doing fieldwork with the Nicaraguan people, which included critical care, community health care, rural health care, and nursing education in Nicaragua. The investigator served as a consultant, health educator, and clinician for the Ministry of Health, hospitals, and university systems in Nicaragua. The researcher has been recognized as a Nicaraguan expert in the United States as validated by presenting at international, national, and local conferences. The researcher has published a number of articles related to Nicaragua's health care and nursing education.

Phase III involved reflection and analysis. The researcher's continued work in rural Nicaragua (La Reforma) allowed him to continue with participant observation, raising questions, and double-checking data. Phase IV involved finalizing the data analysis and findings and writing up the conclusions. The data collection techniques that the researcher used in the study included: participant observation, field notes, genograms, and semi-structured audiotaped interviews.

In summary, the steps used in conducting this ethnographic research approach were dynamic and moved back and forth throughout the study. The first step in data collection was participant observation and making an ethnographic record of the observations. The second step involved conducting semi-structured interviews with both general and key informants. Following each of the interviews, the researcher conducted a domain analysis on the data. Following the domain analysis, categories and subcategories were identified as patterns that were consistently emerging from the data. Final data analysis led to the formation of cultural themes and values. Validation of emerging themes and theoretical typology took place in conjunction with the dissertation committee. The final step involved writing up the ethnography.

Fieldwork

The researcher has worked for 6 years with Nicaraguan families, communities, and health care professionals. Working with the Nicaraguan culture for the past 6 years and having a Nicaraguan live with the researcher and his family for 3 years offered the researcher the opportunity to learn about and directly observe values, beliefs, and practices of the Nicaraguan people and their culture. The researcher's numerous visits to La Reforma allowed a number of participant observation experiences that led to an accurate and detailed description of the life of rural Nicaraguan men. This cultural immersion and participant interaction gave the researcher the opportunity to develop a trusting rapport with the participants.

Routine activities that the investigator observed included but were not limited to the daily routine of these Nicaraguan men, their work routine, their interaction with each other, their interaction with their families, specific interactions with their spouses, their modes of transportation, church services, religious rituals, weddings, funerals, and school activities. Health-related observations included but were not limited to the use of a rural health care clinic, behaviors at the clinic as they waited for care, behaviors during health care, interactions with families at the clinic, participation in health education and screening programs, and decision making at the clinic that involved themselves and family members.

Interviews and participant observations alone will not give richness to the data. However, together they will bring depth of meaning to the phenomena under investigation. Participant observation assisted in validation of data obtained from the semi-structured interview. As such, the data are triangulated to ensure accuracy. The researcher reviewed informant written clinic records to enhance the richness of the data. Participant observation field notes were recorded and analyzed. The researcher interviewed key individuals from MINSA. The purpose of the MINSA interview was to obtain their perception of the health needs of Nicaraguan men. The employees of MINSA, the Ministry of Health, regulate health care in Nicaragua. These notes assisted in validation of interview data.

Genograms

Genograms are drawings of family trees; family trees of four generations were completed for the study but are not included here because they include identifying data. Including them would violate privacy regulations. Genograms were developed for each informant during the introductory phase of the interview process. The genogram was developed using the criteria outlined by McGoldrick and Gerson (1985). Use of a standardized format for the development of the genogram allows for consistent interpretation within and between informants. Genograms allowed this researcher to understand both the family and relational context of rural Nicaraguan men. Family systems theory is based on the assumption that all physical, emotional, and social functioning of family members is interdependent. Any change in one part of the family system affects all other aspects of the system (McGoldrick & Gerson, 1985).

Bowen's (1978) family systems theory employs a longitudinal, trans-generational approach to the study of intra-family dynamics. The focus of Bowen's theory is on the reciprocal family role relationships that develop over time. Bowen's theory states that family patterns are usually repeated from one generation to the next, and the same family issues are generated generation after generation through the transgenerational transmission process (Bowen, 1978). It is through the use of the genogram that the researcher is able to visualize these repetitive family patterns, issues, myths, and rules. The genogram provided a data set on the family dynamics of each informant allowing the researcher to interpret familial illness as well as generational patterns.

Semi-Structured Interview Guide

The researcher conducted open-ended, semi-structured interviews with both general and key informants. The interview guide was not formal but used open-ended questions to assist the researcher in asking valuable questions of the participants. The interview also was used more to prompt participants when defining their personal meaning of health and well-being.

The researcher conducted interviews with general and key informants, because the interview is one of the ethnographer's most important data gathering techniques. The interview consisted of both global and specific questions. The global questions helped to focus and direct the investigation. Specific interview questions and probes assisted in eliciting responses that provided the meaning of health and well-being. The open-ended questions allowed the participant to interpret and elaborate on the question. The open-ended questions allowed the participants time to reflect and express their feelings and allowed the researcher the ability to develop specific questions based upon responses. Interviews were terminated when repetitive domains, categories, subcategories, and patterns were obtained. Saturation is a signal that the essential features of the questions have been gathered.

SAMPLE

Informants included Nicaraguan men who lived in La Reforma, Jinotega, Nicaragua. Inclusion criteria consisted of men who (a) were 18 years of age or older, (b) were willing to share their meaning of health and well-being and experiences with health, and (c) gave informed consent. Both general and key informants participated in the study. Key informants were selected based on their special position of trust, knowledge, and respect within the community. Key informants were helpful in recommending people who meet the study criteria. One of the main roles of key informants was to use their own influence to facilitate trust between the local people and the researcher in the community. The first inclusion criterion, age 18, was selected because it is the legal age for consent. The sample size was determined when data saturation was reached. Data saturation was defined as the sense of closure of categories, themes, and concepts that the researcher experienced when data collection ceased to yield any new information. Consent to participate was completely done on a voluntary basis. Participants were selected based on their willingness to participate in the interview and willingness to talk about their personal meaning of health and well-being.

During the preparatory phase, the researcher had meetings with the Ministry of Health in Jinotega at which time they discussed the research study. The Ministry of Health was very enthusiastic and supportive about the study, offered their assistance in recruiting participants, and offered the researcher an area for data collection. During a December 1999 visit to La Reforma, the investigator met with key community leaders and explained the study, evaluated inclusion/exclusion criteria, and set up the groundwork for data collection, which occurred in February and March 2000.

SETTING

Nicaragua and La Reforma

This study was conducted in the homes and clinic of the rural people who live in La Reforma, Jinotega, about 125 miles north of Managua, Nicaragua. Nicaragua is located in Central America between Honduras and Costa Rica. It is the largest country in Central America and is equivalent in size to the state of Georgia. The population of Nicaragua is approximately 4.3 million, of which 65% live in the more urban areas of the Pacific coast with an urban growth rate greater than 2.6% annually. Almost half of the population (47%) is under the age of 15. *The population is 52% female and 48% male* (PAHO, 1998).

According to PAHO (1998) and the MINSA (1996), the overall mortality rate estimated for Nicaragua in 1990 was 10%, which is higher than the Latin American average of 7%. According to PAHO (1998), the life expectancy of men is 5 years less than women. In the rural areas, however, life expectancy is almost 10 years lower than in the urban areas, with females having a higher life expectancy than males. La Reforma, Jinotega, Nicaragua, is a district equivalent to a county in the United States. There is no real central town or village. White and Johnson (1998), in personal conversation, stated that La Reforma has been described as "six miles from electricity and six miles from nowhere" by those coming to the area, but it is "everywhere for those who live here" The population of the area is approximately 2,700. The average family size is about eight members. Thus it can be projected that there are about 300 family units in the district. From local statistics, about half of the population is younger than age 18.

Access to the district is possible only by four-wheel drive vehicles via dirt roads. The roads are drivable during the four months of the dry season; however, during the remainder of the year, especially the rainy season, access is more difficult. The nearest city to La Reforma is Jinotega, which is located approximately 1 to 1½ hours from La Reforma during the dry season. La Reforma is typical of the western half of Nicaragua with a population largely composed of people of mixed Spanish and Indian descent. The main industry is agriculture. This area produces mainly coffee, bananas, and vegetables as cash crops. La Reforma is entirely agricultural with land owned by individual families who farm plots varying from a few acres up to 50 acres. A plot is insufficient to support a family unless it is about 5 to 10 acres. The terrain is mountainous and difficult to farm.

Residents of La Reforma are poor with an average income of US$1 to $2 per day. This equals $300 to $600 annually. Coffee plantations greater than 10 acres produce more income. Most families live below the poverty level and suffer extreme penury.

The researcher made a number of home site visits within the context of providing health care. These visits also provided the opportunity to directly observe and participate in the homes and family life of rural Nicaraguans. Home visits allowed the researcher to observe family structure and interactions, living arrangements, work distribution and activities, cooking methods, home safety issues, and spiritual artifacts, and enabled the researcher to learn about home remedies. Housing is crude and consists of basic planks on frame structures. Roofs are predominantly wood with tin sheets. Dirt floors are the norm. Furniture is basic and minimal. Cooking is done in iron pots on primitive clay wood-burning hearths in the home. The hearth is usually a simple clay dome as a bread oven alongside the main hearth. There are no chimneys, and smoke is directly vented into the rooms of the house. The kitchen is usually located in the corner of the main family room. This room serves in most cases as the sleeping area, particularly for the children. Hammocks are pulled to the ceiling during the day and lowered at night as family beds. Animals are encouraged to stay outside; however, animals ranging from dogs and cats to pigs and chicken run freely through the house, leading to many disease processes. Despite these conditions, Nicaraguan people are proud, and dwellings are kept as clean as possible. The exteriors of the homes are landscaped with native flowers and plants such as orchids and impatiens. Some families cultivate herb gardens and use many of the plants for medicinal purposes. Eucalyptus and banana trees are found growing on the property. Some families use discarded and recycled jugs and soda cans as hanging planters and wall planters to decorate the outside walls of the home and garden. Frequently, a family would have a cross located in the middle of the gardens. Although poor and with limited resources, Nicaraguan people often try to "beautify" their homes.

Water sources are invariably contaminated, because animals are allowed free access by necessity. There is generally poor disposal of human waste. Some families have constructed pit latrines, but many have not because it is expensive. Human feces are often used for fertilizer. If the water source is a stream, it is often contaminated along its entire length by animals, livestock, and families living upstream. Poor sanitation and contaminated water are two important causes of disease.

The nutrition of La Reforma is similar to other parts of the country. Rice and beans are the dietary staple. The blend of nutrition for this community is varied based on the families' livestock and crops, but the researcher's initial cursory opinion is that it is suboptimal in general. Families may have a pig or a cow, but most have chicken.

Predominant health problems of La Reforma include intestinal diseases, respiratory diseases, and subtle malnutrition. These account for 60% of the population's health problems. If problems of childbirth and sexually transmitted diseases are included, then 80% of health issues faced in the region can be accounted for (MINSA, 1996). Other problems include bacterial infections of the skin due to poor personal hygiene, accidental injuries, and burns. Hypertension and diabetes exist and need to be addressed, but these are secondary issues. Eye and dental problems are prevalent among the residents and need to be addressed by health care professionals. As part of the preparation for this study, the researcher participated in providing vision screening and dental hygiene education to the residents of La Reforma.

The Roberto Clemente Clinic

Built by the Pittsburgh Rotary Club in collaboration with the Rotary Clubs of Managua-Tiscapa and Jinotega, the Roberto Clemente clinic is situated in a compound shared by the local two-room school. The clinic was established in 1998 in response to the overwhelming need for health care and community health education for the people of La Reforma. The clinic is well constructed with concrete walls and a tin sheet roof on steel rafters. The clinic was the first solar building in the country. It has four main areas: a central receiving room that usually serves as a reception area and a general history taking and examination area for children and adults. There is a consultation room that usually serves as a private examination room. There is a large examination room that is suitable for emergencies, minor surgery, and delivery of infants. The fourth room is often used as living quarters for two resident health care workers. The sleeping room has two beds, a hand basin, a small countertop gas cooker, and simple furniture. There is a small area that is used for laboratory specimen analysis, distribution of medication, and administration. This area houses a rudimentary filing system. There is a bathroom with a nonfunctioning toilet and shower. There are minimal cooking and eating utensils and a pot for cooking rice. There is no two-way communication system at the clinic. The clinic has a front porch that serves as a cool waiting area for patients.

The Roberto Clemente Clinic provides health care for nine communities, comprising a total population of 2,797. The nine communities served by the clinic are Anita, Los Angeles, Naranjo, La Florida, Dolore, La Reforma, Santa Rosa, San Visente, and Santa Fe, Corona. The Ministry of Health staffs the clinic with two auxiliary nurses or a nurse and physician. These health care professionals are fulfilling a 1-year clinical training obligation. Thus the clinic is staffed by those fulfilling their social service requirement following the completion of their formal education. The staff are hardworking, intelligent, and dedicated health care professionals. The staff identify individual as well as community health problems. They conduct health education programs addressing identified health problems. Visiting doctors from the city of Jinotega may be sent to the clinic to provide care to more complex patients.

DATA COLLECTION AND ANALYSIS

Ethnographic research helps develop understanding of the people and their lifeways in their natural setting. Data collection and analysis were performed simultaneously. The data were analyzed according to domains, categories, and finally cultural themes. Further data analysis revealed themes, categories, and concepts related to the perceived meaning of health and well-being of rural Nicaraguan men.

Procedure for Data Collection

The following procedure was used for data collection:

1. Approval to conduct the study was obtained from the IRB of Duquesne University and the Ministry of Health of Nicaragua prior to initiating the study.
2. Participant observation was continuous during and after data collection.
3. Once a general informant was identified, the researcher explained the study and offered to read or ask the informant to read the consent form. Due to the high level of illiteracy, verbal, as well as written consent was available. Both consent forms were available in Spanish. During the December 1999 trip to La Reforma, the consent form was tested to ascertain the reading level. Once all questions were answered, the informant was asked to sign the consent form.
4. All informants received a copy of the consent form.
5. The researcher conducted the semi-structured interview in Spanish with the help of two Nicaraguan male translators who were fluent in English. Once the interview was initiated there were no interruptions.
6. The semi-structured interview was audiotaped as identified in the consent form. These taped interviews offered the researcher accurate recall of the discussions that occurred during the interview.
7. The researcher kept field notes for reference during analysis of the data. All audiotaped interviews were transcribed verbatim by two Nicaraguan male translators who were natives of Nicaragua. The translators signed a confidentiality agreement before participating in the research.
8. Because of time constraints and the difficulty of revisiting the informants, the researcher continuously clarified any questions or unclear meanings before terminating the interview. However, during a follow-up trip, the researcher made all possible attempts to contact the informants to validate their interview.

Procedure for Data Analysis

Ethnographic analysis is a dynamic process of moving back and forth between global cultural themes and more-specific analysis. All data were analyzed according to the methods of ethnographic research. Data were analyzed in a four-phase process. Phase I of data analysis consisted of collection, recording, and transcription of data from interviews with the general and key informants. During Phase II the researcher grouped, coded, and classified the raw data according to the domain of inquiry. The researcher used a three-column format when transcribing and analyzing the interviews. The three columns were content interaction, process, and themes and patterns.

Following the identification of themes and patterns, the researcher used different colored index cards to represent the domains and categories. The reason for the use of the index cards was to assist in identifying connectedness between domains, categories, and subcategories. The domain of inquiry was the health care meaning, values, expressions, lived experiences, and practices of rural Nicaraguan men. Phase III involved searching the data for recurrent patterns of meanings and saturation. Phase IV involved finalizing the patterns to develop universal and diverse theme statements. These theme statements made the components of an abstracted model that will assist nurses and other health care professionals in promoting health and well-being among Nicaraguan men. According to Spradley (1980), "ethnographic data analysis is a search for patterns and these patterns make up the culture" (p. 3).

Rigor

The researcher conducted "member checks" to ensure credibility. The researcher has done and will continue to do extensive fieldwork with the population under study to enhance credibility to the study. Credibility in this study was achieved by having the informants validate the researcher's interpretation of their interview responses and observations. Audiotapes of each informant was transcribed verbatim by two male Nicaraguan translators, and field notes were taken to enhance credibility. White and Johnson (1998) support the use of a male Nicaraguan translator and identified that, when gender differences exist between researchers and participants, researchers can miss or misinterpret a vital aspect of data because its relevance is not identified. In the positivistic paradigm, credibility would be equated with internal validity.

Consistency of the research findings was achieved by validating and clarifying emerging data as the study progressed. The researcher kept a list of evolving concepts as well as a journal documenting data analysis decisions. Only the researcher conducted all the interviews with the help of Nicaraguan translators. A doctorally prepared nurse, who was a member of the dissertation committee and experienced in qualitative data analysis, served as the mentor to ensure credibility. This ensured accuracy of data analysis by the researcher by validating the researcher's interpretation and decision trail. In the positivistic paradigm, consistency would be equated with reliability. Neutrality was achieved in this study by consistently validating and clarifying data. The researcher made all efforts to separate any preconceived notions or biases by keeping a journal on any ideas that may evolve during the research process.

Procedures

Gaining Access and Acceptance

When the researcher decided to conduct the ethnography in La Reforma, the next step was to gain access and acceptance into the culture. Although any resident of La Reforma will speak to strangers with a respectful greeting or a pleasant comment, more substantive conversation begins only after the residents accept the person. Because ethnography requires the intimate study of people, the activities in which they are involved, and the places in which they live, the researcher needed to gain access and acceptance from the residents of La Reforma in order to collect these data. The researcher did fieldwork for 1.5 years, during which time he became familiar with key individuals of the community and hired a translator and a driver, who were originally from the La Reforma area. The primary persons were the supervisor of La Reforma, the two schoolteachers of La Reforma, and the deacon of the local church.

The supervisor has responsibilities much like a mayor in the United States. He is responsible for running community meetings, seeking out assistance for the community when needed, and representing La Reforma in governmental meetings in Jinotega. The schoolteacher is responsible for educating the youth of La Reforma up to sixth grade. There is no secondary education in La Reforma. He teaches in a very small two-room schoolhouse located directly behind the Roberto Clemente Clinic. He holds status in the community because of his ability to read and his general knowledge. He is viewed as a scholar in the community. The deacon of the local church is a significant member of the community because of his religious commitment. His responsibilities include providing weekly religious services to the people of La Reforma because Easter Sunday is the only complete mass available to the people. A main responsibility for the deacon is to bring communion to the ill and those who cannot attend the weekly services. The deacon provides spiritual counseling to individuals, families, and the community.

These key individuals, as well as the driver and the translator, expedited access and acceptance. My association with Duquesne University School of Nursing, which played a vital role in the development of the local clinic, and past work in the Rotary clinic, facilitated gaining access to and acceptance from the people of La Reforma. The researcher had seen patients and taken students to the Roberto Clemente clinic, and the people of La Reforma trusted his commitment to improving their health. Much of the population is Catholic. Because the researcher is a Catholic and frequently participated in church activities by invitation, acceptance into the community was enhanced and a sense of trust was established. Some residents believe that health care providers, by nature of their work, are extensions of God.

Another event that eased the access and accessibility process for the researcher was conducting a pilot study with six informants to validate the validity of the semi-structured interview guide prior to conducting the ethnography. The pilot study assisted with specific factors such as becoming more familiar with strategies of ethnography, ways to approach the men, learning the language, and pacing the interview because time was an issue for these men.

Process of Analysis

In keeping with the ethnographic practice of using "researcher as instrument," data were collected through field notes, participant observation, researcher as participant, and semi-structured interviews with study informants. The researcher interviewed 20 general informants and 4 key informants using a semi-structured interview. Interviews took place in the field, homes, and at the Roberto Clemente Clinic located in La Reforma. Interviews were conducted in Spanish by the researcher and two native speakers. Because of the native Spanish dialect that was spoken, two male Nicaraguan translators fluent in English were used to translate during the interviews.

The interviews lasted from 40 to 80 minutes. The average interview was 50 minutes. The interviews were audiotaped by the researcher and transcribed by the two translators. Interviews were translated into English and then back to Spanish to ensure all meaning was captured in the translation. Daily field notes were written by the researcher to reflect events, conversations, and observations. Field notes were used to validate and enhance the meaning of health and well-being obtained from the informants. Data were then organized into categories, subcategories, and patterns that were constantly compared and contrasted until data were saturated and no new situations occurred.

To ensure credibility, the researcher attempted to conduct second interviews on all informants to ensure the data were accurate. The second interview was conducted to confirm or correct the researcher's interpretation of the significant statements obtained from the first interview. Any new data were included in the analysis. The researcher was able to conduct second interviews on 45% ($n = 9$) of the 20 general informants and 75% ($n = 3$) of the 4 key informants. During the follow-up interview, each man had the opportunity to clarify data and to elaborate on his answers to the questionnaire.

These second interviews were conducted in the field, in homes, and at the Roberto Clemente Clinic and lasted an average of 20 minutes. Categories, subcategories, five themes, and cultural values emerged from the data. Spradley's (1979) category analysis was used to identify common characteristics and common meanings within the culture of rural Nicaraguan men. Data collection and analysis occurred simultaneously.

RESULTS AND DISCUSSION

Description of Cultural Informants

There were a total of 20 general informants, nine of whom were interviewed twice and four key informants, three of whom were interviewed twice. The informants were selected for interviews using the "snowball" method through the key and general informants. The demographic descriptions include age, marital status, utilization of Jinotega hospital, use of Roberto Clemente Clinic, number of children, number of individuals living in same house, and the community. The goal was to obtain a heterogenous group of men who shared their meaning of health and well-being. The demographic data illustrated the heterogeneity of the group. The ages of the men ranged from 19 to 61 years. The mean age was 38.6 years. The marital status of the men included 14 (70%) who were married and 6 (30%) who had a partner that they referred to as their wife but stated they were not married. The mean number of children per man was 4.25. The mean number of individuals living in the same house was 6.9 residents. Seventy-five percent ($n = 15$) of the general informants have never been a patient in the Jinotega hospital. Eighty percent ($n = 16$) of the general informants use the Roberto Clemente Clinic. All participants ($n = 20$; 100%) lived in small pueblos in the area of La Reforma.

Theory of Endurance

A beginning theory of endurance emerged from the analysis of the data. Rural Nicaraguan men live in a world that requires a high degree of endurance. Five main themes that compose the Endurance Model are:

1. Health is being able to function and meet responsibilities for self, family, and community.

2. Health is believing that you will be cared for by God.
3. Health is composed of five dimensions: spiritual, physical, mental, family, and community.
4. Health is withstanding the hardships of poverty, access to health care, and inadequate health care supplies.
5. Health and health care practices are impacted by economic, environmental, work, and worldview factors.

The Endurance Model represents the interrelationships among the major concepts and themes and is a dynamic model. The components of the model are complex and interrelated. The identified concepts impact the way these individuals define their health and well-being and the manner in which they maintain and restore health and well-being. At the center of the model, the main emic definition of health (health as being able to function) is given. The five dimensions of health as described by rural Nicaraguan men are depicted as a circular border with no definitive beginning or end. The significance of this circle is that no one dimension of health can be altered without impacting the other dimensions. Each dimension is equally important in maintaining homeostasis that ultimately leads to health and well-being.

In the Endurance Model, the rural Nicaraguan man and the dimensions of health are surrounded by a halo that represents the health care provider. The majority of rural Nicaraguan men believe that health care providers are extensions of God. Health care providers have the ability to impact all dimensions of health in an attempt to assist these men in attaining, regaining, and maintaining their health and well-being. The rural Nicaraguan man and the dimensions of health are suspended in a triangle representing the limitations of the social situation. The three social structure limitations located at each corner of the triangle are poverty, access to health care, and inadequate health care supplies. Each dimension of health touches the triangle showing that each element of health is impacted by the inherent social structure. An isosceles triangle is suspended in the middle of a circle, illustrating the world of endurance in which the Nicaraguan man lives. The circle's border represents the stable line of endurance. If one would dissect the stable line of endurance, the finding would reveal three interwoven strands representing the dynamic and interrelated properties of these elements by which the rural Nicaraguan man endures.

The three elements inherent in endurance are God, natural medicines, and suffering. The interwoven strand representing God is larger than the strands representing natural medicines and suffering. God is viewed as the main resource for enduring and assisting by providing natural medicines and strength during suffering; the other two elements are associated with enduring. All lines starting from the center of the model outward are connected, showing the interconnectedness of the concepts and comprehensiveness and dynamic relationship of the model. No one concept stands alone in the model. One can follow any line that is connected to the Nicaraguan man and trace it out to the stable line of endurance. The Nicaraguan man is represented by the connection between earth and heaven, and the passion the Nicaraguan man endures is based on the social situation of La Reforma and Nicaragua.

A cultural example illustrating the use of the model became evident during the fieldwork phase of the study. Male participants in the study frequently told me that they would go to the clinic as a result of experiencing pain and burning on urination, and pain located in the flank area lasting approximately 2 weeks. The men would not travel to the clinic immediately because to do so would take them away from their work. When they arrived at the clinic, they encountered one of two situations: either the clinic was closed, or the antibiotics were not available to treat what was most likely a urinary tract infection. If the physician was at the clinic, the doctor would write them a prescription for the antibiotic. As a result of the inadequate supply of medications, the man would have to go to the nearest city, which was about 1½ hours by bus, to purchase the antibiotic. Due to the extreme poverty in the region, these men did not have the money to take the bus or to purchase the antibiotics. As a result, they would return home to suffer further from the symptoms of a urinary tract infection, pray to God for healing and for the strength to endure, and utilize natural medications such as Llanten and Bejuco de sangre. Llanten was taken to alleviate acidic urine and Bejuco de sangre for alleviating kidney pain.

The rural Nicaraguan men have a strong spiritual dimension of health that gives them faith that God will provide them with strength to endure the discomfort in order to continue to work. These men described how they thank God for the natural medicines He has provided them. A strong cultural value of family is seen when one is ill, the nuclear as well as the extended family and the community assist and provide for each other during a time of need. Mental health is maintained knowing that the family and community will assist them until they can return to work.

The model of endurance was generated from the themes and cultural values of Nicaraguan men expressed to the researcher during the fieldwork and the interviews. Table 4.1 lists emerging themes and the cultural values that emerged from the data analysis.

Table 4.1 *Five Themes That Evolved From the Data*

Themes	Cultural Values
Health is believing that one will be cared for by God	God must prevail
Health is being able to function and meet responsibilities for self, family, and community	Acceptance of God's will
Health is composed of five dimensions: Spiritual, physical, mental, family, and community	God knows one's name
Economic, environmental, work, and worldview factors guide health care practices of rural Nicaraguan men	Health and well-being as being able to function
Health is maintained through enduring the hardships of poverty, access to health care, and suffering from inadequate health care supplies	Peacefulness is equivalent to being healthy
	Strong quality of endurance
	Provide for the family
	Community healthiness
	Helping each other
	Natural medicines
	Father as health care decision maker
	Mother as health care informant
	Respect (Santito)

Discussion of Domains, Categories, Subcategories, and Themes

This section contains an abbreviated discussion of the concepts and themes that emerged from the data and that led to the Endurance Model. Due to the space constraints of writing a chapter as opposed to a dissertation, only some highlights are given here. Within the domain of health and category dimensions of health, five subcategories or dimensions of health were identified: spiritual, physical, mental, family, and community. An interdependent association exists among these subcategories. Although these are discussed separately, the men described health and well-being in general as equilibrium among all six.

Subcategory of Spiritual Health

The men of La Reforma commented on the link between God and health. The first and strongest dimension of health is the spiritual aspect of self, and they said they experienced a personal relationship with God. These men viewed

God as a friend, a confidant, and a guide; they believed that God is in total control and that He knows all and that a person cannot fool Him. Some of their comments were:

"We live by the power of God; if God does not move, not even a leaf can move."

"God is over everything including our health."

"What happens to us is God's will."

According to comments made by study participants, God is good, and these men call upon Him not only for strength to function every day but also for strength to endure in times of need and suffering. Comments made by these men included:

God is the main resource that we have to help us with health. God is the only one who can give health and strength to me. He gives strength and health to all people. All you have to do is trust in God and ask him to provide you with good health and strength, and He will do for you what He has done for others. He provides you with what you ask Him for.

Many of the men believe that God knows each of us by one's name. During the researcher's first two interviews, when the men were asked to falsify their name for the purpose of anonymity and confidentiality, they selected animal names such as dog (*perro*) and cat (*gatto*). During the third interview when the researcher asked the man to falsify his name to maintain anonymity and confidentiality, he refused to do so for this reason:

I will not change my name because God is my father and He knows me by name; He knows us all by our names. That is bad luck to change your name. If you need to include my name in your write up, you have my permission to use my real name.

Many of the men believed that all occurrences are a result of God's work, whether favorable or unfavorable. Many of these men viewed the Contra War, the 1972 earthquake, and Hurricane Mitch (1998) as a message from God, reminding them that He is in control. One man stated:

I asked for God's help because it was God's command to have the hurricane affect us, because it was a punishment for us. Sometimes we forget that God is in control, and we think we are, and God has to remind us, and the hurricane was how He reminded us who is in control.

Doctors and nurses were viewed as extensions of God by study participants. The belief is that God gave doctors and nurses their intelligence to help people.

I thank God every day for people like you and our doctors and nurses at the clinic.

The Roberto Clemente Clinic was viewed as a gift from God and the doctors and nurses as extensions of God. One's relationship with God was viewed as an essential element of good health. All the general and key informants commented on this balance between their relationship with God and health. Field notes and observations were used to validate this relationship between God and these Nicaraguan men. Many of the men wore religious artifacts around their necks such as rosary beads, crosses, and icons of saints. All the homes that the researcher visited had religious pictures hanging on the walls, and one area of the home was specifically designated as a prayer area. This area usually consisted of a kneeling area, a statue of the Virgin Mary, rosary beads, and burning candles.

Each community was proud to show the researcher their church. One community invited the researcher to participate in mass on Miercoles de Ceniza (Ash Wednesday). Children's spirituality combined with respect was demonstrated when the children approached the researcher. Children approached the researcher with their hands folded as in prayer, and the researcher was instructed to touch the child's hand and say, "santito" (little saint), allowing the child to continue on with a blessing from God. During earlier visits to the Roberto Clemente Clinic, the researcher had brought rosary beads for the residents. The residents were frequently seen wearing the rosaries around their necks; the rosaries were also seen on the necks and wrists of their children.

The men who participated in the study reported that God had influenced many aspects of their life. Prayer was the most frequently observed and reported religious practice. Men were also observed praying in their homes, churches, and cemeteries. A small church is located close to the La Reforma clinic. Many of the men were seen leaving the clinic and going over to this adjacent church to pray. Blessing themselves with the sign-of-the-cross was a common practice of the men prior to performing daily activities.

The men reported a strong belief that God was in control, and if you ask Him for help, He will provide it.

We all communicate with God through prayer at Mass. Mass is a celebration of God's word. The priest unites us with God.

In summary, spirituality was an integral component of all aspects of life, including health and well-being. Spiritual health involved living a life dedicated to God, relying on their trust in God, recognizing that God is in control, and following God's command. Nicaraguan men reported maintaining their relationship with God through prayer. They told the researcher that they believe they should help each other because they all are brothers and sisters and God is their father. These men demonstrated commitment to their faith through church activities and spiritual customs carried out in the family and the community.

Subcategory of Physical Health

Informants described health as being able to conduct daily activities, and they related it particularly to work. All men defined health as not having problems that kept them from working. Consistent with this definition was that the men referred to health as not being ill.

> Health is knowing your body and being able to recognize symptoms that prevented you from working.

Being healthy means being able to conduct daily functions, especially being able to work every day. Consistent with this definition of health, health care is defined as sick care. Most of the informants in the study described health care as sick care. Sick care enables them to function again. Many men commented on the need for medications to rid their bodies of symptoms that may impede them from working. All the men defined health as being able to function and work to provide for the family and the community. When asked "How do you know you are healthy?" all the men commented that they felt healthy when they were able to work and provide for their family and community. The second most common remark made was that they felt healthy when their body didn't feel bad.

> I am not healthy when I feel a change in my body different than a healthy feeling. I feel heavy and have no intentions of working.

> Work and health are equal.

> It is very important for me to work, and God has put me here to work, and being able to work means to be able to live.

> I think health is being able to work well and to feel good with no problems in the body. It is important for me to work every day for the necessities. One is always healthy and peaceful when one is able to get food, money for his children, and himself.

Healthy is being able to get medicines when we need them for the illness. This is important! When I am healthy, I can work without any pain. I am happy when I can work and buy my food. When I am sick, I can't work.

One of the informant's comments illustrates health as being able to function and that rural men must continue to work even when some symptoms of illness are present.

When I don't feel sick and I go to work peacefully without any pain, I feel healthy. Sometimes, you have to go to work with a headache or some sickness, but it is necessary to work to provide for your family, so you go regardless of how you feel.

In summary, the informants in the study experienced health as the ability to function. The emphasis was on being able to conduct daily activities, not to become sick, and to seek health care only when the ability to function was impaired. The major concern for health care providers is that, with this perception of health, early symptoms may be ignored until functioning is impaired. How rural Nicaraguan men define physical health and ways they stay healthy will be the focus in the following discussion.

Subcategory of Mental Health

No major mental illnesses were obvious during fieldwork. However, during the interviews emotional statements emerged. Many of the men commented that:

Health is being peaceful; where peaceful is being happy with your life, family, and community; and being able to provide for your family and community.

Many of the men voiced a feeling of frustration with the lack of medications and services provided by the clinic. One informant stated:

When I come to the clinic to obtain medications for my child and they don't have any, I become frustrated. That means that I have to go into the city, and I don't have the money or the time from work to do so, but I do because the medications are necessary for my child.

It is significant for me to work every day for the necessities. One should always be healthy and peaceful when they are able to get food and money for their family.

Nicaraguan men defined health as being peaceful. In La Reforma "peaceful" has a literal connotation, the absence of war. La Reforma was one of the regions where much of the contra war transpired. The residents of La Reforma suffered immensely from much of the combat that occurred during the contra war. The word "peaceful" was used by several informants in their definition of health. The majority of the men referred to being peaceful when one can work and provide for the family and community and when one is able to eat every day. Peacefulness was frequently referred to as doing God's will or following His command. A strong theme running throughout the study was that, when these men were able to work and provide for the family and community, they are in peace. This was identified as equivalent to being healthy. For example, one informant said:

> When I am able to work, I live happy and with peace of mind, and I am able to think clearly. I live peaceful because I can work every day. I don't feel any pain in my body and I eat normal. When I am sick, I don't have an appetite, and when I go to my house for a break from work, I can't relax because I am not peaceful.

Several of the men referred to experiencing peacefulness when they go to the clinic or bring their family to the clinic and find it open.

> I am peaceful when I go to the clinic and see the same nurses. It is not peaceful to go to the clinic for medicines that I need or my family needs and find the nurses not there.
>
>> One principle I live my life by is being healthy which makes me peaceful. When I am sick, I am not peaceful.

Some informants referred to being "peaceful" as a result of their ability to do things in the community, being with other people, and assisting the family and community.

In summary, changes in emotional mental health occurred in response to physical health, and influencing variables appear to be due to the individual's financial situation and lack of medications. One goal of these Nicaraguan men is to achieve and maintain internal peacefulness in order to function or work, thus remaining healthy.

Subcategory of Family and Community Health

Family and community were the fourth and fifth subcategories of health identified. Several Nicaraguan men defined health as being able to provide for one's family. Family data were obtained through field notes, participant observation, and genograms. Families that live in La Reforma care for themselves through cooperative efforts of the family members. During one of the researcher's visits, a 5-year-old girl was observed cooking a banana in the hot coals for her 2-year-old sister. After cooking the banana, she peeled it and fed it to her sister. Frequently older children were observed watching their younger siblings, allowing time for the mother to do her chores. Younger generations were expected to show respect to adults. Children approached adults with their hands folded and waited for the adult to touch their folded hands saying, "santito." Younger generations always addressed the older men and women as Senora and Senor as a way of showing respect.

Appropriate use of words also demonstrated respect; for example, when younger individuals spoke to adults, they used the formal form of "usted" in the place of "tu" when referring to the pronoun "you." When children were told to do something for the father, mother, and adults, they would respond by saying, "Si, senor" or "Si, senora." During home and clinic visits, many of these respectful behaviors were implemented when meeting the researcher.

The Nicaraguan family unit varied considerably from home to home. The man lived with his wife, or significant other, and their children. Data obtained from genograms identified that more information was known about the man's family than the woman's family. The reason for this was that the woman left her family and began her new life with the man's family. As a result of distance and travel issues, the women would frequently lose contact with their families. It was not uncommon to have relatives of the man living in the house along with girlfriends and boyfriends of their children. The average number of individuals living in a one- or two-room house was 6.9. The men referred to the members living in their house as their nuclear family. The extended family referred to relatives such as brothers, grandparents, aunts, and uncles who lived close to the man. They all worked the same fields to provide food for their families. They were very proud of their relatives and frequently invited the researcher to visit their relative's home in order to be introduced. One informant and the researcher walked a mile and a half to meet the informant's 100-year-old (approximate age) grandmother.

Many times, the men referred to members of their church as spiritual brothers and sisters. Godparents (padrinos) were frequently referred to as members of the family. Close family members have frequent contact and a sense of obligation to other family members.

Sunday was referred to as a day of rest. Following mass on Sunday, families and close friends gathered at a particular home for a day of eating and relaxing. Prior to gathering at the identified home, families visited ill members of the family and community. Many of the men referred to themselves as the community supporters. Community supporter was used with reference to the agricultural work that needs to be maintained to keep the community healthy. Many families in the community shared their livestock and crops. The men of the community verbalized a strong value committed to helping provide food for all members of the community. Many of the men served on community councils and church councils. The men were very active in developing and setting up community programs usually associated with the church and the Roberto Clemente Clinic.

A strong value of "we are one" supported the strong community commitment of these men.

"Our community has an agreement to help each other."

"I am healthy when I know I could help someone when she or he needs it."

"My family and my community . . ."

"For me, health is important for the community and the family."

"Being healthy is when not much sickness is in the community, and my family and community is eating well."

Many interviews began in crop and coffee fields. The majority of the time the informants asked the researcher to accompany them to their house where the interview continued. The researcher observed women carrying wood to start the fire. All homes had fires going all day and the day's supper cooking. Once the research team arrived at the house, the man asked the researcher and translators in to sit at the table to continue the interview. During the health history component of the genogram, all the men would refer to their wives or significant others to answer questions about the family's health history. It was found that the men made the families' health care decisions and the women were the health care historians. When women and children were seen in the clinic and needed to be referred to the city for treatment, the wife would seek out the husband and allow him to make the decision. The main reason the man would not permit them to travel was the fear of losing work time because he would have to care for the remaining children at home.

Domain of Health

Ways to stay healthy was identified as a category under the domain of health. The majority of the comments made regarding ways to stay healthy focused on God, medicine, sleeping and eating well, natural medicines, family members caring for them when they were sick, and the use of the clinic only when experiencing symptoms.

Even though the diet seemed suboptimal, families seemed to have adequate amounts of food, which they had grown within the community. The nutrition in La Reforma consisted of rice, beans, plantains, fruit, and occasionally red and white meat. Women in some of the homes were making tortillas. Much of the food was cooked in animal grease. Cabbage stew was a popular meal. The researcher observed cabbage stew boiling in many of the homes. Knowing that their family and community had what they considered good food created a sense of well-being among the men.

Many men admitted to using the clinic in an attempt to obtain medications to rid the body from bad symptoms. They strongly expressed their concerns and frustrations with the Roberto Clemente Clinic. Two main issues that kept surfacing during the interviews were (a) frequently finding the clinic closed after they had walked hours to be treated and (b) the clinic not having adequate medications needed to treat their illnesses.

> I go to the clinic to see the doctor, and I hope they have the medications to give me. I say in the name of God that this medication will resolve my illness. If I don't ask God to help me first, the medicines will not work. God is first and then man. Without God, there is nothing.
>
> When I do not have the intention to work, I know my body is not right; so I look for medicines to help me get better. I look for a way to get healthy.
>
> When I feel unhealthy; I look for medications and try to eat correctly.

None of the men interviewed indicated he had regular health checkups for disease or for health promotion purposes. The local Roberto Clemente Clinic was only used for sick care and not for illness prevention or health promotion. During participant observation a number of these men brought their significant others and children to participate in health promotion activities at the clinic; however, they would not routinely participate. The main reason for using the clinic was for obtaining medications to relieve symptoms that prevented them from working. Many times the clinic did not have medications, and they would be given a prescription. This troubled the men because they had to then travel to Jinotega to get the prescription filled. These men lacked the money needed for the medications; they did not have the money required to take a bus to Jinotega. Many of these men reverted back to enduring through

God, natural medicines, and suffering as a way to stay healthy. These remedies were substances used to prevent, heal, or cure an illness. Most of these natural remedies were botanical in nature, and their identification, knowledge, and uses have been shared from generation to generation by storytelling. Natural medicines were in the form of tablets, drinks, lotions, rubbing solutions, and bathing solutions. The most common natural medicines and their uses identified by these rural Nicaraguan men are listed in Table 4.2.

Not every informant believed in natural remedies; however, the majority stated they used these remedies. The doctor and nurse who worked in the Roberto Clemente Clinic agreed that the use of natural remedies is widespread. Many of the men told the researcher that, as a result of the lack of medications at the clinic and money to purchase medications, they must use natural remedies as they endure to restore health, because that is all they have in the mountains. One informant commented that he has always tried to treat the pain in his body.

Table 4.2 *Natural Medicines Identified by Informants*

Natural Medicines	Conditions and Uses
Aquacate (avocado)	Hypertension, kidney infections, diarrhea, headaches, fever, gallbladder, source for vitamins A, B, D, E
Arnica	Calms nerves
Bee stings	Arthritic pain
Bejuco de sangre	Kidney pain
Gavilon leg	Itching
Eucalyptus	Coughs, sinusitis, fever
Junta/ion (icy/hot)	Muscular pain
Zacate de limon (Lemon grass)	Bronchitis, coughs, colds, headaches, stomachaches, sleep
Llanten	Skin infections, liver infections, antiseptic, cleanses the blood and lungs, alleviates acid
Manzanilla (chamomile)	Calms stomach infections, regulates digestion, assists with sleeping, calms nerves
Pelo de maiz (corn hair tea)	Kidney infections
Ruda	Nerves, sore throat, intestinal parasites, menstrual discomfort, prevents heart attacks and epilepsy,
Savila (aloe vera)	Gastritis, colitis, hemorrhoids, burns, prostate inflammation, fever
Naranja acida (sour orange juice)	Colds, flu, stomach ache, diarrhea

> When I have a fever, I boil the lemon grass and savila with sugar and take it and then cover myself up to get rid of my fever.
>
> I use sour orange juice and lemon leaves to help people with stomach aches, and when I can't get medications from the clinic, I use lemon grass, savila, avocado, and ruda.

In summary, men would attempt to eat and sleep well in order to remain healthy. Once one identified himself as unhealthy because of the development of some symptoms, he would first ask God for strength to regain his health. A second way to stay healthy and to restore health was to seek out medications at the clinic. If medications were available, these men would take them appropriately. However, many times these men found that the clinic did not have the medications needed to treat them. Because of the lack of medications at the clinic and lack of money needed to pay for the travel to Jinotega, these men reverted to natural medicines. Many of the men told the researcher that they believed in *curanderos* (natural healers); however, since the one in La Reforma died approximately 6 years ago, there are no others. The closest Curandero is in Jinotega.

Endurance

Enduring is a means to maintain or regain health; it is the result of the daily challenges of work, poverty, lack of access to health care, and inadequate health care supplies. Endurance refers to the ways a person "gets through" extraordinary physiological or psychological assault. In this study, endurance was an internal psychic as well as a physical process that these men go through when they are unable to obtain necessities needed to resolve the problems of everyday life. Many informants identified endurance as an internal feeling that one experiences to sustain one's self, family, and community.

> I hurt when one of my family is hurting, not physically, but deep inside I have the pain in me. We are all brothers, God is our Father. We all have pain, and we all suffer together.

> When someone in our community suffers, we all suffer too.

> If we go to the clinic, most of the time, they don't have the right medications or they don't have enough of it. So they give us prescriptions and expect us to go to Jinotega for the medications. We are poor and do not have the money to go to Jinotega; so we have to endure the problem. God is the only medicine we have. That is all we have.

I have to use natural medicines like manzalla. This means for me, I just have to endure.

We endure because we don't have the money to buy medications, therefore we endure the pain. God cares for me first when I am enduring and then my family.

When enduring I pray to God, I believe in God, God is the first to help us when we are enduring, the best medicine is to pray to God.

Endurance means that my body suffers, and I don't have the strength to go to work.

SUMMARY

The goal of this ethnographic study was to uncover, identify, and understand the cultural meaning of health and well-being among rural Nicaraguan men. This ethnographic approach explored the emic meaning of health and well-being, variables that influenced health and well-being, and identified self-care behaviors of rural Nicaraguan men. This study involved 20 general informants and four key informants, who volunteered to participate in the study. The sample was limited to Nicaraguan men who lived in La Reforma, Jinotega, Nicaragua. The results of this study contributed to the generation of a theory of endurance that can be used by professional nurses who care for rural Nicaraguan men. The five themes that were revealed through analysis of the data will be presented in light of the current literature related to each theme.

Review of the Research Literature Related to the Emerged Concepts

Following the data analysis the researcher returned to the literature in search of additional research exploring the concepts of God, health as the ability to function, endurance, family and community impact on health, and the use of folk remedies. Review of the literature revealed a number of articles addressing the identified concepts; however, the majority of the literature studied Mexican Americans living in the United States. Few articles addressed the concepts related to Hispanic men, and no studies were identified addressing concepts regarding Nicaraguan men. When a Hispanic family member is ill, family members usually provide the family member with physical and emotional support. Hispanics have a commitment to the extended family which becomes even stronger during illness. In addition to valuing the family, many Hispanics have traditionally valued religion, especially Catholicism and the celebration of the mass. Because of this deep religious faith, many Hispanics believe in self-sacrifice, giving rather than taking, enduring hardships, and accepting fate. Hispanics typically value the present over the future.

Coffin-Ronig (1997) conducted a study that investigated the sociocultural factors that play a role in the process of ending an abusive relationship among Latinos. Dimensional analysis was the method employed for the development of a grounded theory. Enduring emerged from this study as pivotal in gaining an understanding of the process of ending an abusive relationship for Latinos. Participants indicated that personal and religious beliefs, the importance of family, and needs of their children were reasons for enduring the abuse.

Martinez (1999) conducted an ethnographic study to gain a definition of health as perceived by a group of Hispanic older adults. The major domains of health, which were identified, were family, God, and community. Spiritual aspects of life played a major role in their health. Caring for self was lived through caring for others for whom one has responsibility. A strong emphasis on natural remedies emerged from this study.

A focused ethnography conducted by Higgins and Learn (1999) discovered the patterns and variability of health practices used by Hispanic women aged 20 to 40 years. These women were interviewed about their health practices. A theme that emerged from the data was an emphasis on the importance of spirituality and integration of the spiritual dimension as important to healthy living.

Rehm (1999) explored Mexican American family experiences with chronic childhood illness, from the perspective of parents, and reported findings about the influence of religious faith on families' spiritual and secular responses to illness. Following in-depth interviewing for data collection, six unifying dimensions of religious faith were related to parental caretaking and decision making for the family. The six dimensions were (a) God determined the outcome of the child's illness; (b) God and health care for the child were closely linked; (c) parents took an an active role in facilitating God's will; (d) families had obligations to God; (e) intercession with God by others was often sought by or offered to the family; and (f) faith encouraged optimism.

Villarruel (1995) conducted an ethnographic study to discover Mexican American cultural meanings, expressions, self-care, and dependent-care actions associated with experiences of pain. Data were collected from 20 general informants and 20 key informants. Thematic and pattern analysis was used to examine meanings, expressions, self-care, and care of others related to experiences identified by informants as painful. The six themes identified included (a) pain is an encompassing experience of suffering that transcends the individual and affects others in the family and community; (b) pain is an accepted obligation of life and one's role within the family, a burden one must bear so as not to inflict pain on others; (c) to endure pain stoically is expected and esteemed; (d) a folk system of beliefs related to causes and care for illness and pain has been transmitted across generations and is used with other health systems in care of self and others who are experiencing pain; (e) the primacy of caring for others is the essence of the family; and (f) variation in gender expressions of pain and patterns of care are context specific. The acceptance of pain as part of life, expectations to hide the pain, and the centrality of care by and for the family were among the patterns that have been transmitted from generation to generation.

Additional literature that identified health as the ability to function was reviewed following data analysis. Purnell and Counts (1998) identified that, among Appalachians, health was perceived as the ability function. In the Appalachian culture, health is defined as involving the body, mind, and spirit. Disease is a problem if it interfered with one's daily life or functions.

Suarez, Raffaelli, and O'Leary (1996) investigated the use of folk healing practices used by HIV-infected Hispanics. Anonymous individual interviews were conducted with 58 male and 18 female HIV-infected Hispanics aged 23 to 55, primarily of Puerto Rican origin. The majority of the informants believed in good and evil spirits (73.7%); among the 56 believers, 48% stated that the spirits had a causal role in their infection. Two thirds of the informants engaged in folk healing (spiritualism and/or Santeria). The main desired outcomes of folk healing included physical relief (44%), spiritual relief (40%), and protection from evil (26%). A number of the respondents stated that they hoped to effect a cure by engaging in folk healing.

Conclusions

1. The informants (all rural Nicaraguan men) of this study had faith that God will provide them with strength to function or endure.
2. The informants of this study defined health and well-being as being able to carry out responsibilities for self, family, and community.
3. The informants of this study viewed health care as sick care.
4. The informants of this study viewed professional health care providers as extensions of God.
5. The informants of this study are restricted to health care access due to socioeconomic variables.
6. The informants of this study had a strong quality of endurance.

The rural Nicaraguan men of La Reforma live health by creating a homeostasis within their spiritual, physical, mental, family, and community lives. Their faith allows them to develop an intimate relationship with God and to believe that God's plan is the natural process. Between this relationship with God and their value system, they will be guided to make appropriate decisions. Many of life's daily struggles, social inequities, natural disasters, and war are viewed as tests or challenges for the men to live their faith. The community shares responsibility and accountability for individual and group well-being. Men define health as the ability to function to meet the responsibilities of family and community. One is never alone in this world was a common theme among the study participants. A strong commitment to "we are one" was described frequently by the men in relation to how the family and community support each other. God, family, and community must, therefore, be recognized as important extensions of the individual within this culture.

This attempt to understand the lifeways and worldview of rural Nicaraguan men was driven by three research questions. First was the need to understand the meaning of health from the perspectives of Nicaraguan men. Men shared their cultural meaning through defining their meaning during the interview. The responses assisted the researcher with the emic definition of health and well-being. Study participants consistently referred to health as the ability to function in order to meet their family and community responsibilities. To maintain well-being, informants identified five dimensions of health: spiritual, physical, mental, family, and community. Well-being was defined as a homeostasis among all five dimensions of health. The rural health clinic and health care providers were viewed as gifts from God.

Rural Nicaraguan men have traditionally valued religion, especially Catholicism and the celebration of the mass. Mass was a time to be united with God, a time for prayer, and a time for forgiveness. Because of this deep religious faith, these men believe in self-sacrifice, giving rather than taking, enduring hardships, and acceptance of fate. One man offered an entire banana branch full of bananas to the researcher, knowing how much that could provide to his family. Observation of the lifeways of these Nicaraguan men allowed the researcher to appreciate the self-reliance of the rural Nicaraguan people. The strength to endure the social limitations was beyond the researcher's comprehension, but for the rural Nicaraguan, it was a way of life. The rural Nicaraguan men value the present over the future. The present is viewed as a gift from God, and the future is viewed as the will of God. They work to live for one day at a time. What will be will be God's will. Many of the natural disasters were viewed as a reminder from God that He is in control.

In addition to valuing religion, the researcher found that many of these Nicaraguan men value the development and nurturing of close personal relationships. When a man's family member was ill, family members were observed providing their sick member with physical and emotional support. Both nuclear and extended family members were involved with the ill person's care. The people of La Reforma have a commitment to the extended family, which becomes stronger during illness.

During fieldwork and interviews, the researcher observed and identified variables that impacted the health of rural Nicaraguan men. It became evident how social restraints, such as poverty, access, and inadequate health care supplies, influenced the health of rural Nicaraguan men. The majority of rural Nicaraguan men who participated in the study verbalized how important the Roberto Clemente clinic was to their health. The clinic was used predominantly for sick care. The men would travel to the clinic in response to a health problem, but once they arrived at the clinic, the men would be told that the medication needed to resolve the health problem was not available. The lack of necessary medications is one of the biggest deterrents to the health and well-being of these Nicaraguan men. When medications are not available the clinic physician or nurse gives the men a prescription for the medication and informs them that they need to go to Jinotega to purchase the medication. Most of these men do not have the money, time, or transportation needed to obtain the medication in Jinotega. Men are beginning to lose faith in the clinic because most of them have found the lack of medications at the clinic to be the norm rather than the exception.

As the men answered the researcher's questions during the interviews, it became evident that self-care behaviors of rural Nicaraguan men were influenced by the inherent social structure. Men care for themselves with natural medications learned from past generations . They believe that nature holds the ability to restore health and well-being; it provides natural remedies. The men only use the clinic when they believe that the illness threatened their ability to function/work. The men described the illness process as follows: when one becomes ill, they first pray to God because he is the only definite cure they have in the mountains. Then once they feel their ability to function is impaired, the men would travel to the clinic in the hope of receiving medications to get rid of the illness. The majority of the time, the lack of medications causes the men to revert to enduring through God, natural medicines, and suffering.

The theory of endurance provides an understanding of the cultural meaning of health and well-being among rural Nicaraguan men. As social and environmental factors impinge on the health and well-being of these rural men, multiple interventions need to be implemented to promote an optimal goal of well-being. Health education programs focusing on health promotion and illness prevention need to be developed and implemented. Health policy changes need to address the issue of supplying medications to the rural areas. As a result of the poverty level of these men and lack of transportation, health policy agendas that address transportation issues to larger health care centers must be a priority. Tapping into international drug companies and asking them to assist with the medication situation in La Reforma can be a solution to the medication problem.

As health care professionals, we must reach an understanding that culturally specific beliefs and behaviors of clients need to be an essential and fundamental component to practice. Nurses who care for Nicaraguan men in Nicaragua and the United States must be open to extending the concept of "client" to include family, community, and perhaps extending or redefining our concept of health care providers to include informal healers, religious leaders, and family and community members who are highly regarded.

IMPLICATIONS FOR NURSING

Acting as a client advocate is a fundamental responsibility of nurses. To effectively perform this duty, nurses need an accurate understanding of the client's needs from their perspective. Nurses must be aware of the uniqueness of cultures and their responses to health and illness to ensure that appropriate health care interventions are designed to meet the needs of specific cultural groups such as Nicaraguan men. Health care providers will need to intervene with Hispanic clients and communities in culturally sensitive ways such as viewing culture as an enabler rather than a resistant force, incorporating cultural beliefs into the plans of care, stressing familismo, and involving the community in preventive health care programs. Such interventions require nurses and other health care providers to be knowledgeable about the culture, customs, and beliefs of the Hispanics within their practice area. Nurses will need to take a leading role in health care policy development that will improve health care for the growing Hispanic population.

The family was consistently identified as a main element in the health and well-being of Hispanics. It is essential for nurses, as health care leaders of the community, family, and other health care providers to develop better models of family-centered care. The importance of understanding individual values, beliefs, and health care practices is emphasized in the nursing literature (Leininger, 1991). Once values, beliefs, and health care practices are identified, appropriate health policy, health education programs, and research can be designed and implemented. As agents and advocates for consumers of health care, nurses need to be aware of information about the meaning of health and well-being of specific populations in order to provide culturally congruent nursing care. When health education programs and interventions are developed according to the individual's belief systems, compliance to such interventions are most likely to transpire.

The findings of this study support the need for nurses to gather more information on this vulnerable population. An understanding of the themes and the conceptual model of endurance that evolved from the study will help nurses to plan and provide culturally competent care to rural Nicaraguan men. The clinic nurses working with these rural Nicaraguan men can play a key role in the education of other health care practitioners involved in caring for these rural men. One important member of the community health care team in Nicaragua is the *brigadistas*. Currently, the brigadistas are trained to care only for women and children. As a result of this study, nurses can provide health education programs that incorporate men's health issues into the health care role of the brigadistas.

This study supports the inclusion of information on cultural variances in nursing and other health care curriculums. The findings of this study with regard to the definition of health and well-being among rural Nicaraguan men, the variables that influence their health and well-being, and their self-care behaviors indicate a need for understanding of the culture and the definitions of health across nursing and other health care curriculums. Culture plays a large role in how one defines health and well-being as well as health care. Therefore, an understanding of the culture of populations provides insights into the needs of these specific populations.

RECOMMENDATIONS FOR RESEARCH

Nursing is a practice-oriented discipline. The focus of research, then, needs to capture the response of the person as the person interacts with the environment and the social structure the person lives under. Nurses need to gain knowledge that emerges from the emic perspective. These experiences are not quantifiable; nurses need to implement qualitative research findings to gain insight into the meaning of human experiences, thereby improving the approach to health care by providing culturally congruent nursing care.

The role of waiting during the enduring experience should be further investigated. Waiting is prominent during the experience of enduring as the individual waits to return to health. How long do these men endure? Enduring and suffering is viewed as an expected life process because God's son in the Roman Catholic faith had to endure and suffer. How much time is enough time needed to move through this enduring process? What is the specific time frame that elapses, if any, that causes the stable line of endurance to break down causing these men to seek out further health care or death?

Additional research is needed to assist with the ongoing development of the theory of endurance. This research should focus on identifying related attributes and concepts of enduring. Morse and Penrod (1999) identified hope and uncertainty as related concepts of endurance when caring for spinal cord injury clients. What are the related attributes and concepts, if any, that these rural Nicaraguan men identify? These cultural attributes and concepts should be investigated qualitatively and added to the beginning model of endurance developed as a result of this study.

Additional ethnographic research studies are needed to understand whether this is the experience for all Nicaraguan men and if women share this same meaning. The meaning of health and well-being of men who are not in the rural areas is needed to build on and expand the developing theory. Further studies are needed to explore the impact of culture on the meaning of health and well-being of different cultural groups in the United States and internationally.

In summary, based on the results of this study, further research is recommended in the following areas:

1. Replication of the study using different settings
2. A comparative analysis of rural men and rural women to identify if the themes uncovered in this study are a result of the rural environmental context or gender
3. A comparative analysis of rural men, their families, and communities to identify consistency among the identified themes
4. Developing and implementing health care to rural Nicaraguan men using the developing model
5. Investigation of the waiting period that is involved during the endurance process
6. Investigation of the other attributes and concepts that might be related to the process of enduring and incorporating these concepts into the model of endurance
7. Studies that would test the developing theory of endurance

REFERENCES

Artinian, N. T., & Duggan, C. H. (1995). Sex differences in patient recovery patterns after coronary artery bypass surgery. *Heart & Lung: Journal of Critical Care, 24*(6), 483–494.

Bowen, M. (1978). *Family therapy in clinical practice.* New York, NY: Aronson.

Coffin-Ronig, N. (1997). *The process of ending domestic violence among Latinas: Aguatando no Mas* (doctoral dissertation). San Diego, CA: University of San Diego.

Goetz, J. P., & LeCompte, M. D. (1984). *Ethnography and qualitative design in educational research.* Orlando, FL: Academic Press.

Higgins, P., & Learn, C. (1999). Health practices of adult Hispanic women. *Journal of Advanced Nursing, 29*(5), 1105–1111.

Lane, P. (1995). Economic hardship has put Nicaragua's health system on the sick list. *Canadian Medical Association Journal, 4*(152), 580–582.

Lawton, N. (1988). Health care in Nicaragua. *Nurse Practitioner, 13*(1), 1–10.

Leininger, M. (1985). *Qualitative research methods in nursing.* Orlando, FL: Grune & Stratton.

Leininger, M. (1991). *Culture care diversity and universality: A theory of nursing.* New York, NY: National League for Nursing.

Leininger, M. (1995). *Transcultural nursing: Concepts, theories, research & practices* (2nd ed.). St. Louis, MO: McGraw-Hill.

Lustig, M. W., & Koester, J. (1993). *Intercultural competence: Interpersonal communication across cultures.* New York, NY: HarperCollins.

Martinez, R. J. (1999). Close friends of God: An ethnography of health in older Hispanic people. *Journal of Multi-Cultural Nursing and Health, 5*(1), 40–45.

McGoldrick, M., & Gerson, R. (1985). *Genograms in family assessment.* New York, NY: W.W. Norton.

Ministerio de Salud (MINSA). (1996). Prioridades del programa de subsidios de investigacion de la Organizacion Panamericana de la Salud. *Buletin Epidemiologico, 1*(1), 10–14.

Morse, J. M., & Penrod, J. (1999). Linking concepts of enduring, uncertainty, suffering, and hope. *Image: Journal of Nursing Scholarship, 31*(2), 145–150.

Pan American Health Organization (PAHO). (1998). *Health in the Americas I.* Washington, DC: Author.

Purnell, L. D., & Counts, M. (1998). Appalachians. In L. Purnell & B. Paulanka (Eds.), *Transcultural healthcare: A culturally competent approach* (pp. 107–125). Philadelphia, PA: F.A. Davis.

Rehm, R. (1999). Research, religious faith in Mexican American families dealing with chronic childhood illness. *Image: The Journal of Nursing Scholarship, 31*(1), 33–38.

Spradley, J. P. (1979). *The ethnographic interview.* Fort Worth, TX: Holt, Rinehart, & Winston.

Spradley, J. P. (1980). *Participant observation.* New York, NY: Holt, Rinehart, & Winston.

Suarez, M., Raffaelli, M., & O'Leary, A. (1996). Use of folk-healing practices by HIV-infected Hispanics living in the United States. *AIDS-Care: Psychological and Socio-Medical Aspects of AIDS-HIV, 8*(6), 683–690.

Villarruel, A. M. (1995). Mexican-American cultural meanings, expressions, self-care and dependent-care actions associated with experiences of pain. *Research in Nursing and Health, 18*(5), 427–436.

White, A., & Johnson, M. (1998). The complexities of nursing research with men. *International Journal of Nursing Studies, 35,* 41–48.

CHAPTER FIVE

HOW TO DO ETHNOGRAPHY

Ditsapelo M. McFarland

Nurses use a variety of methodologies to answer a research question. Ethnography is one such methodology. This chapter provides definitions of ethnography and its origin, describes different types of ethnographic designs, and explains how ethnography differs from other qualitative designs. Finally, the chapter describes the steps of the ethnographic methodology.

I am an associate professor at the Adelphi College of Nursing and Public Health, a position I have held since the fall of 2009. Born and raised in Botswana, in the southern part of Africa, I received my bachelor of education (BEd) in nursing from the University of Botswana and diploma in midwifery from the National Health Institute. I then earned my master of nursing science from Russell Sage College in Troy, NY, and PhD from Boston College, MA. My professional experience includes teaching nursing both in diploma and graduate programs in Botswana and in the United States. My specific subjects include medical-surgical nursing and research. In addition to teaching and clinical practice in both Botswana and U.S. hospitals, I have made presentations in Botswana to several groups on the impact of cultural diversity in health care and cervical care, both at the urban and village levels. My research, which started with my doctoral dissertation, focuses on women's use of the cervical cancer screening services, and I have published a few articles that address women's screening practices in Botswana. Consistently, the findings of my studies have shown low utilization of the Pap smear screening services either because women do not have adequate information about the services or they simply are not motivated to screen or they do not regard Pap smears as important to them (McFarland, 2003, 2013). To a greater extent, these findings shaped my understanding that traditional beliefs and values strongly influence health and illness behaviors of many Batswana (the people of Botswana), both at urban and tribal levels. It is on the basis of this understanding and the writings of foreign researchers (McDonald, 1996; Staugard, 1985) that I find ethnography important for nurses in Botswana to understand the ways of the local people, their heath belief systems, and their values and develop service that is effective in a culture-specific way. It is also my goal to further understand women's health beliefs and expectations using ethnography.

WHAT IS ETHNOGRAPHY?

Ethnography is a type of qualitative research methodology that is used to study cultures. Culture basically refers to beliefs, values, and attitudes that influence behavior patterns of a specific group of people. The word ethnography comes from Greek words *ethnos*, which means "the people" and *graphis*, which means "to write." As such, Harris and Johnson (2000) described ethnography as a written portrait of a people's customs and beliefs, collected through fieldwork. Ethnography has many other definitions. Fetterman (1998) defined ethnography as both art and science; it describes a people's culture, whether it is of a small tribal group or of a suburban classroom. The term ethnography can mean both research technique and product of research technique (Creswell, 1998). As a method, ethnography includes participant observation by a fieldworker who spends a year or longer living with the people (van Maanen, 1996).

Origin of Ethnography

Ethnography originated from anthropology as a mechanism for studying cultures (Denizen & Lincoln, 2000; Marsvasti, 2004). Its beginnings date back to the late 19th and early 20th centuries, when famous anthropologists, such as Margaret Mead, explored several non-Western cultures to understand the lifestyles of the people within those cultures. Over the years, ethnography evolved further to involve social sciences such as education and health-related studies (Marvasti, 2004). In health care, ethnography provides access to health beliefs and health practices of a specific culture or subculture. For example, Madeleine Leininger (1985), the nurse anthropologist, developed a field of transcultural nursing based on the anthropology tradition. Present-day researchers conduct ethnographies in organizations and communities.

Types of Ethnographic Research

There are two types of ethnographic research: macro-ethnography and micro-ethnography. In macro-ethnography, ethnographers focus on broadly defined cultures such as the Maori culture of New Zealand (Polit & Beck, 2010). Micro-ethnography, also referred to as focused ethnography, is used by ethnographers to study narrowly defined cultures such as the culture of an intensive care unit (Polit & Beck, 2010). Ware and colleagues (2000) used focused ethnography to evaluate cultural and other factors influencing cancer pain management in South Africa. Ethnographers assume that every group eventually evolves a culture that guides the members' view of the world and the way they structure their experiences. In ethnography, the ethnographer is both the researcher and the research instrument.

STEPS IN ETHNOGRAPHIC RESEARCH

There are several approaches to conducting ethnographic research. Each design is intended to perform a specific task as determined by the researcher. The steps of ethnography presented in the following sections draw largely from those described by Burns and Grove (1993) as well as other authors.

Identification of a Culture

This initial step includes background information about the country, the health belief systems, the health care systems, and the health care providers. As an example, Soengas (2009) conducted an ethnographic study of the Bakoya Pygmies in Gabon, Central Africa. The author gave a full description of the Bakoya culture, which included the historical background, residential patterns, social organization, political organization, and the economy and subsistence of the Bakoya tribes.

Defining the Research Question

The ethnographic research starts with a guiding question. The research question should convey a general theme rather than a specific hypothesis because prediction of behavior is not intended. An ethnographic question is explicitly stated and is usually open ended. The research question can be implied in the purpose statement or explicitly stated. For example, the ethnographer might ask, "What is the culture of an intensive care unit?" The research might also state that the purpose of the study is to explore health care seeking beliefs and behaviors of Mexican men living in a state (Sobralske, 2006).

Literature Review

Before contacting the individual for study, the researcher must do a literature review about the subject under study. The review of literature provides background for the study and enables the researcher to gain a broad understanding of the variables to be considered in a specific culture. Furthermore, the researcher will be able to identify the gaps in the topic under study in the literature as well as avoid repeating what other researchers have already done.

Gaining Entrance

After gaining a broader understanding of the culture through review of the literature, the researcher needs to enter the field to access members of a culture to be studied. This step involves negotiating permission with people in power, such as the heads of the organizations or the village chief, to enter the research field. Permission to enter the research field can be negotiated at different levels. Negotiating permission may involve writing a letter requesting permission to observe certain events. The researcher needs to provide a clear explanation of the study purpose and methodology and draw on his or her interpersonal resources and strategies (Hammersley & Atkinson, 2007).

Acquiring Informants

Once the researcher has gained entry into the research site and become familiar with the culture, he or she solicits the help of key informants. Informants are people the ethnographer spends most time with during the fieldwork to learn more about the culture under study. Informants are usually colleagues and are not research subjects. They are the ethnographer's link to the culture. A good key informant is one who is well informed about the culture, is willing to talk about it, and can communicate about his or her culture in a nonanalytic manner (Moore, 2008). Informants are usually few in number as dictated by the need for thick description of the data, which requires time. In her ethnographic study to evaluate factors influencing cancer pain management in South Africa, Beck (2000) enlisted the help of 33 key informants who represented multiple stakeholders in a variety of settings.

Participant Observation

The ethnographer must become familiar with the culture being studied through participant observation or fieldwork. Participant observation is a process in which an ethnographer makes observations about the culture under study while participating in its activities. It is regarded as the core of ethnographic research during which the ethnographer becomes immersed in the culture being studied. In this cultural immersion, the ethnographer spends time in the setting, asking questions, observing, and collecting documents about the group in order to understand their culture, beliefs, and language. The purpose of fieldwork is to understand life from perspectives of the people in their own setting or social group, which is the area of interest to the researcher (Bailey, 2007). Participant observation is also useful in that it allows the researcher to gauge the difference between what people do and what people say they do. It also enables the researcher to see the culture without imposing her or his own social reality on that culture.

The ethnographer makes field notes, which are written accounts of what the researcher observes in the field. These include observations of what the researcher has seen and experienced. Field notes should be written immediately or as soon as possible after leaving the field site so that important details observed are not forgotten. In her study of Llembula culture in Tanzania, for example, Juania participated in the nursing activities while observing and taking notes. Field notes should be written immediately or as soon as possible after leaving the field site so that important details observed are not forgotten. During and after participation, the researcher will reflect on what he or she has experienced and observed in the field. Fieldwork is not without disadvantages. It is time consuming, and it requires commitment and sacrifices. It takes months or years for the researcher to learn about the cultural groups of interest, sometimes under unfavorable conditions.

Data Collection

The ethnographer relies on a variety of techniques to collect the data. These techniques include observation, examination of records, photographs, artifacts (what members of the culture make and use), diaries to understand their meaning and significance to the culture, and listening to and interviewing focus groups and informants. Many ways of collecting both quantitative and qualitative data are used in ethnography but the primary methods are observation, interview, and collection of objects and artifacts.

In addition to observing the activities of the culture, the ethnographer conducts interviews with members of the culture to gain deeper understanding of what people believe is important to them. The researcher also uses interview technique to validate what was obtained through participant observation. The interviews generally last an hour or more to capture participants' perspectives and are audiotaped. Interviews can be formal or informal, structured or unstructured.

During interviews, the researcher collects both emic and etic perspectives of the culture. An emic perspective, also referred to as the insider's view, is the way members of a culture regard their world. The emic perspective includes the local language, concepts, or means of expression that are used by the members of the group under study to name and characterize their experiences. The emic perspective is regarded the heart of the reality of the culture by most ethnographers (Fetterman, 1998) because it provides information that may not be obvious to the researcher. The etic perspective is the outsider's (ethnographer's) interpretation of the experiences of that culture.

Analysis and Interpretation of the Data

Data analysis starts at the beginning of the project and continues throughout the project. It involves transcription of the interviews to assist analysis. Analysis involves interpretation of what the researcher observed and heard during fieldwork. The process of data analysis involves developing a code book, reading through the field notes to become familiar with the information, identifying emerging themes and patterns of the particular cultural group under study, and interpreting the findings. Spradley (1979) proposed a 12-step demographic data analysis. Leininger and McFarland (2006) developed a four-phase ethnoscience data analysis.

Ethnographic Report

An ethnographic report includes clear and thick description of research methodology, including of people who participated in the study and the experiences and processes observed during the study. Quotes are used to represent the experiences of the participants in their own words. The researchers' prejudices and biases are also highlighted. An ethnographic report may be shared with others through journals, books, and conference presentations.

Ethical Consideration

Ethnographers are generally people from outside the culture. Furthermore, ethnography involves human beings. As such, it involves a number of ethical considerations involving the protection of the cultural group under study, the protection of the rights of participants through informed consent, and maintaining the privacy and confidentiality of their responses. It is also important for researchers to make sure that the research poses no harm to the people involved in the study.

CONCLUSION

Ethnography is a research methodology that is used by ethnographers to study cultures. It lends itself to the study of subcultures, such as intensive care units. Unlike other qualitative methodologies, ethnography takes place within a natural setting where relevant events and behaviors can be easily observed. The ethnographer uses the technique of participant observation to become immersed in the culture to be studied. The outcome of ethnography is thick description of the data collected during the fieldwork.

REFERENCES

Bailey, C. A. (2007). *A guide to qualitative field research* (2nd ed.). Thousand Oaks, CA: Pine Forge Press.

Beck, S. L. (2000). An ethnographic study of factors influencing cancer pain management in South Africa. *Cancer Nursing, 23*(2), 91–99.

Burns, N., & Grove, S. K. (1993). *The practice of nursing research: Conduct, critique, & utilization* (2nd ed.). Philadelphia, PA: Saunders.

Creswell, J. W. (1998). *Qualitative inquiry and research design: Choosing among five traditions.* Thousand Oaks, CA: Sage.

Denizen, N. K., & Lincoln, Y. S. (2000). *Handbook of qualitative research* (2nd ed.). Thousand Oaks, CA: Sage.

Fetterman, D. M. (1998). *Ethnography step by step: Applied social research methods series* (Vol. 17). London, UK: Sage.

Harris, M., & Johnson, O. (2000). *Cultural anthropology* (5th ed.). Needham Heights, MA: Allyn and Bacon.

Hammersley, M., & Atkinson, P. (2007). *Ethnography: Principles in practice* (3rd ed). London, UK: Routledge.

Leininger, M. M. (1985). *Qualitative research methods in nursing.* New York, NY: Grune & Stratton.

Leininger, M., & McFarland, M. (2006). *Culture care and diversity: A worldwide nursing theory* (2nd ed.). Sudbury, MA: Jones & Bartlett Publishers.

McDonald, D. S. (1996). Notes on the socio-economic and cultural factors influencing the transmission of HIV in Botswana. *Social Science Medicine, 42*(9), 1325–1333.

McFarland, D. M. (2003). Cervical cancer and Pap smear screening in Botswana: knowledge and perceptions. *International Nursing Review, 50*(3), 167–175.

Marvasti, A. B. (2004). *Qualitative research in sociology: An introduction*. London: Sage.

McFarland, D. M. (2013). The Associations of demographic data and Pap smear use in urban Botswana women. *International, Journal of Women's Health, 5,* 709–716. Retrieved January 18, 2014, from http://www.ncbi.nlm.nih.gov/pubmed /24179380

Moore, Q. (2008). Doing ethnography: Some preliminary steps. Retrieved from http://blogs.cofc.edu/expressiveculture/

Polit, D. F., & Beck, C. T. (2010). *Essentials of nursing research: Appraising evidence for nursing practice* (7th ed). Philadelphia, PA: Lippincott, Williams and Wilkins.

Sobralske, M. C. (2006). Health care seeking among Mexican American men. *Journal of Transcultural Nursing, 17,* 129–138.

Soengas, B. (2009). Preliminary ethnographic research on the Bakoya in Gabon. African Study. *Mongraphs, 30*(4), 187–208. Retrieved from http://jambo.africa .kyoto-u.ac.jp/kiroku/asm_normal/abstracts/pdf/30-4/30-4-2%20Soengas.pdf

Spradley, J. P. (1979). *Ethnographic interview*. New York, NY: Holt, Rinehart and Winston.

Staugard, F. (1985). *Traditional healers*. Gaborone, Botswana: Ipelegeng.

Van Maanen, J. (1996). Ethnography. In A. Kuper & J. Kuper (Eds.), *The social science encyclopedia* (2nd ed., pp. 263–265). London, UK: Routledge.

Ware, L., Epps, C., Herr, K., & Packard, A. (2000). Evaluation of the revised Faces Pain Scale, Verbal Descriptor Scale, Numeric Rating Scale, and Iowa Pain Thermometer in older minority adults. *Pain Management Nursing, 7*(3), 117–125.

CHAPTER SIX

IMPLEMENTING A NEEDLE EXCHANGE PROGRAM: AN ETHNOGRAPHIC ANALYSIS

Jeri A. Milstead

*I*n the 1980s, HIV/AIDS became pandemic. Little was known at the time about how the disease was spread, and no treatments were available to cure or even slow the progress of the disease. The causal factor appeared to be the exchange of human blood and body fluids, and the first groups that exhibited symptoms were intravenous drug users (IDUs) who shared needles and syringes, and homosexual men. As officials at the Centers for Disease Control and Prevention (CDC) became aware of an alarming increase in the numbers of cases, they set about to alert the public and to seek assistance from the federal government. Often government addresses serious health threats by providing legally sanctioned programs for research, prevention, and treatment. However, because possessing needles and syringes without a prescription (e.g., for injection of insulin for diabetes) and the use of heroin and other IV drugs were illegal in most states, and homosexual activity was not accepted in U.S. culture as a topic of discussion, government policy makers were reluctant (even adamantly opposed) to providing solutions.

Government funding in the United States was limited until research reported that the disease was known in heterosexual populations and was labeled by CDC as a "communicable disease." This designation took away some of the stigma, and legislators could discuss the growing problem in a more neutral framework. Early research was focused on discovering the cause and means of transmission. Treatment options were harsh and focused on preventing death; drugs were developed to arrest the disease but often left the patient with a poor quality of life.

In the meantime, patients and friends of patients who were dying of the disease took a pragmatic approach and created an innovative, although illegal, response through the establishment of needle exchange (NEX) programs. These programs surfaced along the coastal cities of the United States, especially in big cities and metropolitan areas where drug users had access to imported heroin for IV use.

HIV/AIDS was not restricted to the United States—it was becoming pandemic across the globe. The concept of NEX programs in the United States was borrowed from the Netherlands. In the 1970s the Dutch had experienced an outbreak of hepatitis. A causative factor was sharing needles and syringes by IDUs. Some public health experts and IDUs thought that providing for an exchange of "dirty" needles and syringes (i.e., those that had been used for IV drug use, thus contaminated by blood or body fluids) for "clean" ones (i.e., unused sterile needles and syringes) would reduce transmission of hepatitis. The Dutch government established NEXs as a response and the incidence rate of hepatitis dropped. By extrapolation, the Dutch government applied the same logic to the issue of HIV/AIDS and, again, set up officially sanctioned NEXs; there were no laws against possessing needles and syringes in the Netherlands. People could insert a "dirty" (i.e., unsterile or used) needle and syringe into an apparatus that resembled a vending machine (available at many sites throughout the country) and obtain a sterile (i.e., "clean") set. No financial charge was incurred. The idea was to reduce the incidence and prevalence of HIV/AIDS. The government responded to a major health problem quickly.

This chapter provides a brief overview of the research followed by a discussion of what issues the author considered in preparing a qualitative design, the challenges faced while conducting the study, and lessons learned from the process.

RESEARCH CONSIDERATIONS

Conceptual Framework

At the time the researcher entered the program there were only four programs in the South that conferred a PhD in nursing, none in the state in which the researcher lived and none within driving distance. Part of the former job of the researcher was as a lobbyist to a state legislature. The process was intriguing and, without many other options of interest to a nurse, she applied to the department of political science at a major state university about an hour and a half from her home. Although the university was in another state, a consortium existed among seven universities at the time to which all had agreed that if a university in which the prospective student did not offer a specific doctoral degree, the student could enroll in the closest program and not pay out of state tuition. Two of the four areas of concentration within the department were comparative politics (comparing nations) and public policy. These are the two areas the researcher chose to focus on health policy.

The process of seeking government assistance for a problem and obtaining a response (usually in the form of a law or program) is called the policy process. This process is composed of agenda setting, government response (usually in the form of a program or law), program/policy implementation, and evaluation. The process is not linear and has been conceptualized by Kingdon (1984) as a "garbage can" of problems, politics, and solutions that connect, disconnect, and reconnect in a "policy soup" in which elected government officials and career bureaucrats and their staffs, and "street level bureaucrats" (i.e., those people who actually implement programs) discuss issues. A "window of opportunity" may occur as problems and solutions are deliberated, and the two may be joined to appear as a program or law.

Although Kingdon's research focused on the agenda-setting process, this author proposed that the garbage can model could also be used in the implementation process, especially since she viewed the two components as fluid and interacting. Concepts and practices inherent in the garbage can model were used as a framework for a qualitative study of NEXs in two sites in the United States and one site in the Netherlands. The research became this author's dissertation research toward a PhD in political science with a focus on comparative politics and health policy (Milstead, 1993).

METHODOLOGY

A qualitative study was proposed to establish information about what appeared to be a rational, but controversial, approach to slowing the spread of the disease. An extensive literature search indicated a gap in governmental and cultural acceptance of NEXs between the Netherlands and the United States. The Netherlands was chosen because of the researcher's prior experience in that country and her familiarity with NEXs there. Literature suggested the two sites in the United States: Tacoma, Washington, and New York City (NYC), New York. Using a snowball approach, personal interviews, and participant observation, the researcher interviewed 41 policy makers and service providers and several individuals and groups of clients from three different NEX programs in Rotterdam, the Netherlands, NYC, and Tacoma, Washington. Data analysis revealed several emergent themes and a program design that was unique to each of the programs. Barriers and facilitators to implementation in all of the programs were determined. A new model of program implementation was identified in the Tacoma program.

Rationale for Three Sites

This author had created a course for master's students in nursing in which she and they lived in the Netherlands for one month during the summer and studied the Dutch health care and nurse education systems. Four to six students enrolled each summer; college credit was awarded for successful completion of the course. As a result of personal contacts with nurses in the Netherlands made during the courses, a contractual agreement was established between an academic university in the United States and a hospital in the Netherlands. Dutch hospital personnel (e.g., director of nursing and staff) organized a program in which the class met with health care professionals and others in every part of the country and in an extensive range of sites. Initial information about NEXs came from personnel who worked in drug rehabilitation locations. The author realized that NEXs were legal in the Netherlands and were illegal in the United States and decided to analyze sites in both countries to determine issues in implementation.

NYC was chosen as one site based on knowledge from the literature that there were many cases of HIV/AIDS reported. An NEX had been established on two street corner venues (in the Bronx and Harlem) where volunteers provided services every Saturday morning at a specified time and in the same specified locations. Through extensive research of New York newspapers and a discussion with a contact at CDC, this author talked with one of the initial eight originators of the NYC program who invited me to visit the area and also agreed to help me contact others who were involved in the issue.

By chance an official at CDC, during a phone conversation with this author (who was seeking information about HIV/AIDS and NEXs at the early stage), shared a flyer from his desk announcing the "Second Annual Needle Exchange Seminar" in Tacoma, Washington. I called the contact in Tacoma and registered immediately for the 3-day weekend seminar. The meeting provided initial information and tacit approval to investigate that NEX as part of my research. The NEXs in NYC and Tacoma were implemented illegally; the NEX in the Netherlands was a government-sanctioned program.

In the 1990s, 11 U.S. states had laws that prohibited sale or possession of drug-related equipment without a prescription, and most states specifically prohibited possession of a needle and syringe without a prescription. In contrast, the Netherlands provided legal exchange programs and did not have restrictive laws about possessing needles and syringes.

SUMMARY OF THE STUDY

HIV/AIDS came to the attention of the CDC during the mid-1980s and quickly reached pandemic proportions. Little was known about how the disease was transmitted, but it was observed most often in IDUs and homosexuals. Congress was not moved to allocate funding for research or treatment in such "distasteful" populations but, because of the widespread extent and pressure from affected groups such as the American Foundation for AIDS Research (AMFAR, a private organization) and the Gay Men's Health Crisis (GMHC, the largest AIDS organization at the time) funded some initial research to find the cause.

Small clusters of individuals realized they or their friends were contracting the disease and dying quickly. In an effort to stem inevitable death, they searched for what little information was available. One man in Tacoma, Washington, discovered NEX programs in the Netherlands while reading during a prolonged rehabilitation after an accident. The Tacoman realized the importance of the disease and understood that HIV/AIDS occurred most often in the United States in large cities along the east and west coasts. After his hospitalization, he initiated a conference held in Tacoma, developed a flyer, and invited anyone who had knowledge or who was involved in programs that addressed the disease. Nearly 200 people gathered over a 4-day weekend to discuss what was known, what research was needed, and the status of treatment. The session became an annual event.

At the same time, the Tacoman and some friends pooled their money and bought an old van that they parked on a suburban street in the same location once a week. They distributed 2-ounce bottles of chlorine bleach and small plastic bags of clean cotton balls (to clean "the works"), clean needles/syringes in exchange for dirty needles/syringes, condoms, and information about HIV/AIDS. Volunteers drove the van and posted pictures of abcesses from IV use and rashes and other manifestations of sexually transmitted diseases (STDs) from medical textbooks on the outside walls of the vans as visual aids for IDUs to compare any health problems they may have had. Suggested referrals to local physicians, the health department, and other clinics where treatment could be obtained also were posted.

In contrast, the NEXs in NYC grew out of the activism of a small group of men who were former addicts, were not health care professionals, and who were self-educated about HIV/AIDS. They could not interest government or public health officials to provide funding for a NEX that, instinctively, they believed was the "right" thing to do and at least was something practical that they could do. They pooled what money they could gather and planned their own version of a NEX. Every Friday night, the activists met in the basement of an old building in the southern tip of Manhattan to prepare for the next day's NEX. They filled 2-ounce bottles with clean water from a spigot (clean water was not easily accessible on the streets of NYC in contrast to Tacoma) and 2-ounce bottles of chlorine bleach, packaged small plastic baggies with clean cotton balls (all to clean "the works"—IV equipment), and put clean needles/syringes, condoms, and information about HIV/AIDS into plastic grocery bags. Every Saturday morning this group took the subway and set up a card table at the same street corners in the Bronx and Harlem and offered the material to anyone who would exchange a dirty needle/syringe. The activists were adamant that they were not interested in identifying the IDUs by name or in any other way—the transfer was strictly anonymous. The IDUs indicated they would not reveal any personal information about themselves. No information was recorded in any way. Weather did not deter the activists—they took pride in noting that they "were there" even, as one volunteer noted, if snot was freezing on their noses.

The Netherlands situation was entirely different. The Dutch government provided large vending machines filled with clean needles/syringes that could be accessed in many places around the country. The machines originally were designed and built to release one needle/syringe in response to accepting another needle/syringe. Some IDUs inserted ballpoint pens into the machines in lieu of a needle/syringe, but the machine "ate" the pens. The IDUs then hammered on the machines and damaged them. The United States manufacturer re-engineered the machines to reject any items other than needles/syringes. Dutch IDUs could obtain drug rehabilitation if they chose, but pressure to participate was not applied by government workers. Methadone, a heroin substitute used to treat IV drug use, was available through an electronically linked system so that participants were able to obtain the drug only at prescribed levels, no matter where in the country they obtained it.

The author found a nurse whose practice focused on prostitutes, many of whom were IDUs, who worked in the area of the railroad station in central Rotterdam. The nurse helped the women identify, treat, and prevent abcesses from IVs and sexually transmitted diseases. She also provided tips on safety (e.g., do not wear long dresses or scarves that could be caught in car doors to prevent escape and always keep one leg in your jeans in case of needing a sudden escape from a car). One vicar convinced his "kerk" (church) to convert the basement to a café so that IDUs would have a place to stay off the streets during the day. The church provided coffee and newspapers (for sale) and, although they did not allow users to "shoot up" in the café, they created a closet-type room where users could inject IV drugs before they entered the café.

Policy Communities

Tacoma had a tight-knit group of elected and appointed officials. Most went to high school together, many also attended college together and then returned to live in Tacoma. Long-term relationships allowed easy discussions to take place among the policy makers. The Tacoman who started the NEX was a friend of the chief of police, director of the local health department, city government officials, and others; they shared an easy camaraderie. They all were aware of the illegal NEX but had agreed to not make any official reference to it or to arrest the participants or volunteers at the exchange. Activists decided to educate members of the Board of Health on what HIV/AIDS is, how it is transmitted, and how it is treated (as far as was known at that time). The activists held 1-hour information sessions prior to each board meeting, a tactic that informed the members, established initial relationships between the groups, and kept the issue from fading on the policy agenda.

At one point, city and county leaders agreed that the local health department would hold a NEX on its premises as a program that was paid for by the city. This allowed the county to issue a civil suit (important that it not be a criminal suit as in NYC) against the health department for violating the state Drug Paraphernalia Act (i.e., permitting an illegal program). After much testimony by HIV/AIDS experts, the judge ruled that the NEX did not violate the Act because of an exemption for any authorized state, county, or city official engaged in the legal performance of one's duties. The health director was determined to be an authorized "officer." The court decision reframed the definition of "officer" beyond the usually-thought-of police officer, which allowed the director of health to take extraordinary measures to slow an epidemic through the NEX.

On the other hand, the policy community in NYC was fragmented. In the 1970s NYC was in a financial crisis in which the city nearly went bankrupt. City administrators relinquished several services to the state, including drug treatment services, in an effort to reduce costs. Although NYC is the largest city in the state, jurisdictional tension existed between state and local officials related to the administration of several services, including health care services. The NYC mayor, after pressure from activists and some officials, approved a pilot NEX that had many problems. The NEX was located near "the tombs" (the NYC court buildings) where IDUs who carried needles/syringes were at great risk for arrest. Transportation was another problem, because most IDUs were unemployed, did not live in or near Manhattan where the NEX was located, and could not afford even the subway system. City and state officials openly expressed their opposition to the exchange. State and local African American leadership opposed loudly, stating that linking HIV/AIDS to IDUs was an attack on people of color and compared the health problem to the Tuskegee Project. Religious leaders opposed the NEX because of a belief that HIV/AIDS affected mostly homosexuals and homosexuality was forbidden in the writings of the Bible and other religious books. State officials reduced the budget for the program several times. After a limited trial period, only 300 people participated, and the program was closed and labeled a failure.

The policy community in the Netherlands is decentralized; officials in the large cities control budgets and services for regional implementation. Methadone and other drug treatments are available to IDUs if they choose to participate. Although drug use is not legalized, all regional governments provide NEXs through the vending machines. There is little stigma to IV drug use; the Dutch focus on a model of harm reduction, not criminalization.

Language and the Media

Language became important on several levels. Early on, Tacomans insisted the program was called an "exchange" program so that the public would not perceive NEXs as condoning or expanding drug use, a common fear. The term "exchange" seemed to lessen the fear. The Tacoma policy entrepreneur also used metaphors and challenging statements (e.g., "AIDS is a holocaust in slow motion" and "This is a new world order with disposable humanity") for the shock value and to confront people with the emotional characteristic of the disease. This deliberate use of challenging language also ensured media attention and kept the issue from fading on the policy agenda. NYC IDUs were confronted often with slurs and other negative phrases aimed at them. Personnel at one NYC hospital yelled to each other to prepare for another "SCHPOS" (subhuman piece of shit) whenever an IDU was spotted in the emergency department waiting room. All of the NEX workers in both countries took pains to refer to IDUs as "users" rather than "addicts"—a term they considered much more pejorative. Language was also used repetitively to establish public familiarity with terms. Dutch officials were aware of the official U.S. drug policy known as the "War on Drugs" but noted that in reality it was a "War on Drug Users." The Dutch did not criminalize IDUs and were openly contemptuous of the American phrase.

Themes That Emerged From Research Findings

After extensive interviews of 41 government officials and volunteers in NEX programs, this author uncovered the impact of HIV/AIDS on individuals and governments. Interviews were conducted in Tacoma, New York City, and Rotterdam. This author also read newspaper and journal articles and CDC briefs related to the status of the disease and treatment.

This author identified five themes that emerged from the study, although number 4 is more a disbelief that the early Dutch study on the efficacy of NEX produced such positive results.

1. Conflict between U.S. policy and NEXs
2. HIV/AIDS as an intractable problem
3. Conflict in drug treatment philosophies between the United States and the Netherlands
4. U.S. policy makers question Dutch study
5. Influence of the policy community

HOW RESEARCH-RELATED DECISIONS WERE MADE DURING THE STUDY

Qualitative or Quantitative?

A qualitative study was decided by the dissertation chair and committee—rare for an academic department that was highly quantitative. Qualitative research was coming into its own in the early 1990s, and members of the department were interested in this approach. The department had offered no courses on qualitative research, and the faculty and students were schooled in quantitative methods. Nearly all of the students were male; two female students were highly enthused to conduct qualitative studies. All five members of this researcher's dissertation committee were male and were highly qualified quantitative researchers. Committee members were not comfortable with qualitative methods being used by the researcher, such as elite interviews conducted only by the researcher. They recommended confirmation of information obtained in interviews through triangulation with information from at least two other sources of documentation, specifically, newspaper articles and journal articles, for each oral data point. The researcher followed this recommendation, even though she believed this approach was not true to heuristic, qualitative methods. There were many newspaper articles about NEXs because of the uniqueness and notoriety of the plan or the participants, so the researcher was able to gather material that satisfied the committee.

During the process of the dissertation research, one committee member left the university and was replaced by a female professor from another college within the university. The replacement committee member was selected by the chair of the committee because of her expertise in qualitative methods. By this time the researcher was deep into writing the final draft; there was very little communication between the new committee member and this researcher. The final dissertation document does not read like a typical qualitative study; it is a combination of qualitative and quantitative methods.

This author wondered about the motives of the chair but felt impelled to move forward, so sought out a nurse colleague who was an expert in qualitative research, read books and articles about qualitative methods, and became self-taught (although on a limited basis). The objective at that time was to complete the program in as short a time as possible and with at least a basic understanding of the methodology.

An ethnographic approach was chosen, because little was known about how NEXs were established and implemented in the United States. The researcher decided to conduct interviews with people who were knowledgeable about HIV/AIDS and NEXs in three sites. The process was elite interviewing as described by Dexter (1970) that focuses on the situation from the point of view of the person being interviewed. The author chose to conduct all of the interviews herself to ensure consistency in process and identify early themes. She also was funding the study from personal savings and could not pay others to interview. The researcher was an expert clinical nurse specialist in psychiatric–mental health nursing with years of experience in interviewing clients. She wanted to let the interviews move in any direction the subject wanted, rather than in a structured direction, depending on how the subjects responded. She realized early that the interviewees had stories to tell so she encouraged this approach. She did construct an open-ended, semi-structured interview document to satisfy the dissertation committee. She agreed that the interview questions helped focus her own thoughts but did not want to manipulate any subject's narration of events and information. The tool was not needed during the interview process. All subjects were asked to sign a consent form so that they were aware of the reason for the interview, possible risks involved, and protection of the information obtained.

The researcher tape recorded each interview and simultaneously wrote notes (verbatim and paraphrased) during each interview as it seemed appropriate. Usually the taped interviews would be transcribed by a person knowledgeable about this process and reviewed by the researcher for correctness and omissions, then compared with the written notes of the researcher. The researcher did not have the money to pay for a transcriber, so she did not use this step. The transcription process is important and adds credibility to a qualitative study, especially since the impact of the research does not use terms such as "generalizability" to a greater population.

Interview Process

The researcher used a snowball method of selecting people to interview. That is, she found one person at each site who then would provide the names of others who were involved in the topic, until the names became duplicative or were exhausted. She kept a careful list of all persons suggested that included name, address, phone number, title, and any alternative information. She started with the person in Tacoma who had originated the now-annual NEX conference. He agreed to be interviewed and gave the names of others with whom he worked on the issue. The researcher spent 1 week in Tacoma interviewing subjects every day. She also visited the Chamber of Commerce for publication about the city and the region. She took time to meander through the downtown area to get a "feel" for the city and its culture. For example, she found an outdoor cultural arts festival that contributed to the flavor of the area. The researcher also visited the NEX site and talked with volunteers and any clients who would speak with her anonymously (she and the volunteers agreed that anonymity had to be protected at all times).

Government officials in NYC were identified through newspaper articles and offered a list of other officials and volunteers. The researcher spent 1 week in NYC talking with officials and others. Officials were not hesitant to discuss the HIV/AIDS issue (some acknowledged they had the disease) and the NEXs. They freely shared names of others who were knowledgeable and could offer substantive input into the study. The researcher was also invited to meet with the volunteers on Friday night as they prepared the packages for distribution. The researcher met the volunteers on Saturday at the subway station and accompanied them to the NEX in the Bronx where she observed the 2-hour NEX. During the wait in the subway, one of the volunteers dropped a grocery bag full of needles/syringes that scattered all over the ground. The researcher quickly told them to put down their bags of material and that she would shield it so that they could gather up the spilled needles/syringes. It was very important that they retrieved all of the material immediately so that none would be left on the subway platform. This rapid decision contributed to trust between the researcher and the volunteers who had only known her for a few hours and insisted on keeping the clients' anonymity.

The author had taught a graduate course for nurses in the Netherlands for several years for a month every summer and studied the health care and nurse education systems. Through the many sites the class visited, the researcher was known and trusted by the workers. From the United States, the researcher contacted one person at a drug rehabilitation site in Rotterdam who agreed to point her in the direction of others who could be helpful after she arrived in the city. The plan was to complete work in Rotterdam in 1 week and then spend a second week in Belgium where the researcher's daughter, son-in-law, and grandson were living. Through the son-in-law, the researcher had access to a phone in Belgium and called the single contact in Rotterdam as soon as she arrived only to discover that he was ill and would be out of work all week. The researcher decided to reverse her plan and to spend the first week with her family in the hope that her contact would be available the next Monday. Luck held and she was able to interview the initial contact who subsequently provided names of several people who also provided several names until the researcher could discern duplication. She was able to conduct face-to-face interviews with all the people whose names were provided except one whom she interviewed by phone. The last subject did not supply new information but confirmed information already obtained.

In total, 41 persons were interviewed—all of the persons on every contact's list. The researcher was prepared to stay in each city as long as it took but hoped that a full schedule of 8 to 10 hours every day would limit her work to 1 week in each city.

Language and Culture

One concern in conducting qualitative research is that the researcher should recognize and understand the language and culture. Subjects in Tacoma spoke English; those in NYC spoke English (a few spoke Spanish but conversed with the author in English). The subjects in Rotterdam spoke excellent English (they learn English, Dutch, German, and French in elementary and secondary school) although there usually was one of their colleagues nearby who could provide interpretation if needed. Despite the Dutch felicity with the English language, there were a few occasions in which Dutch words or phrases were not easily interpreted. In those instances, the researcher asked for clarification or for the interviewee to rephrase the response or have a second person explain.

There were subtle differences in the culture encountered by this researcher who, although born and reared in the midwest United States, was living and working in an academic setting in a southern state. The researcher was comfortable in Tacoma and found the language and habits similar to those of her own. Although New Yorkers have a reputation for being impersonal and at times rude, this researcher found all subjects provided time for interviews and were very eager to help the researcher understand what they were saying. The Dutch culture was not unfamiliar to the researcher because of the time she had spent previously with her class. If conducting research in a site or venue is very different from one's own, this researcher recommends reading about the area and talking with people who live there or have had recent experience there or using an interpreter and/or translator who is fluent in the language. Untangling subtle cultural meanings during interviews could skew understanding of content and meaning and could distract both the interviewer and the interviewee.

When living in a culture that is different from one's own, there may be a danger in becoming "native" (i.e., in immersing oneself so deeply in the new culture that one loses the original perspective). The Netherlands is a developed country with many similarities to the United States; the researcher did not become "native." Acknowledgment of cultural customs is important, and the researcher was careful to demonstrate respect for all people she met, even if she discerned differences of opinion or culture. For example, during a hot afternoon in Rotterdam when the researcher was talking with people at a local drug rehabilitation office, one of the IDUs brought in a watermelon, cut it up, and offered all the people there a slice. Although the researcher does not like watermelon, she accepted the slice and ate it so that she would not be perceived as a "bad American" or fearful that she would contract HIV/AIDS by sharing food. It was an issue of trust.

Funding Issues

The author was faced with limited personal funds but made a decision to be responsible for funding, even though the research included trips to the east and west coasts of the United States and to Europe. A friend provided frequent flyer miles to obtain a plane trip to Tacoma for the initial NEX conference.

During the interview phase, the researcher was able to stay in Tacoma with the daughter of a colleague. The daughter's Army husband was stationed overseas and she was glad to share the apartment. In NYC the researcher stayed in a hotel in Manhattan for 1 week; in Rotterdam, she stayed in a hotel for 1 week with her son who accompanied her. He feared that his mother would be at risk of harm due to the content of her research. However, the researcher felt safe in all situations and she sent her son off to visit several parts of Holland while she was working. She ate at cheap restaurants or street food trucks and suffered no ill effects. She was alert to the surroundings and did not put herself in risky situations. She dressed casually, carried a purse that held a small tape recorder. She wore her passport, credit card, money, and any other valuables in a pouch around her neck inside a t-shirt. She did not wear expensive jewelry that might put her at risk for robbery in any of the cities. The researcher conducted all interviews during daylight hours in places where there were other people around. During a trip to The Hague in which she interviewed two members of Parliament, she was careful to dress appropriately, although one male member was dressed in jeans. The researcher did let the United States consulate in Rotterdam know when she would be in the country and for what purpose before she left the United States. She did not visit any personal friends outside the interviewees during the time she was in any of the cities—she was there to work, not to visit. Therefore, her attention was focused on the most efficient use of her personal funds.

CONCLUSION

Policy implementation theory was advanced by extrapolating Kingdon's model of agenda setting and by raising additional questions for future research. Facilitators and barriers for implementing NEXs were identified and were available to policy makers to consider in planning and implementing NEX programs. The value of a shared philosophy about drug use, drug users, and implementation strategies was clearly important as an implementation strategy to the policy community.

Lessons Learned

1. The qualitative researcher has to be rigorous and informative. In spite of the exclusive quantitative training in the doctoral program that may have presented a bias against qualitative research, this researcher gained

immense respect for qualitative methods. With better training in qualitative methods, this researcher believes the final dissertation could have been written better.

If interviews are a major part of the investigation process, a researcher must be an expert at listening, clarifying, questioning, and other communications techniques. This researcher believes that nurses have a unique felicity for conducting interviews because of the coursework, especially in psychiatric–mental health courses, required during their nursing education. An interview guide may assist those researchers who do not have expert skills in this area.

2. Influence of the policy community was strong and both negative and positive. In Tacoma, the local political leaders were a tight-knit group who supported NEX even if it was not within written agency policy. In NYC, policy leaders were divided: many supported NEX openly and some only covertly; others opposed NEX loudly. In the Netherlands, political and health care workers were supportive of NEX as a strategy to combat a huge social disease. The Dutch did not make loud noises in either opposition or support—they just made policy decisions related to NEX as a rational response.

3. Conflict existed between U.S. laws that prohibited possession of needles and syringes and government sponsorship of NEXs. Proponents of NEXs in the United States had to work outside the law. They put themselves at personal risk by ordering sterile needles and syringes, by accumulating supplies, and by actually conducting the NEXs. Law enforcers took personal risks by not arresting those who participated in the exchange.

4. Conflict in drug treatment philosophy existed between the traditional drug rehabilitation model and the harm reduction model. The traditional model used terms such as "addict" and "drug abuse" and "recovery." Drug addiction was seen as a disease state, and treatment was abstinence and a twelve-step model of rehabilitation. Any indication of drugs found in the blood or urine signaled that the person was to be dropped from the rehabilitation program. The fact that there were not nearly enough treatment slots available for the number of "addicts" had little impact. On the other hand, the harm reduction model assumed a person is responsible for his or her own health. Multidrug use was accepted and not considered a disease; treatment programs were available if a user chose but were not mandated. In the Netherlands, methadone was available at most drug treatment centers. Harm reduction advocates provided education on proper injection techniques, how to spot and care for abcesses from IV drug use, and how to stay healthy in spite of drug use.

Personal Reflection

There was strong, personal commitment, and creativity of volunteers in NEX programs in the United States. Since possession of needles/syringes was illegal, volunteers (usually those with HIV/AIDS or those who had friends with the disease) staffed NEX programs in a variety of layouts, on a consistent weekly basis, and in all kinds of weather. In Tacoma, the NEX occurred in a battered old van that was parked on a street one day each week in an area in which there were likely to be IVDs. Volunteers pasted pictures that showed abcesses, rashes, and symptoms of STDs and HIV/AIDS and suggested whether, how, and where treatment could be obtained. NYC volunteers worked during the week to prepare packages for distribution on a street corner where IVDs congregated and made the NEX available every Saturday morning, rain or shine. These activists often had little money of their own to take the subway.

Creativity Flourished

Volunteers were faced with a problem of how to dispose of dirty needles and syringes. In Tacoma, "sharps" boxes (used in hospitals and other health care sites to hold contaminated/dirty sharp instruments) were accepted at the local health department without question. In NYC, volunteers filled large empty water jugs with needles and syringes, hid them under their beds, and then and surreptitiously left the jugs outside health department offices just before the offices closed. A person caught with a jug full of dirty needles and syringes was subject to prosecution. The volunteers were very careful to not leave the dirty "works" where they could do harm. They considered this an ethical issue and were quite verbal in discussing it with this author. Needles/syringes often were ordered by mail in the United States. In completing the order application, there usually was a signature line for the physician's name. The volunteers did not write in a name on that line, and the distributor did not deny the order.

Unanticipated benefits occurred with NEX in all three sites. Regardless of where IDUs injected their drugs, prior to the NEX the needles/syringes often were thrown on the ground or street or wherever the IDU was at the time. When IVDs could exchange their needles/syringes for clean ones, there were fewer found in parks, yards, and other places. Also, police had fewer inadvertent sticks from dirty needles while doing pat-downs in IDUs during arrests. The environment and police became safer. Other research reported that the use of NEXs did not result in an increase in IV drug use, a fear held by some officials prior to NEXs.

There were great differences in police attitudes in Tacoma and NYC and between the United States and the Netherlands. Most often, the police did not arrest the IDUs in Tacoma. The police would park their cruisers around the corner from the van but made arrests only if there were obvious offensive behavior (e.g., loud oral outbursts or fights). In NYC, police were less tolerant. Eight activists were arrested in 1991 for possession of needles at the NEX site. After a very widely publicized trial, a Manhattan Criminal Court judge acquitted all eight defendants and ruled that possession of needles at the NEX was a medical necessity that was intended to prevent a greater harm to society. Although this was a landmark decision, it did not reverse the law that declared possession of needles/syringes without a prescription illegal. Since there were no similar Dutch laws, there were no arrests in the Netherlands for possession of needles/syringes.

Language and media were important. The Tacoma policy entrepreneur deliberately used colorful, challenging words and sentences to get media attention to highlight the immediacy of the disease. Because of his high profile, his colleagues suggested he should not testify in court to reduce emotion surrounding the issue, to which he acceded. He and his colleagues recognized that the media could be friendly or could have a negative impact on the work they were doing. NYC volunteers had to contend with slurs and other negative attitudes and phrases even when testifying in court for NEXs. The eight defendants in the NYC trial used the media to gain support for their position and to enlist the action of certain policy makers to visit the NEX and see for themselves what was occurring. Early information about HIV/AIDS centered around homosexuals and IDUs, and the media focused on inflammatory comments from policy makers, religious leaders, and the general public that made sensational press. The term "sound bites" was coined and was used by reporters to capture startling remarks and also by NEX volunteers to further their own perspectives. Dutch language related to IDUs was not pejorative, and there was little media attention. Dutch people who worked in drug rehabilitation services expressed dismay and disappointment that HIV/AIDS and NEXs in the United States were so volatile.

In spite of some negative issues that occurred during the planning and execution of the dissertation, the researcher believes the study was well-done. The researcher serendipitously found four other nurses who also had master's degrees in nursing and PhDs in political science. All had conducted their dissertation research on different aspects of the policy process. These researchers provided the foundation for a textbook, *Health Policy and Politics: A Nurse's Guide*, which is preparing for its fifth edition.

REFERENCES

Dexter, L. A. (1970). *Elite and specialized interviewing.* Evanston, IL: Northwestern University Press.

Kingdon, J. W. (1984). *Agendas, alternatives, and public policies.* Boston, MA: Little, Brown.

Milstead, J. A. (1993). *The advancement of policy implementation theory: An analysis of three needle exchange programs.* (Doctoral dissertation, University of Georgia, 1993). Dissertation Abstracts International, 54, 2311A.

CHAPTER SEVEN

EXPERIENCES OF A NURSE ETHNOGRAPHER: FROM STUDENT TO FACULTY

Pamela J. Brink

DOING ETHNOGRAPHY

Learning to Do Ethnography

As a graduate student in anthropology at Boston University in the 1960s, I was hard pressed to discriminate between the terms ethnography and fieldwork, as ethnography was used conceptually as well as descriptively. Ethnography is a specific form of fieldwork among an indigenous people with a culture and language totally foreign to the anthropologist. It was understood that to be an anthropologist one must survive culture shock (Oberg, 1960) and live to tell the tale. There was no course on "Anthropological Fieldwork" or on "How to do Ethnography." Anthropology students were expected to absorb the meaning of ethnography by reading ethnographies. The actual process of doing fieldwork was learned by listening to the stories of faculty and returning graduate students at departmental parties. Ethnography was part reality and part mystique.

Books available on doing ethnography were sparse. Eleanor Bowen's (pseudonym for Laura Bohannan) *Return to Laughter* (1961) candidly admits that her preparation and advice for fieldwork consisted of the admonition by her major advisor to "be sure and take leaky tennis shoes." Beatrice Whiting spearheaded the massive "Six Cultures" project, in which married pairs of graduate students went to six different field settings to document child-rearing practices. The teams were trained in child-rearing theories, in the interviews they were to conduct, and the specific observations they were to make. An extensive correspondence between faculty and students during the fieldwork period helped to clarify issues in the field. A compilation of the findings of the Six Cultures Project was published under Whiting's name as *Six Cultures: Studies of Child Rearing* (1963). In addition, a small volume contained the protocol, including the interviews and observations used as the basis for the ethnographies, which came out in 1966 (Whiting, Child, & Lambert, 1966).

I was accepted by Boston University in 1963, under a United States Public Health Service (USPHS) grant designed for nurses to earn their doctorates in fields useful to nursing. The grant was for a maximum of 5 years and consisted of a monthly stipend and tuition fees. The only requirement was that the recipients return to nursing for a period of at least 2 years after completing the doctorate. The candidate was expected to remain on campus for the duration of the training. To do a "proper" ethnography, therefore, special dispensation needed to be obtained to leave Boston to live on a Northern Paiute reservation in Nevada. Otherwise, the field site, as chosen by my classmates, would have been an urban neighborhood (Ragucci, 1972) or hospital (Govoni, 1970) in Boston.

I have conducted several ethnographies since beginning my doctoral work in anthropology. In 1964, under the supervision of Richard Kluckhohn (son of the famous team of Clyde and Florence Kluckhohn), I made my first foray into fieldwork by spending my summer in a small depressed county in Eastern Kentucky. (The county seat had a population of 2,000 people.) In 1967, I moved to the Pyramid Lake Paiute Reservation in northern Nevada, for the fieldwork for my dissertation on child-rearing patterns among the Northern Paiute (Brink, 1969). After receiving my degree, I was hired by the School of Nursing at UCLA and was given a sabbatical leave for the academic year 1974 to 1975. I traveled to eastern Nigeria and lived with the rural Annang in what later became the Cross River State. I wanted to know just what it was that made the Annang decide between traditional medicine and Western medicine as they had both options available with no coercion from either (Brink, 1977). I made two subsequent trips to the Annang in 1982 and again in 1989 looking at different questions.

Each fieldwork experience posed different challenges, problems, and solutions. The major lesson that needs to be learned when doing ethnographic field research is that the researcher is not in control of the field site, the kind and amount of data to be collected, or even what will be done on any given day. Unlike tightly controlled laboratory experiments or sociological studies of urban populations who are familiar with questionnaires and interviews, the fieldworker comes to realize that it is the indigenous population that is in control. It is only through their good will and courtesy that the fieldworker will learn anything at all.

The Kentucky Experience

I spent two months in Paintsville, Kentucky, trying to puzzle out what I was supposed to be doing as an ethnographer. I had my pads of paper and pencils (there were no computers at the time), and the department chair had bought me a Dictaphone from the USPHS grant to record interviews. (I needed a tape recorder, but he needed a Dictaphone.) I was informally adopted by an older couple who treated me as one of their granddaughters. I ate with them, went out into the country to buy beans and potatoes with them, went to church and revivals with them, and sat with them on the front porch shucking beans. Mam-ma and Pop-eye shared their histories and the history of Paintsville and Johnson County. They had a grown daughter living nearby who worked nights in the hospital. She was the only nurse at night and I shared some of those hours with her. Her boyfriend, who worked for the county roads department, drove me around the county and taught me how to find my way by the size of the trees and rocks because there were no road signs. The county librarian took me with him in his bookmobile when he went up into the hollers. We usually chatted with whoever was home, but the only words I ever understood were "hell" and "damn." These mountain folk spoke Elizabethan English with a Kentucky twang. He took me to meet the out-of-work destitute coal miners and their families. The contrast between town, country, and hollers was often startling. I was accepted only because I was "J. V. Stambaugh's granddaughter." Otherwise I would have been ostracized as an uppity northerner. My way was eased by having a built-in family who sheltered me from harm and gave me a kinship role in the community.

The Northern Paiute Experience

In contrast, for my dissertation research, I was alone. I was in an unfamiliar area of the United States with unfamiliar people. I had only one desire, to be able to observe and talk to the people of the Pyramid Lake Paiute about their child-rearing patterns (Brink, 1971a, 1971b) following the Whiting protocol. There was little literature on the Northern Paiute. I had written to the Tribal Council requesting permission to do research on their reservation. They sent me an invitation to come to the next Tribal Council meeting and put my request to the members of the council. So I got a room at a motel in Wadsworth, a small town outside the reservation, and drove the 17 miles to the small general store (the only business on the reservation) to find out where the meeting would be held. As it happened, there was a baseball game in progress, and the meeting did not begin in the gym until after the game was over. I was granted permission to interview people. I commuted from the motel in Wadsworth to the reservation every day and "hung out" at the general store, eventually getting involved with some women who ran a small craft shop. One of them told me of a small house on the reservation available for rent. It had been used by Peace Corps volunteers to learn about "hardship" before being sent to their assignments. Later the schoolmaster of the elementary school offered me one of the houses on the school property. Becuse it had a stove, and the other did not, I decided to move. As I learned later, this placed me in the "camp" of those who favored the teachers as opposed to those who didn't. This immediately cut my target population in half.

It was the older women of the reservation who first befriended me. I would drive them to Reno for doctors' appointments, out in the country to collect willow to make baskets and cradleboards, up in the foothills to collect pinion pine seeds and to various all-night Pow-wows around the state. I went to funerals, funeral lunches, and basketball games. I drafted kinship charts for anyone who wanted one. I was asked to emcee the annual Christmas party.

When I tried to interview young mothers who met my criteria for the child-rearing protocol, I had doors closed in my face. There were 25 families who met the criteria for the Whiting protocol, but only 7 who agreed to be interviewed. I had alienated some because of my friendship with the schoolteachers, some were just naturally reticent to be interviewed, and others were not friends with some of those who had befriended me. Because I was not able to get a large enough sample, I was told to change the topic of my dissertation research after I passed my dissertation exam, which would be supervised by my committee.

Fieldwork With the Annang of Nigeria

Nigeria offered an entirely different field setting. A colleague asked me to join him in his "research area" among the Annang: he would do the archaeology, and I, the ethnography. Our unrealized dream was to coauthor books, monographs, and articles. Getting a Nigerian visa for the sabbatical year posed the first obstacle. Learning the language was important as few spoke English. I found a linguist at UCLA who had written a book on Ibibio, a related language (similar to the differences between Spanish and Portuguese). Both languages are tonal. There was little literature on the Annang, but some on the Ibibio. When I finally got to Nigeria (my trunk containing all medications, clothing, and film was lost at the airport and not recovered until I left the country), my colleague provided me with a car in need of repairs, a place to live, an interpreter/informant (a young Annang man of the village), and a young girl of a nearby village to serve as my cook–housekeeper.

Our house was beside the main road between Abak Town and Ikot Ekpene and consisted of two rooms with a kitchen between them. There was a cement squatting toilet out back, and a bathtub was brought in for me so I did not have to bathe in the river. Eventually a mat was erected around the tub so I could bathe in relative privacy. My house was next to a large open field used for the market held every 8 days. A little further down the road was a Catholic boarding school for girls and in the opposite direction, also on the main road, was the Catholic junior seminary that offered Sunday Mass for the community. Otherwise all was dense vegetation interspersed with narrow, rutted dirt roads and bicycle tracks cut through the trees. Guides were necessary to find residences. Recognizing a village square (a widening in the road with perhaps a small storage hut made of palm fronds) was a challenge.

Because I was a "Prof" (an assistant professor), I was accorded very high status/seniority. I was also accepted because of my archaeologist friend and my informant. I was introduced to "important people," and others would drop by and visit. I soon realized that my shoestring budget of $5,000, which had to last for my entire 7-month stay, could never meet their expectations because of their notion that I was a professor and therefore wealthy. Wherever I went, I was expected to pay the expenses of everyone present. At ceremonial occasions, I was expected to donate large sums of money, announcements for which were made out loud to the crowd. Customs and expectations were unfamiliar.

Two incidents prompted my early departure from the field. The first was a bad bout of malaria that had settled in my liver (the antimalarial was not effective), and the second was the psychotic breakdown of my chief interpreter/informant.

Two subsequent trips to Annang-land in Nigeria provided excellent material on culture change over time. Each field visit was piloted by a different chief informant/interpreter; each time had different housing and faced different challenges. The last visit included a graduate student collecting data for her master's thesis.

LITERATURE REVIEWS

It was important for an anthropology doctoral student to find an isolated group of people who had never been studied before. Failing that, the student/ academic was expected to find a group having the least amount of published information. Literature reviews would consist of ethnographies on neighboring peoples who might or might not share similar traits. In addition, as there was no expectation of a "research problem" prior to entering the field, problem-oriented literature reviews were not expected. The "problem" was to emerge from the field experience with enough data to cobble together a dissertation topic.

This loose field strategy was beginning to change with the federal funding of research projects. As finding literature on the population was a problem, literature reviews might focus on methods or some culture trait or category such as adolescent initiation rites. The human relations area files (HRAF) at Harvard University was extremely helpful for finding other culture groups and studies with similar traits. (Fortunately, Harvard University was just across the river from Boston University, and the universities had reciprocal library privileges, so I was able to go to the room that housed the files and sort through all the ethnographies contained there.)

Child rearing was becoming of great interest, especially when the Western world discovered that the child-rearing practices considered basic or essential did not exist in other cultures (thanks to the work of Margaret Mead). Although child rearing was the focus of my literature review prior to going to the Pyramid Lake Paiute Reservation, culture change became the focus of my literature review for the dissertation itself because my doctoral defense committee, most of whom were sociologists decided my sample was too small for a decent report.

For the initial Nigerian field trip, I looked at the literature on patient decision making both in the United States and elsewhere. How do patients make choices for where they seek care? What kinds of symptoms drive people to seek professional help? What kinds of care are available? What is the difference between traditional or indigenous medicine and Western medicine in Nigeria? Are there government sanctions against choosing one alternative over the other (Brink, 1977)?

For the second Nigerian field trip, I was interested in the Kluckhohn and Strodtbeck (1961) value orientation theory and its instrumentation, so the literature focused on values and cross-cultural comparisons of cultural values (Brink, 1984).

The last trip to Nigeria was to clear up some issues raised in the first field study in which I was introduced to the concept of "the fattening room" (Brink, 1989a, 1991, 1993, 1995). What was it about the value on fat and fatness in Nigeria that differed from the Western value on thinness as being healthy and beautiful? What physiological basis might there be for the fattening room? What happened in a fattening room? Was it always associated with initiation into a secret society or were there other reasons?

METHODOLOGY

For an ethnographer, participant observation is the basic method of data collection. It is slower than interviews and questionnaires, but without that period of observation and informal questioning, errors based on preconceived notions will occur. For example, there was a question in the Whiting and colleagues (1966) child-rearing schedule that dealt with masturbation. The question as written was: "Do you allow your children to play with themselves?" I asked the question as written. Invariably, the Northern Paiute mothers responded: "No, I would rather they play with other children. It's not good for children to play alone." (Although I asked my dissertation chair what I was to do about this situation, he did not respond. In fact, I received only one letter from him while I was in the field and that was during the past month of data collection.)

Getting involved in community life to the degree possible and asking about customs is simply the first step. Although Kentucky is an American state and English is the primary language, there were some customs and beliefs that were different from those of California or Massachusetts residents. For example, Johnson County was a dry county. Those wishing to buy alcohol had to drive to West Virginia. This law created the practice of Country Clubs providing the mix, but the client providing the alcohol and leaving the bottle at the club for the next visit. A black market for alcohol was acknowledged. Men earned their living making and/or selling illegal liquor they bought in West Virginia. Feuding was still in practice, and men living in the hollers routinely carried shotguns. Church was a central organizing principle. Each of the 27 Protestant churches had its own congregation. Each congregation had its own rules for proper behavior; the punishment for violating the rules was banishment from the congregation. This often meant a shunning of the individual from their own nuclear families. It was a social death. On the other hand, the churches supported members in illness and health. If anyone was in trouble, their church was there to help.

In Nigeria, social customs are dictated by age, gender, and wealth. The older a person, the more senior they are. No matter how uneducated, an older man would be obeyed over a younger well-educated man. It is the senior's advice that would be listened to even if he was clearly in the wrong. Everyone in a village knew where they stood in terms of age and seniority. Men had more status than women, but a young man must show respect to an older woman. Many social decisions were made on the basis of gender and age. Boys were always given an education as that increased the status of a family. Because girls would marry outside the village, their education was not as necessary. The wealthy who could afford it would educate all their children. The less wealthy had to decide who was to receive an education or health care. Most of this information becomes apparent over time. It is rarely, if ever, elicited in an interview.

Sampling

Unlike sampling issues in urban populations or where population data is known, sampling is not as straightforward in rural areas with no population records. In Nigeria, among the Annang, there was a major women's revolt against a proposed population survey. The women stormed the government offices shouting that they were not cattle to be counted! "Count the men, if they don't mind, but don't count us." So from that time all government census data is only of men.

Although Catholicism was the major Christian religion in the area, there were other faiths such as Mormonism. The Annang were polygamous. Even among Catholics, a man might have more than one wife if his senior wife had not borne him a son. This fact, however, was withheld from the priest. Although there was an estimate of the number of men, there was no way of knowing how many women and children lived in an area.

Houses were separated by dense bush, so knowing which house belonged to which village was something a stranger could not know. There were no maps of the area. In fact, village boundaries were known only by those living in the village. Even an aerial photograph would simply show treetops. Sampling, in this situation, was not straightforward. In fact, sampling was totally dependent on the help of informants, word of mouth, and amount of time in the field.

For the value orientation schedule, I was looking for an equal number of men and women as informants. I would be invited to a home only to find that when I arrived, many others came to look at this strange White woman. Every interview would be conducted with an interpreter in the presence of at least 15 people. The women tended to defer to their husbands and agreed with whatever they said if they were asked questions first. So, in this public situation, the women were asked their opinion first. Sometimes the questions elicited a group discussion.

In trying to find a sample of knowledgeable women to interview about the fattening room, I soon discovered they were all old women who spoke no English and were major players in women's secret societies. No one knew how many of these women were there. Each village had at least one secret society. Did I have a right to hear this information since it was secret (Brink, 1993)? Probably not. At one interview, a man came storming into the compound shouting and waving his machete at me, saying I had no right to talk to his mother! I had to pay for the information! He was going to speak to the chief! Get out! Get out! Sampling was not always easy.

Once, at dusk, as I was driving home with a car full of people, someone pointed out a fattening room girl walking home from a village market with a basket on her head and carrying a stool. I wanted to turn around and take a photograph but was told I could not do that. At another time, a friend came to tell me she had found a fattening room girl and I was to come and meet her. I went with my young informant, met the fattening room girl and asked her many questions. I was hesitant to take a picture of her or her hut and was in fact chased away when her mother arrived and found us there.

Interviewing the old women, who were in charge of women's secret societies, was a challenge, as no man could hear these stories, nor could a woman who had not been through the experience themselves. Because they spoke no English and my Annang was abysmal, I needed an interpreter who met their specifications. Once we made the appointment, the old women were quite voluble and indeed allowed me to photograph them. It helped that I had been adopted, as a sister, by the senior man, the chief, in one village. Because he approved of me and made me a ritual relative, they respected his decision.

Settings for Data Collection

Ethnographers always hang out with people. The ethnographer tries to be wherever other people are gathered. In Kentucky, I hung out at the home of my ritual grandparents going wherever they went. On the Paiute Reservation, my hangout was the general store as everyone came through for their mail or to leave their crafts for sale. The older women discovered that I was willing to drive them wherever they wanted to go. We would dance all night at pow-wows or travel to another town for Indian parades and dancing. I felt I had arrived when I was invited into a home, helped in the backyard, and was given by my "old ladies" a going away lunch of traditional foods, a cradleboard they had all contributed to making, and my formal Indian name, before I left the field. Observations and questions happen wherever one is. For the formal interviews, I sometimes stood at the front door, and other times I was invited into the front room.

Hanging out in Afaha Obong just did not happen. In the first fieldwork experience, because I lived beside the main road, people would call on me. They were invited into my room, offered something to drink (either fresh palm wine or Akaikai—a distilled native gin—if my visitor was a man, or soft drinks if it was a woman). They were also offered kola nuts and a knife. Before I gave anyone a glass of anything, I was expected to "kiss it" or take a sip, demonstrating that the drink was not poisoned. These little formal rituals were taught to me by my chief interpreter/informant. I was taken to different places for different events whether a second burial, Mass at the Junior Seminary, a funeral and burial, or just to visit. (A second burial is an expensive funeral celebration for a deceased person when a big party can be afforded. It might be years after the death, but includes drummers and dancers, new clothing for relatives, slaughtering a goat or small calf for a feast, and erecting a memorial such as a sculpted sign post at the road.) At different times of the year, different spirits are in charge of the Annang. Watching the secret societies and their rituals was always by invitation only.

As a White woman in a Black society, I stood out everywhere I went, especially because I was blonde. So I was a great figure of curiosity. During one Catholic Mass, at the Offertory where everyone dances up in procession to leave their gifts at the altar, I danced with the women. Everyone at the back of the church stood up to watch.

Respecting the Rights of Research Subjects

American Institutional Review Boards evaluate the protection of human subjects based on their assumptions about research subject's rights. Approval of a proposal can be based on an ignorance of cultural diversity. In addition, institutional review boards (IRBs) are not consistent in decisions across university departments. What a social science IRB will approve might easily be denied by a medical IRB. Sometimes stringent rules are applied unnecessarily. Anthropologists have found that when they disguise the identity of the people they have lived with and studied, they may please the IRB but offend their hosts. They have been told, "You lived with us for 2 years but did not learn our name!" In addition, many medical IRBs are familiar with the clinical trials or an epidemiology study but are abysmally ignorant of qualitative research methods, especially ethnography, and make judgments based on their ignorance.

One nursing IRB rejected a proposal to use the Kluckhohn and Strodtbeck value orientation schedule on a group of students. The study proposed to test the test–retest reliability of the schedule. The questions being asked were "Are cultural values stable or affected by experience? Which values, if any, are most affected by experience?" The researchers wanted to test the students before and after a 2-month clinical experience in a developing country. The nursing IRB said that unless an interview schedule had construct validity, it could not be used on students. Because students were used as research subjects by other faculty throughout the university using qualitative data collection methods (which do not have construct validity), the decision by the IRB seemed unnecessarily rigid and arbitrary. In addition, the value orientation schedule did have construct validity, but the IRB did not know that. The study had to be scrapped.

Major problems encountered with IRBs involved an inability to specify beforehand the nature of participant observation and what questions would be asked; an inability to specify how many people would be in the sample; and an inability to promise the use of statistical sampling techniques.

Data Analysis

Data analysis is ongoing throughout the fieldwork as well as at home. There are several sets of data that can be used to construct ethnography for publication. The field diary provides an outline of what happened on what day with whom and how much it cost. It helps to document the weather in that it can limit what can be done on a particular day. The field diary is supplemented with more specific notes on observations or conversations, which are referenced in the field diary. Here again, the who, when, what, and why of the observational note are specified.

Because all of my fieldwork occurred before laptop computers were publicly available, I recorded everything in typed and handwritten notes supplemented with still photography. Specific interview schedules and responses, of course, were kept separate from observational data and informal interviewing notes. Visits to a traditional healer in his compound, the nursing center, which was primarily a birthing center, the different markets, the local elementary school, attending Catholic Mass or Protestant services, and visiting the hospital in Abak Town were all documented separately.

One day as I was returning home, I found that the fields next to my house were on fire. The first thing I did was to enter the house and rescue my field notes and typewriter. Only afterward did I discover that it was a controlled fire, an annual event, and my belongings were not in danger.

The first thing to do when back home would be to organize notes according to the primary question being asked. Everything else helps to place the question in context of the culture. The more unfamiliar the culture, the more copious the notes, because the answer to the question must always be in context of the culture group. For this reason, ethnography reads more like a travelogue or a story, rather than a research report. Because ethnographies try to make the culture group come alive for the reader, they rarely follow the academic outline of problem, methods, analyses, findings, and conclusions.

Data analysis for the Northern Paiute followed the protocol suggested by Whiting and colleagues (1966). When the focus of my dissertation was changed, I had to go back and look at the aspects of the culture that I had observed that demonstrated a difference between the culture at the time of initial contact with the culture as it was in the late 1960s. Because field notes were not organized according to that theme, I had to do a search for anything that demonstrated a difference or a similarity. The easiest, of course, was documenting the child-rearing patterns, as that had been the original focus of the study. A decision had to be made on what to look for in the data: Was it to be culture traits, behavior patterns, health and illness, or religious beliefs? These data were necessarily incomplete as they had not been deliberately sought out. As there were no books or articles on how to do data analysis for an ethnography, the process was fluid and intuitive.

The Nigerian data collection and analysis differed according to the research question being asked. The first task, of course, was to try to situate the findings in context of the culture. Second, analysis depended on whatever data had been collected.

The question on health care decision making had no built-in analytic protocol. It also became apparent during fieldwork that direct questions about the decision-making process, gleaned from the literature review, made no sense at all to the Annang. I was, therefore, forced to rely completely on participant observation with subsequent questions. Because I had a car and because it was five miles from where I lived to the nearest hospital, I was asked to transport people to the hospital. On the way, I could ask questions about what was wrong and why we were going to the hospital. The same was true for traditional healing. When someone became ill and either called in the traditional healer or was taken to see the traditional healer and I was allowed to be part of this situation, then I could ask questions so long as I did not interfere. These occasions were rare. Fortunately, a traditional healer found me attractive enough to propose marriage, and as a result was more willing to share his compound, his wives and children, his medicine hut and its contents, as well as the different clothing he would wear for different curing ceremonies. In this way, I was able to discover what symptoms or problems brought people to him for a cure and to learn the process of healing itself.

Quite unexpectedly, as is often true in ethnography, I discovered a third form of health care: the native nurse. This was an untrained individual who had observed the healing practices of a Western-trained person, frequently an employer, and who knew how to give shots. These people were often sought for cures simply because the patient could not afford to go to the hospital or had no transport.

I was able to observe a patient at the local hospital, and had a trained registered nurse friend explain the Western health care system as practiced in that hospital. I also had the privilege of being invited to observe a live birth attended by a traditional birth attendant in her backyard and interviewed another. In addition, I was invited to visit the trained midwives at the health center (Brink, 1982a).

Perhaps an example or two of these observations would help. For my first trip to Nigeria, the young girl who had been hired as my housekeeper and cook suffered a grand mal seizure outside the house at my front door in full view of everyone who passed by on the road. Because grand mal seizures were believed to be caused by witches and evil spirits, we tried to block a view of her from the road as best as possible. When the seizure was over and she had recovered sufficiently, we took her to her father's compound. Because he was himself a traditional healer, he sought the services of a well-known traditional healer from outside his own village. I was then able to observe her first traditional healing, but was excluded from all her other treatments. Only much later did I discover that my sponsor had offered to take her to the university health center in Port Harcourt for treatment, but her father had refused.

In another situation, an old woman had developed an enormous inguinal hernia and was in desperate need of surgery. The village men (all relatives) held a council to decide whether or not they could afford to pay for her surgery. In the end, they decided that she had passed her productive years (she was no longer able to conceive and bear a child), and the money was better spent on someone who still contributed to the family. She did not have the surgery.

In this Nigerian experience, data analysis consisted simply in a compilation of documented situations involving a health issue. These were then separated by the initial complaint, the type of health care sought, the age and gender of the patient, the treatment given, and its and outcome. Then came the problem of teasing out on what basis the decision was made to seek health care and which type of healing had been given (Brink, 1977).

In the study on the Kluckhohn and Strodtbeck value orientation schedule (1961), the data analysis protocol, meticulously described in the book, was part of the method. Just as with the culture groups described in the book, the answers to the questions had to be seen in light of the culture.

The last Nigerian field study was to clarify questions that had arisen on the first field trip. Because I was interested in successful dieters in the United States, I was intrigued by the cultural attitude toward fatness as it was valued and considered beautiful. Placing a girl in a fattening room was prerequisite to marriage. If a married woman could not conceive, she was placed in a fattening room. The fattening room was also part of the entrance requirements for women's secret societies. Were these all part of the same ritual? Did they signify different things or different developmental issues? Who was in charge and what were their qualifications? I had my questions prepared prior to entering the field and discovered, again, that my questions made no sense in the context of the culture. The women who were interviewed had no idea what I was asking, and I was confused by their answers. We were talking past each other. Because I never got the answer to my question, I simply settled on a description of the girls and women who entered the fattening room, what it looked like, what they ate to get fat, why they were in seclusion, and so on.

DISSEMINATION

There was only one nursing research journal in the United States during my early years as a student and later as a faculty member and graduate anthropologist. The preferred type of research report was the experimental design or at least a highly controlled observational study with some statistics. Ethnography was not understood by the editor and, in addition, was too long and too loose for nursing research. The earliest publications were method papers about participant observation (Byerly, 1969) and ethnography (Ragucci, 1972). Nurse anthropologists were limited to presenting papers at invitational nursing research conferences (only nurses with doctoral degrees were invited), which were later compiled into research proceedings or anthropology journals. One early ethnographic study was reported in *The American Journal of Nursing* by Charlotte Gale (1972). In a personal conversation with me, she shared her hurt that so many nurse colleagues discounted her research for her doctorate as mere storytelling and not "real" research. This was a common experience in those early years. Few nurse editors and researchers knew anything at all about anthropology, much less ethnography. It was not until the *Western Journal of Nursing Research* began publishing that ethnographies were published (see Vol. 1, Number 3, the article by Jeannie Kayser-Jones, 1979).

Few of the early nurse anthropologists published their doctoral work, some not even presenting their work at conferences. For example, there is no evidence that Madeleine Leininger, who did her doctoral fieldwork in Oceania, or Oliver Osborne, who did his doctoral research in Nigeria, ever published their doctoral ethnographies in a nursing journal. I didn't either. Instead, we were more interested in trying to convince schools of nursing to accept anthropological theories and principles, especially the concept of culture. Nursing, in general, in the 1960s and 1970s, was more interested in theory than in qualitative methods of research.

Madeleine Leininger founded the Council on Nursing and Anthropology (CONAA) in 1968 under the auspices of the Society for Medical Anthropology as a venue for nurses with doctoral degrees in anthropology to share their research interests. She invited me to be its first secretary for the following year's meeting. In 1972, she announced to the Council that she was forming a new organization to be called transcultural nursing for nurses with no background in anthropology but an interest in culture. In essence, this group was formed to talk about the theories of anthropology and how to implement them into nursing. It was very successful. Only much later did Leininger raise the issue of doing research in transcultural nursing, which she labeled ethnonursing (see Ray, Morris, & McFarland, 2013). She eventually founded the *Journal of Transcultural Nursing* to publish work related to this topic. Few of the early nurse anthropologists were published in this journal.

My own fieldwork was published primarily in conference proceedings (Brink, 1971, 1977, 2000), anthropology journals (Brink, 1982a, 1989b), and chapters in books (Brink, 1982b, 1993, 1995). One paper from my dissertation was published in the *Indian Historian* (Brink, 1971b), the other was a conference proceeding (Brink, 1971a). My only publication in a nursing journal was on the use of the Kluckhohn and Strodtbeck value orientation schedule (1961) and that was because it was primarily hard data (Brink, 1984).

SUMMARY

In the 1970s when I was an assistant professor at UCLA, my anthropology colleagues were expected to publish a book based on their doctoral dissertation as well as at least 12 data-based articles in anthropology journals to be considered for promotion and tenure. In nursing, publication of any kind, whether research based or not, was acceptable for promotion and tenure. Having only one journal available for the publication of nursing research of any kind, coupled with nursing's general ignorance of and lack of interest in ethnography and limited access to publication, most nurse anthropologists did not publish their work.

I was one of the lucky ones. Two of my publications (that I know of) made a difference in the lives of the people I studied. A few years after completing my dissertation, I found that it had been used by the Pyramid Lake Paiute as evidence in a case against the army corps of engineers who kept building more and more dams across the Truckee River thereby significantly decreasing the amount of annual spring runoff to Pyramid Lake. Because the lake contained a rare species of fish, not found elsewhere in North America, and with the lake drying up for want of water, the fish were dying out. I had documented this fact in my dissertation.

The second article that made a difference was the article on traditional birth attendants (TBAs) (1982). The article was used to support the Cross River State's (Nigeria) decision whether or not to fund the training of TBAs. That year, during the annual parade in Abak Town, the TBAs paraded in celebration of their recognition. Ethnographers rarely hear about the impact of their basic research on others, unlike the immediate feedback of applied researchers, so this feedback was gratifying.

Ethnography is a long and intense personal process. It demands immersion into a culture, a suspension of preconceived cultural values and beliefs, and an acceptance that the population is in control of the situation, not the researcher. Data collection is fluid, dependent on the situation. Fact checking is repetitive, comparing one person's perception with another and then another until a broad general agreement is reached (Brink, 1989b). Time is also fluid. Few appointments are made based on the clock. A Westerner will always bump up against this relativism. History is also fluid and not based on a Western calendar. Values and beliefs are most often discovered by bumping up against them. Being a stranger in a foreign culture can be confusing and lonely. It is only through the graciousness of the hosts that the ethnographer survives the experience to tell the tale.

In today's fast-paced world, classical ethnography is rarely the choice of a novice nurse researcher. It is simply too time-consuming and does not fit the requirements of the local IRB, most granting agencies, or publication outlets. When academics can achieve promotion and tenure by publishing many "quick and dirty" quantitative studies, very few will opt to conduct "down and dirty," long, drawn out ethnography. Ethnographic fieldwork for 2 years in an isolated island community is no longer the norm, even in anthropology. The sad commentary on this is that so many are barred from an experience of self-discovery and an appreciation of another's culture.

Finally, ethnography teaches the researcher that most people are unaware of what prompts their decisions or their behavior. What a person says in an interview about what they believe or what they would do in a situation is not always borne out by their behavior in a given situation. Only through observation can the researcher judge the strength of the belief. What a person does or says, day in and day out, may or may not be reflected in the answers to a questionnaire or interview. Ethnography is enriching for both the researcher and the data.

REFERENCES

Bowen, E. S. (1961). *Return to laughter*. Garden City, NY: Doubleday.

Brink, P. J. (1969). *The Pyramid Lake Paiute of Nevada*. (University Microfilms 69-18, 440).

Brink, P. J. (1971a). Some aspects of change in Northern Paiute child rearing practices. In C. Melvin Aikens (Ed.), *Great Basin Anthropological Conference 1970: Selected Papers* (pp. 167–175). University of Oregon Anthropological Papers, No. 1.

Brink, P. J. (1971b). Paviotso child training: Notes. *The Indian Historian*, 4(1), 47–50.

Brink, P. J. (1977). Decision making of the health care consumer: A Nigerian example. In *Communicating nursing research: Nursing research in the bicentennial year* (pp. 351–362). Boulder, CO: Western Interstate Commission for Higher Education.

Brink, P. J. (1982a). Traditional birth attendants among the Annang of Nigeria: Traditional practices and proposed programs. *Social Science and Medicine: Medical Anthropology, Part B*, 16(21), 183–189.

Brink, P. J. (1982b). An anthropological perspective on parenting. In C. B. Hughes, J. A. Horowitz, & B. J. Perdue (Eds.), *Parenting reassessed: A nursing perspective* (pp. 66–84). Englewood Cliffs, NJ: Prentice-Hall.

Brink, P. J. (1984). Value orientations as an assessment tool in cultural diversity: Theory, method and examples. *Nursing Research*, 33(4), 198–203.

Brink, P. J. (1989a). The fattening room among the Annang of Nigeria. *Medical Anthropology*, 12(1), 131–143.

Brink, P. J. (1989b). Issues of reliability and validity. In Janice M. Morse (Ed.), *Qualitative nursing research: A contemporary dialogue* (pp. 151–168). Rockville, MD: Aspen.

Brink, P. J. (1991). The fattening room in Nigeria. *The Canadian Nurse*, 87(9), 31–32.

Brink, P. J. (1993). Studying African women's secret societies: The fattening room of the Annang. In Claire M. Renzetti & Raymond M. Lee (Eds.), *Researching sensitive topics* (pp. 235–248). Newbury Park, CA: Sage.

Brink, P. J. (1995). The fattening room in Nigeria. In N. Pollock (Ed.), *Social aspects of obesity*. Victoria University of Wellington, NZ: Gordon & Breach.

Brink, P. J. (2000). Values and conflict in clinical settings. In Kurt W. Russo (Ed.), *Finding the middle ground: Insights and applications of the value orientations method* (pp. 109–118). Yarmouth, ME: Intercultural Press.

Byerly, E. L. (1969). The nurse-researchers as participant observer in a nursing setting. *Nursing Research*, 18(2), 230–238.

Gale, C. (1972). Walking in the Aide's shoes. *American Journal of Nursing*, 73(4), 628–631.

Govoni, L. (1970). *A method of analyzing the value system of a general medical-surgical hospital.* Unpublished PhD dissertation. Boston, MA: Boston University.

Kayser-Jones, J. (1979). Care of the institutionalized aged in Scotland and the United States. *Western Journal of Nursing Research, 1*(3), 190–200.

Kluckhohn, F. R., & Strodtbeck, F. L. (1961). *Variations in value orientations.* Greenwood Press Evanston, IL: Row, Peterson.

Oberg, K. (1960). Cultural shock: Adjustment to new cultural environments. *Practical Anthropology, 7,* 177–182.

Ragucci, A. T. (1972). The ethnography approach and nursing research. *Nursing Research, 21*(6), 485–490.

Ray, M. A., Morris, E., & McFarland, M. (2013). Ethnonursing method of Dr. Madeleine Leininger. In C. T. Beck (Ed.), *Routledge international handbook of qualitative nursing research* (pp. 213–229). New York, NY: Routledge.

Whiting, B. B. (1963). *Six cultures: Studies of child rearing.* New York, NY: John Wiley and Sons.

Whiting, J. W. M, Child, I. L., & Lambert, W. W. (1966). *Field guide for the study of socialization.* New York, NY: John Wiley and Sons.

CHAPTER EIGHT

USING MALARIA RAPID DIAGNOSTIC TESTS IN GHANA: A FOCUSED ETHNOGRAPHY

Nana Yaa Boadu and Gina Marie Awoko Higginbottom

*F*ocused ethnographies (FEs) evolved in the field of sociological ethnography and are rooted in classical anthropological ethnography. FEs concentrate on specific elements of society. They are therefore suitable for studying cultural perspectives surrounding specific issues among defined subgroups of society. FEs generate specific knowledge to address specific research questions and are useful in applied research that aims to inform policy and practice. They are therefore a fitting approach to understand health and illness beliefs, behaviors, and attitudes among specific providers or patient populations to improve health care delivery processes and outcomes. Traditional ethnographies are time extensive and experientially rich. FEs, on the other hand, are *data intensive,* in that large volumes of data from multiple sources are collected and analyzed within a relatively short time period. From the standpoints of time and funding constraints, FEs adapt suitably to modern health care and policy research studies. The growing representation of focused ethnographical studies in the health care literature underscores their importance and legitimacy in informing policy and practice.

This chapter presents a practical overview of a focused ethnographical study in health care. Against this backdrop, the chapter aims:

1. To outline the theoretical underpinnings and overarching principles of FE;
2. To demonstrate the congruence between the underlying philosophical assumptions, the methodological approach, and the research objectives presented; and
3. To elucidate the suitability of an FE for investigating health care providers' perspectives regarding compliance with guidelines for malaria diagnosis in a limited resource setting.

The outline is context-specific. The principles, however, are broadly applicable to the use of FEs across a diverse spectrum of research disciplines.

FOCUSED ETHNOGRAPHIES IN HEALTH CARE RESEARCH

FEs evolved from classical anthropological ethnography, particularly among sociological ethnographers (Knoblauch, 2005). Consequently, they maintain several distinctive features of traditional ethnography (Cruz & Higginbottom, 2013; Muecke, 1994). However, FEs are guided by a specific research question and are conducted among a small group of people within a particular context. FEs elicit specific information, which is useful for decision making regarding a distinct problem (Knoblauch, 2005; Mayan, 2009). Based on their *focused* nature (Morse, 1987; Richards & Morse, 2007), such studies are also termed mini-ethnographies (Leininger, 1985) or microethnographies (Werner & Schoepfle, 1987a). FEs employ anthropological research methods to generate targeted information in a shorter time frame than traditional ethnographies (Knoblauch, 2005). This makes the approach suitable for studying cultural perspectives, behaviors, and beliefs surrounding health care issues, to inform policy or practice perspectives in a timely manner (Higginbottom, Pillay, & Boadu, 2013; Roper & Shapira, 2000; Thomson, 2011). The World Health Organization (WHO) has successfully adopted and developed the FE approach (Table 8.1) in their study of behaviors and perceptions related to the management of infectious diseases in developing country contexts (Cove & Pelto, 1993; Hudelson, 1993; Stewart, Parker, Chakraborty, & Begum, 1993).

Table 8.1 *Examples of FE Studies on Behaviors and Perceptions Surrounding the Management of Illness in Developing Country Contexts*

Primary Author(s) (Year of Publication)	Study Title
Cove and Pelto (1993)	Focused ethnographical studies in the WHO program for the control of acute respiratory infections
Hudelson (1993)	The management of acute respiratory infections in Honduras: A field test of the focused ethnographic study (FES)
Stewart et al. (1993)	Acute respiratory infections (ARI) in rural Bangladesh: Perceptions and practices
McElroy (2011)	Navigating a way forward: using focused ethnography and community readiness to study disability issues in Ladakh, India

Table 8.2 *Examples of FE Studies Demonstrating a Range of Methodological Uses in Health Care Research*

Primary Author(s) (Year of Publication)	Study Objectives	Participants/context
Daarck-Hirsch and Gamboa (2010)	*Beliefs* regarding the causes, prevention, and treatment of cleft lip	Cleft-lip patients in the Philippines
Higginbottom (2008)	*Meanings* and *consequences* of hypertension	People of Afro-Caribbean descent living in the United Kingdom
Spiers and Wood (2010)	*Experiences, perceptions,* and *actions* engaged in during brief therapy with patients	Community health nurses
Wilkinson and Callister (2010)	*Perceptions* of childbirth	Child-bearing Ghanaian women

Higginbottom and colleagues (2013) demonstrated the versatility and usefulness of FEs in health care research (Table 8.2).

THE STUDY

Research Title

Using malaria rapid diagnostic tests (RDTs) in Ghana: Understanding health care providers' compliance with guidelines for malaria diagnosis in peripheral facilities.

Research Objectives

This study aimed to explore health care providers' perspectives regarding guideline compliance for rapid malaria testing in peripheral health facilities in Ghana with the specific objectives being:

1. To identify the factors influencing health care providers' compliance with guidelines for rapid malaria testing in peripheral health care facilities in Ghana
2. To understand health care providers' perspectives regarding compliance with guidelines for rapid malaria testing in peripheral health care facilities in Ghana

3. To determine how health care providers' perspectives regarding compliance with guidelines for rapid malaria testing influence case management of malaria in peripheral health care facilities in Ghana

Research Background

Significance of Malaria in Ghana

Malaria is the leading cause of morbidity and in-hospital mortality in Ghana, with over 3 million cases each year (Ghana Health Service [GHS], 2009; WHO, 2012). Over 40% of all hospital outpatient department (OPD) visits and 30% of hospital admissions are attributable to this disease. Malaria is a major cause of death among pregnant women, and accounts for 30% of all-cause mortality among children under 5 years of age in Ghana (Ghana Statistical Service (GSS)/GHS, 2009). The entire country experiences stable, year-round transmission and is considered hyper-endemic for malaria (GHS, 2009). However, peaks in annual transmission are found during the rainy seasons: from March to July and from August to mid-November (Baiden et al., 2012a, 2012b, 2012c; Dery et al., 2010). Under the auspices of the Ministry of Health (MOH) and the GHS, the National Malaria Control Program (NMCP) provides direction and oversight to nationwide malaria control activities. Key intervention areas for malaria control in Ghana are (a) prevention using insecticide-treated bed-nets; (b) active case detection, using microscopy or rapid diagnostic tests (RDTs); and (c) effective treatment with artemisinin-based combination therapies (ACTs; GHS, 2009).

The Importance of Accurate Diagnosis of Malaria in Ghana

The WHO currently recommends confirmatory testing prior to treating suspected malaria cases of all ages in endemic regions (WHO, 2010a). The objective of this policy guideline is to curb irrational consumption of anti-malarials and to reduce the emergence of parasitic resistance to effective drugs (English, Reyburn, Goodman, & Snow, 2009; WHO, 2010a). Prior to the policy revision, symptom-based diagnosis of malaria, based largely on the history of fever, was common in Ghana. The practice is also widespread across sub-Saharan Africa, where health-system resources are typically limited (Ansah et al., 2010; Baiden et al., 2012b; Chandler, Whitty, & Ansah, 2010; GHS, 2009). Presumptive treatment of fever as malaria seemed practical to ensure prompt delivery of effective treatment, particularly for young children and pregnant women in endemic areas, who are vulnerable to complications and fatality from severe malaria (English et al., 2009; WHO/ UNICEF, 2005). Presumptive treatment practices were further entrenched as a result of inadequate laboratory infrastructure in rural and remote areas and the availability of inexpensive antimalarials, which have since succumbed to parasitic resistance (Drakely & Reyburn, 2008; WHO, 2006).

Ghana adopted the WHO-recommended "test-before-treat" approach for managing malaria in 2010 (GHS, 2009). Despite national guideline adoption, only a third of all reported malaria cases in Ghana are laboratory confirmed (GHS, 2009; WHO, 2012). The persistence of presumptive treatment practices among many practitioners in Ghana leads to routine misdiagnosis of nonmalarial fevers and overconsumption of antimalarials (Ansah et al., 2010; Reyburn et al., 2004). This delays appropriate treatment of nonmalarial fevers and worsens health outcomes (Amexo, Tolhurst, Barnish, & Bates, 2004). Inappropriate antimalarial consumption further contributes to the spread of parasitic resistance and drains household, health system, and donor resources (Ansah, 2010; Bell & Perkins, 2008; Chandler, Whitty, & Ansah, 2010; Reyburn et al., 2007). Prompt treatment with effective antimalarials is an essential component of the WHO Global Malaria Action Plan (WHO, 2010a; WHO/RBM, 2008). Emerging antimalarial resistance therefore poses a significant threat to global malaria control initiatives (WHO, 2010b). Parasitic resistance is particularly a matter of concern, considering the fragile state of development of new antimalarials (Grimberg & Mehlotra, 2011; Wells, 2011).

The Research Problem

RDTs are simple, field-ready test kits used to detect the presence of malaria parasites in fresh blood (WHO, 2003). RDTs do not require laboratory infrastructure or specialized health care provider skills (WHO, 2003, 2010a). Despite wide RDT deployment to enable parasitological diagnosis in peripheral facilities in Ghana (Ansah et al., 2010; Baiden et al., 2012c; GHS, 2009), a trial conducted in one region of the country identified almost 45% of RDT-negative cases being prescribed antimalarials (Ansah et al., 2010; Chandler et al., 2010). Other studies conducted in Africa have reported rates as high as 80% (Msellem et al., 2009; Onwujekwe et al., 2009) of antimalarial prescriptions that are inconsistent with RDT results. The practice is rampant in under-resourced peripheral facilities, which serve as gatekeepers to the health system for more than half of the populace, including the rural poor (Ansah et al., 2010; Baiden et al., 2012a). Success with implementing current malaria diagnosis and treatment guidelines, as well as cost-effectiveness for test-based management of fevers in general, hinges on the health care providers' commitment to *comply* with the guidelines. Guideline compliance in this regard implies that a health care provider tests and, consequently, treats or otherwise manages suspected cases of malaria consistently on the basis of test results (Chandler et al., 2010; English et al., 2009; Lubell et al., 2008). Poor health care providers' compliance is widely documented across sub-Saharan Africa, including Ghana (Ansah et al., 2010; Chandler et al., 2010); Sudan (Abdelgader et al., 2011); Uganda (Asiimwe et al., 2012; Kyabayinze et al., 2010; Tusiime et al., 2010); Nigeria (Uzochukwu et al., 2012); and Tanzania (Chandler et al., 2010). Nonetheless, the underlying causes of poor guideline compliance are barely understood. Moreover, research to inform strategies that effectively address this challenge is limited (Abdelgader et al., 2012; Ansah et al., 2010; Chandler et al., 2010; Lubell et al., 2008).

The Significance of Research

Understanding health care providers' compliance is essential to facilitate guideline implementation for test-based malaria management in Ghana. We aimed at generating information that is applicable to policy and strategies for improving guideline compliance for malaria diagnosis at the primary health care level in Ghana.

METHODOLOGY

Research Design

Crotty (1998) suggests four elementary processes in any research study. These involve the specific methods used to address a particular research objective, which are governed by particular methodological principles. The choice of which methodological principles to apply is influenced by the researcher's theoretical perspective or philosophical assumptions. These assumptions are embedded in the epistemological and ontological perspectives held toward knowledge and reality. He further explains that ontology refers to "what is," the nature of existence, and the structure of reality, whereas epistemology addresses the nature and basis of knowledge (or reality), its scope, and possibility (Hamlyn, 1995). Epistemology is concerned with providing philosophical grounds for decisions on the adequacy and legitimacy of knowledge (Carter & Little, 2007; Crotty, 1998; Maynard, 1994). Therefore, ontological perspectives describe assumptions about reality, whereas epistemological perspectives involve assumptions about how to make meaning of such reality based on the primary assumptions surrounding reality in the first place (Dew, 2007; Mayan, 2009).

Cresswell (2003) defines the researcher's philosophical assumptions or "worldview" as a set of basic beliefs that guide action (Guba, 1990). Worldviews are also referred to as paradigms (Cresswell, 2003; Lincoln & Guba, 2000) or epistemological and ontological perspectives (Crotty, 1998) in the literature. These describe the researcher's general orientation about the world (the nature of reality, or *ontology*) and the approach to discovering and constructing, or making sense of, this reality (*epistemology*) (Carter & Little, 2007; Crotty, 1998; Guba & Lincoln, 1994). Cresswell (2003) describes a framework for research design as the researcher's plans and procedures for conducting a study. The design is informed by the researcher's worldview (philosophical assumptions), the procedures of inquiry (strategy or methodology), and the detailed methods of data collection and analysis (Carter & Little, 2007). The research design is further informed by the nature of the research problem, the researcher's personal experiences, and the target audience for the study findings (Cresswell, 2003; LeCompte & Schensul, 1999; Mayan, 2009). In this regard, the researcher's philosophical assumptions, methodology of choice, and methods prescribed within the selected methodology form the elemental pillars of a qualitative research study (Carter & Little, 2007; Dew, 2007). Their significance within this FE study is outlined in the following section.

Epistemological Perspective (Pillar One)

A constructionist epistemology is founded on the assumption that meaning is *constructed*, rather than discovered, through social interaction (Cresswell, 2003; Crotty, 1998; Mertens, 2005). Cresswell (2003) explains this assumption as the need of people to understand their daily living and working worlds and develop subjective meanings of their life experiences. These meanings are attached to certain objects or things, are many and varied, and are formed through social interactions as well as through cultural and historical patterns that are part of their daily lives (Lincoln & Guba, 2000; Schwandt, 2001). Furthermore, different people construct different meanings about the same phenomenon (Crotty, 1998). In this regard, a constructionist epistemology acknowledges multiple realities and multiple truths (Denzin & Lincoln, 2005; Mayan, 2009; Nicholls, 2009a).

A constructionist epistemological perspective was viewed to be consistent with the aim and objectives of this study. This standpoint was consistent with eliciting perspectives of guideline compliance among different cadres of health care providers, as well as local health administrative and policy officials. In addition, a constructivist epistemological perspective holds the view that meaning is directed toward certain objects or things (Cresswell, 2003), which necessitates that a researcher identify and understand the social, cultural, and historical contexts that are significant to these meanings (Cresswell, 2007; Crotty, 1998). A comprehensive review of the literature identified RDTs as existing tools for malaria testing to support the implementation of revised malaria-testing guidelines in Ghana (Abdelgader et al., 2011; Ansah et al., 2010; Baiden et al., 2012a; Bell & Perkins, 2008; Chandler et al., 2010; Drakely & Reyburn, 2008). Implicit assumptions in the study design led to the expectation that among health care providers in this study, RDTs are symbolic of the guidelines governing malaria diagnosis. Health care providers would therefore attach specific meanings to RDTs and their use in their management of patients suspected of having malaria (Chandler et al., 2010, 2012). This study investigated health care providers' perceptions surrounding RDTs that influence guideline compliance.

Theoretical Perspective (Pillar Two)

This study attempted to access the internal beliefs, perceptions, and knowledge of the health care providers (Lincoln & Guba, 1985) to understand guideline compliance from their point of view. Conducting the study in the natural practice settings for malaria management was consistent with the *interpretivist* theoretical perspective, particularly that of *naturalistic inquiry* (Lincoln & Guba, 1985). Interpretivist research looks for "culturally derived and historically situated interpretations of the social life world" (Cresswell, 2007; Crotty, 1998). An interpretive paradigm was important in this study to identify the cultural, social, and historical influences (Cresswell, 2007; LeCompte & Schensul, 1999; Lincoln & Guba, 2000; Schwandt, 2001) of malaria and its diagnosis on health care providers' compliance. Within interpretivist traditions, naturalistic inquiry acknowledges multiple realities (Nicholls, 2009a; Schwandt, 2001) and postulates that phenomena can only be understood within their natural setting (Cresswell, 2007; Lincoln & Guba, 1985). Previous research has established the importance of historical experiences, beliefs, and traditions in shaping the cultural significance of malaria in Ghana. These factors tend to be reflected in the meanings behind various methods of malaria diagnosis and treatment (Ahorlu, Dunyo, Afari, Koram, & Nkrumah, 2007; Asase & Oppong-Mensah, 2009; Chandler et al., 2010). Emphasis on these factors was essential, considering that the patient–provider milieu, within which malaria diagnosis occurs, is a microcosm of the health system. The health system is itself embedded in the cultural, historical, political, and socioeconomic rubric of Ghana as a nation (Ghana Health Service, 2007).

Methodology (Pillar Three)

Research methodology describes the "strategies of inquiry" (Cresswell, 2003) or the "strategy, plan of action, process, or design" underlying selection and use of specific methods to address research objectives (Crotty, 1998). The methodological approach must be consistent with the epistemological (pillar one) and the theoretical (pillar two) perspectives underlying the research. Methodological and theoretical coherence ensures that appropriate methods are used, which enhances the quality of data produced (Cresswell, 2003; Crotty, 1998; Schwandt, 2001). FE is a methodology that employs anthropological research methods to investigate specific elements or subcultures within discrete communities or contexts of contemporary society (Cruz & Higginbottom, 2013; Knoblauch, 2005) (see Table 8.3). FEs have been used in applied research (Cruz & Higginbottom, 2013; Higginbottom, 2011) to generate specific knowledge that addresses specific problems (Cruz & Higginbottom, 2013; Higginbottom et al., 2013). Mayan (2009) defines FE as "a targeted form of ethnography . . . led by a specific research question, conducted within a particular context or organization, among a small group of people to inform decision-making regarding a distinct problem" (p. 39). The social, cultural, and professional differentiation and fragmentation pertinent to contemporary society necessitates focused studies (Higginbottom et al., 2013; Knoblauch, 2005) with a specific knowledge yield to inform problem solving (Higginbottom et al., 2013). Within health care disciplines, FEs are useful for investigating specific beliefs, behaviors, or perceptions among patients or providers regarding particular health conditions or processes (Magilvy, McMahon, Backman, Roark, & Evenson, 1987; McElroy et al., 2011; Muecke, 1994). Several studies commissioned by the WHO in developing countries have used this method to elicit information for infectious disease program planning (Cove & Pelto, 1993; Hudelson, 1993; Stewart et al., 1993). The evidence underscores the relevance of FEs as a qualitative approach in health care research that aims to inform policy and practice perspectives within resource-constrained environments (Morse, 2010).

The FE approach was appropriate for investigating guideline compliance among health care providers in peripheral facilities. This study aimed to elicit and to understand health care providers' perspectives and beliefs about guideline compliance within their natural practice settings. The FE approach was consistent with the constructionist epistemological (pillar one)

Table 8.3 *Characteristics of Focused Ethnographies—Applications Within Health Care Research Studies*

Characteristic	Guideline Compliance Study
1 Problem focused	Poor guideline compliance among primary health care providers
2 Context-specific	Rapid malaria testing and case management in primary health care settings
3 Focus on a discrete community, organization, or social phenomenon	Primary health care providers in a selected district, involved directly in malaria case management; the district health management team responsible for facilitating policy guideline implementation throughout the district; health policy officials knowledgeable on the issue of health care providers' compliance and other challenges to primary health care delivery in Ghana
4 Requires extensive background knowledge	The conceptual framework, and the research questions were informed through:
	A priori literature review of RDT use and guidelines for rapid malaria testing in Ghana and sub-Saharan Africa as a whole
	Experiential knowledge of malaria control policy development through a policy research internship with the National Malaria Control Program (NMCP) in Accra, Ghana
	Close interaction, consultative discussion, and feedback with local experts and key stakeholders throughout the duration of the study
5 Conceptual orientation of a single researcher	Although informed from several perspectives, the guiding conceptual framework was presented by the researcher and was not a joint community initiative
	Guideline compliance occurs as a composite interaction involving: Technology—RDTs; Policy—the guideline for rapid testing; and Practice—primary health care providers, at the frontline of malaria case management in Ghana

6	Typically involves a limited number of participants	50 overall 21 interviewees 30 interviews
7	Participant observation is episodic	April–May, 2013 2, 3, and 5 days a week based on facility size, patient volume, and traffic
8	Participant knowledge is usually specific	Health care providers were knowledgeable in case management, nature and risk of infection, diagnosis, and treatment, and could inform the research question based on their perspectives regarding revised case management guidelines
9	Used in academia	Field investigation supported the primary author's doctoral thesis
10	Used for the development of health care services	The research aim was to generate information to improve the implementation of test-based management of malaria (TBMM) in Ghana. Knowledge translation activities will target different levels: Local: to inform practice at local levels of health care delivery by way of feedback; National: to generate discussion toward developing and testing interventions to improve TBMM International: To expand current knowledge and inform policy/practice debates regarding health care providers' compliance with guidelines for rapid malaria testing in limited resource environments

and interpretivist theoretical (pillar two) perspectives outlined earlier. It supported the overall aim of eliciting specialized knowledge (Muecke, 1994) to inform policy and practice (Higginbottom et al., 2013; Mayan, 2009) to strengthen guideline implementation for malaria diagnosis in Ghana. FEs share several characteristic features of traditional ethnographies, particularly with respect to methods of data collection and analysis (Knoblauch, 2005; Muecke, 1994). This FE employed trademark ethnographic methods, including (non)participant observation, interviews, focus groups (group interviews), and document analysis (Cruz & Higginbottom, 2013; Mayan, 2009).

Alterity in FEs

Anthropological ethnography focuses on discovering new cultures, with which the researcher is unfamiliar, and strives to describe the experience from the "natives' point of view" (Malinowski, 1922). The anthropological ethnographer is confronted with the issue of "strangeness" in unfamiliar cultures (Richards & Morse, 2007), earning the fitting description of a "professional stranger" (Agar, 1996). Sociological ethnographies, a tradition to which FEs align (Knoblauch, 2005), are conducted in familiar (rather than unfamiliar) societies and cultures (Higginbottom et al., 2013). Focused ethnographers confront another issue—one of alterity. Knoblauch (2005) describes alterity as a phenomenon in which a common, shared, implicit and explicit knowledge of the larger society or culture facilitates the researcher's access to the specific participants, settings, and situations of interest. Against this backdrop of commonality, FEs attempt to uncover specific differences among settings and participants, which are meaningful within the study context (Knoblauch, 2005). To the extent that "strangeness" is the hallmark of anthropological ethnography, Knoblauch (2005) suggests alterity as a necessary prerequisite for FEs.

Issues of alterity in this study revolved around shared Ghanaian heritage, upbringing, and knowledge of cultural and societal norms between the researcher and the health care providers. Moreover, a common interest in improved malaria diagnosis in the study setting was central to alterity in this study. Consistent with Knoblauch's (2005) description of alterity, in spite of shared commonality, differences existed between the researcher and the participants. These differences related to the roles played regarding the common interest in malaria diagnosis. Alterity in this study therefore involved a delicate shared identity, comprising sameness and differences simultaneously. A quote from a health care provider in this study aptly conveyed this sentiment. At the beginning of the interview, the researcher expressed gratitude for the health care provider's time and knowledge, considering their busy schedule. The health care provider responded: "you know, *we* are all doing *the same work*" (Health care provider, Atwima-Nwabiagya district, personal communication). The researcher's reflexive reflections on the use of *"we"* and *"the same work"* identified a shared commonality related to the present study objectives. This transcended common Ghanaian heritage or differences related to the researcher living and being educated outside of Ghana.

Background Knowledge in FEs

FEs are time- and data-intensive and require extensive background knowledge of the field of study to enable meaningful investigation (Knoblauch, 2005). A comprehensive review of relevant literature, prior to field investigations, provided useful information regarding the context of guideline compliance for rapid malaria diagnosis in Ghana. The review established the significance of the research. Although providers are on the frontlines of guideline implementation in their facilities, there is a scarcity of studies investigating health care providers' perspectives on guideline compliance (Ansah et al., 2010; Chandler et al., 2010). The researcher also conducted a policy research internship with the NMCP in Ghana, which facilitated close collaboration with key stakeholders. Discussions with key stakeholders were instrumental in distilling the specific research objectives, and validating their significance in Ghana. A resulting relationship with a local advisor led to the choice of the study setting as the Atwima-Nwabiagya district within the Ashanti Region of Ghana.

Research Methods—Pillar Four

Research methods are the specific techniques and procedures used for data collection, analysis, and interpretation (Brewer, 2000; Cresswell, 2007). Several possible methods can be employed within a given methodology (Carter & Little, 2007; Crotty, 1998; Mayan, 2009). The appropriate use of methods and techniques standardizes the researcher's perceptions and ensures the integrity of the data (Cresswell, 2007; Crotty, 1998; Dew, 2007; Fetterman, 2010). Data collection in this study involved nonparticipant observation, interviews including focus groups, and document analysis. These methods are consistent with ethnographic traditions (Mayan, 2009; Nicholls, 2009c; Roper & Shapira, 2000) and the principles of naturalistic inquiry (Guba & Lincoln, 1988). Moreover, nonparticipant observations generated data that were used to corroborate information gathered during participant interviews (Fetterman, 2010; Roper & Shapira, 2000). Triangulation involves the use of two or more data sources, methodological approaches, or theoretical perspectives, or analytical approaches within the same study (Lincoln & Guba, 2000; Thurmond, 2001). This allows verification of the data using the different sources or of the interpretation (Kimchi, Polivka, & Stevenson, 1991). Triangulation was essential to recognize dissonance between observed (or actual) and reported behavior (LeCompte & Schensul, 1999; Thurmond, 2001) as it related to guideline compliance among health care providers' in this study. This enhanced data completeness and confirmation in this study (Thurmond, 2001).

Study Setting

Atwima-Nwabiagya is the third largest among 27 districts in the Ashanti Region of Ghana, comprising 157,181 residents in 92 communities (GHS/Atwima-Nwabiagya District Directorate, 2012). The district is peri-urban (semi-rural), with many communities inaccessible by road transportation, particularly during the rainy seasons (March to July and August to mid-November). Malaria is the leading cause of morbidity and mortality in the district. Malaria transmission in the area is stable and hyperendemic, with peaks in intensity experienced during the rainy seasons. Twi-speaking Akans form the predominant ethnic group (77.4%). Christianity is the major religion (75.7%), followed by Islam (13.2%). Traditionalists (1.3%), other religions (0.9%), and those who do not identify with any particular religion (9.0%) constitute the remainder of the population. Agriculture is the dominant sector in the district and employs over 50% of the labor force, the industrial sector engages 17.4% of the labor force and various trades and services employ the remainder of the labor force (GHS/Atwima-Nwabiagya District Directorate, 2012; GSS/GHS, 2009). The Nkawie-Toase Government Hospital is the main referral facility. Health care provider density in the region reflects problematic access to quality care. The doctor-to-population ratio in 2011 was 1:30,000, whereas the nurse-to-population ratio was 1:2,015. Medical assistants, who numbered only eight in the entire district in 2012, are in charge at most of the health facilities in the area (GHS/Atwima-Nwabiagya District Directorate, 2012; GSS/GHS, 2009).

Sampling and Recruitment

Sampling Frame and Unit Selection

Rather than size and generalizability, qualitative research studies espouse smaller sizes and characteristic samples that provide the requisite depth and detail to address the research objectives (Higginbottom, 2004; Miles,

Huberman, & Saldaña, 2014; Patton, 2002). Consequently, sampling (size, frame, and strategies) decisions for this study were predicated on the purpose of the study (Ezzy, 2002; Tuckett, 2004). The sample was therefore purposefully selected. Crookes and Davis (2004) describe purposeful or purposive sampling as a researcher's judgmental and conscious selection of participants and other sources of data to include in the study (Higginbottom, 2004). Purposive sampling is common in ethnographic studies, in which judgments regarding participant selection are based on the participants' membership within the group or subculture being investigated. This strategy is useful for determining a pragmatic sample size to address research objectives within time and funding constraints (Higginbottom, 2004). Key informants are individuals, or gatekeepers in the study setting, who are able to expedite or simplify the process of gaining access to the study population (Fetterman, 2010; Higginbottom, 2004; Roper & Shapira, 2000). Key informants in this study assisted with identifying sampling units from which to recruit participants for this study.

Choice of Study Setting

The choice of the study district was practical (Miles, Huberman, & Saldaña, 2014), based on recommendations from the field advisor, whose support was secured through prior networking with stakeholders in Ghana. The field advisor is a medical practitioner, familiar with malaria case management in the region. He is also an established researcher, well known to providers and various leaders in the study communities. He identified three key informants who were knowledgeable in different aspects of community life within the district. These included a primary health care provider, a local community opinion leader, and a representative of a local chief. Having established a study advisory group comprising the field advisor and the three key informants, this study benefited from pooling and leveraging their unique and collective knowledge and influence in the district. This facilitated access to gatekeepers (Higginbottom, 2004; Roper & Shapira, 2000), including representatives of the district health management team, and heads of facilities that the group recommended for inclusion in the study. Practical considerations that informed the selection of health care facilities included geographical and logistical feasibility of access. This was important because certain areas within the district are inaccessible by road during the rainy season (GHS/Atwima-Nwabiagya District Directorate, 2012).

Sampling units comprised six purposively selected peripheral health facilities, from a frame of 17 district facilities. Five of the district facilities are government-run, and the remaining 12 are privately owned. These include five maternity homes at the community sublevel, seven health centers and a clinic as subdistrict facilities, and four hospitals providing care at the district level (GHS/Atwima-Nwabiagya District Directorate, 2012). The sample included two facilities representing each of three sublevels within primary health care delivery, namely community, subdistrict, and district sublevels of primary health care (GHS/GSS, 2009). Each pair was complementary, comprising a government-owned and a privately owned facility. Purposive sampling across the spectrum of available primary health care facilities reflected the existing diversity with respect to health care delivery infrastructure, staff cadres, and basic amenities at the represented sublevels of care (GHS/Atwima-Nwabiagya District Directorate, 2012; Ghana Health Service, 2007). To explore the full extent of possible perspectives (Higginbottom, 2004; Roper & Shapira, 2000) surrounding guideline compliance, it was important to identify potential differences in a perspective that might relate to specific provider roles, cadres, or characteristics represented within the different practice settings. A wide range of participants ensured substantial heterogeneity or within-sample variation (Higginbottom, 2004; Miles, Huberman, & Saldaña, 2014) to facilitate this purpose. Within-sample variation in qualitative research studies allows representation of the full range and extent of a phenomenon under study. This is termed maximum phenomena variation (Higginbottom, 2004; Mays & Pope, 2000; Miles, Huberman, & Saldaña, 2014). This ensured that richer meanings were derived during data interpretation. It also assisted in determining when data saturation had been achieved. Data saturation is said to occur when additional data collection does not shed any further light on the issue being investigated (Charmaz, 2006; Walker, 2012). Purposeful selection of sampling units in this study enabled data collection strategies to elicit the participants' informed perspectives (Higginbottom, 2004). The knowledge generated was therefore specific for addressing the research objectives (Ezzy, 2002; Pope & Mays, 1995; Richards & Morse, 2007).

Participant Selection

The sample comprised 50 health care providers recruited on-site at the selected facilities. The sample size was based on the available numbers of providers directly involved in malaria management at the study sites. Previous qualitative studies involving RDT use in malaria management in Ghana (Chandler et al., 2010) and elsewhere in Africa (Moonasar, Goga, Frean, Kruger, & Chandramohan, 2007; Tavrov et al., 2000) have demonstrated the ability to produce useful findings from similar sample sizes and to reach data saturation. Malaria is hyperendemic across the country (Ansah et al., 2010;

GHS/NMCP, 2009). District facilities are the gatekeepers and the operational unit of the health system in Ghana (Baiden et al., 2012a; Ghana Health Service, 2007). Consequently, health care providers in peripheral facilities are familiar with routine malaria diagnosis and management. RDT use is also widely promoted in peripheral facilities in Ghana (Ansah et al., 2010; Baiden et al., 2012a) and across malaria-endemic areas in Africa (Drakely & Reyburn, 2008; English et al., 2009; Williams et al., 2008). Health care providers in peripheral facilities were appropriate participants, as they are on the frontlines of guideline implementation, which involves RDT use for malaria diagnosis in Ghana (GHS, 2009; WHO, 2006).

Nonparticipant (Direct) Observation

Ethnographic studies involve participant and nonparticpant observation (Roberts, 2009). Participant observation is a form of data collection made possible by participating in, and "becoming a part of" the daily lives of the group being studied (Richards & Morse, 2007; Roper & Shapira, 2000). In nonparticipant observation, the researcher purely observes and records happenings in the setting (Denscombe, 2003; Roberts, 2009). Weekly observations involving at least 3 hours per day, at each study site, elicited information regarding the participants' behavior that may not have been available through other methods of investigation (Roper & Shapira, 2000). This provided an opportunity to verify observed and reported behavior, and to identify and explore any related dissonance (LeCompte & Schensul, 1999). Several factors, including the nature and specific needs of the study, the setting, and the extent allowable by the participants, determine the extent of a researcher's participation in ethnographic observations (Bogdewic 1999; Roper & Shapira, 2000). Ethical and practical considerations influenced the decision to use *non*participant or *direct* observations (Brink, 1982; Roper & Shapira, 2000) of health care providers in daily clinical encounters with suspected malaria patients at their facilities. The researcher is not a trained clinician. Furthermore, the researcher's role was conspicuous to the providers, as well as to patients or caregivers of younger patients being observed. This called for continuous negotiation of informed consent (Richards & Morse, 2007; Roper & Shapira, 2000) and ensured transparency and trustworthiness in the data collection process (Lincoln & Guba, 2000; Nicholls, 2009c).

Observations began with more detailed descriptions including the activities and issues of interest in the practice settings. With time and repeated visits, observations became more focused and more selective to generate specific information (Miles, Huberman, & Saldaña, 2014; Spradley, 1980).

Previous studies have successfully used nonparticipant observations to elicit useful information regarding (providers') observed, rather than reported, practices (LeCompte & Schensul, 1999) in the context of malaria diagnosis and treatment in other settings in Africa (Chandler et al., 2008a, 2008b, 2010). These studies did not document significant changes in providers' behavior as a result of having an observer present.

Audio-recorded and handwritten notes during observations provided documentation (Davies, 2007) to distinguish between actual observations and the researcher's perceptions regarding these observations (Bryman, 2008; Roper & Shapira, 2000). The researcher is the human instrument in ethnographic data collection (Richards & Morse, 2007; Roberts, 2009; Roper & Shapira, 2000). Grounding interpretation of the data and the participants' meanings is essential in naturalistic inquiry, to ensure credibility of the findings (Guba & Lincoln, 1988). This required recognition and documentation of personal perceptions and biases both prior to and during field research (Doyle, 2013). This promoted trustworthiness, as both the researcher and other readers can independently assess the extent to which personal beliefs or perceptions may have influenced data collection and interpretation (Carter & Little, 2007; Lincoln & Guba, 2000).

Interviews

Interviews are commonly used for data collection in qualitative research (Mason, 2002). They are primary data-gathering techniques that provide context and explanation to observations made in the field (DiCicco-Bloom & Crabtree, 2006; Kvale, 1996). Interviews allow the researcher to ask questions regarding observations of interest or about those observations that may be unclear (Roberts, 2009). General interview types include informal, in-depth, and focus group interviews (DiCicco-Bloom & Crabtree, 2006), all of which play specific roles in eliciting information (Bogdan & Biklen, 1992; Kvale, 1996) to understand guideline compliance.

Informal interviews involved laboratory personnel who primarily conduct malaria testing with RDTs in the setting, as well as clinicians who are expected to use RDT results for diagnosis and treatment. These interviews encouraged a natural environment for eliciting information, by embedding interview questions in routine conversation (DiCicco-Bloom & Crabtree, 2006). This helped to build rapport before introducing potentially sensitive discussions (Fetterman, 2010) related to observed differences in the prescribed and actual uses of RDTs in malaria diagnosis. Based on earlier observations, the researcher could ask insightful questions during informal interviews. This allowed participants to provide clarification and enhanced the credibility of data interpretation by representing the participants' point of view (Bogdewic, 1999; Cresswell, 2007). Frequent interactions with these providers over time provided a general understanding of the setting and of interactions that were relevant to the research (Bogdewic, 1999; Roper & Shapira, 2000; Spradley, 1980). Informal interviews produced data to inform a topic guide for in-depth interviews (Richards & Morse, 2007; Roper & Shapira, 2000) with selected participants directly involved in malaria diagnosis at their facilities. By creating a comfortable environment for natural dialogue, this method also proved useful for eliciting information (DiCicco-Bloom & Crabtree, 2006; Fetterman, 2010) from health administrative and policy officials, which might otherwise have been difficult to obtain. These officials had limited availability, with frequent schedule changes that would have posed substantial challenges to scheduling formal interviews. They may also not have been willing to formally discuss matters that involved government perspectives on health policy implementation in the setting.

In-depth interviews are particularly useful for exploring complex social issues that are relevant within health care settings (DiCicco-Bloom & Crabtree, 2006). This method was appropriate for exploring issues related to the challenges that health care providers faced when implementing guidelines for malaria diagnosis using RDTs. Attentive listening (Bogdewic, 1999) and gentle probing such as repeating unfinished participant responses encouraged further information (Roper & Shapira, 2000). In-depth interviews generally lasted 90 minutes and continued across all the facilities until no new information was being added to the data previously collected.

Topics suitable for further exploration were identified through iterative data analysis and review, and informed a topic guide for focus group interviews (Barbour, 2005). To accommodate the various definitions of focus groups, Barbour (2005) suggests that these are any group discussions where a researcher actively encourages and is attentive to group interaction. This study included one small (4 persons) and two mid-size (6–8 persons) focus group discussions, at selected participating facilities to further explore commonly cited perspectives surrounding guideline compliance. These perspectives provided natural starting points for comfortable conversation in the group discussions. Groups included different cadres of health care providers based on their availability at the facility on the scheduled date of the discussion. Group interaction during these discussions allowed exploration of rationale and consensus building (Barbour, 2005; Belzile & Öberg, 2012; Morgan, 1988) among the health care providers regarding their perspectives on guideline compliance.

Document Analysis

Documents, much like oral traditions in non-Western cultures, preserve and provide a record of activities, events, and practices that hold cultural, historical, and political significance in society (Nicholls, 2009c). This information enhances the ethnographic researcher's understanding of the context. Document analysis in qualitative research involves a review of any culturally significant text in the setting. *Documents,* in this regard, can be in written or image form among others. These can include government policies, photographs, or even poetry (Nicholls, 2009c). Documents analysis in this study included Ghana's national 7-year strategic plan (2008–2015) for malaria control (GHS, 2009), case management guidelines for malaria (GHS, 2009), and instructional materials related to malaria diagnosis in the setting. The review also included district directorate reports indicating allocation and distribution of RDTs to health care facilities. This information was useful for understanding health care providers' perspectives and knowledge surrounding guidelines, and the provision (or lack thereof) of existing health-system resources to implement these guidelines accordingly. District health directorate records were also useful for confirming health care provider reports of long stock-out periods for RDTs and for identifying gaps in RDT distribution and delivery to the facilities.

Preliminary and iterative analysis of the data distilled primary areas for which a health policy perspective would better inform analysis. Key informants and local experts facilitated access (Agar, 1996; Fetterman, 2010) to local, regional, and national health policy representatives of relevant institutions. Through informal discussions, these individuals provided additional perspectives that clarified the data (DiCicco-Bloom & Crabtree, 2006; Gilchrist & Williams, 1999) earlier obtained through health care provider interviews and focus groups sessions.

Data Analysis

In-depth interviews and focus group discussions were audio-recorded, transcribed verbatim, and checked for accuracy shortly after each interview (Richards & Morse, 2007). Preliminary analysis of transcripts identified areas needing further investigation through follow-up interviews (Miles, Huberman, & Saldaña, 2013). Ethnographic analysis followed Roper and Shapira's (2000) outline. This began with coding, which identified and labeled key words and recurring phrases relevant to guideline compliance. Coding facilitated the process of sorting the relevant data segments into categories and subcategories where appropriate, based on commonalities or differences. It also indicated potential associations between the categories (Roper & Shapira, 2000) and how these were relevant in addressing the research objectives (Miles, Huberman, & Saldaña, 2013). Similar analysis of focus group data revealed patterns between shared rationale and collective actions or perceptions regarding guideline compliance (Barbour, 2005). Further analysis identified patterns and established relationships within and across the different categories, which identified major themes that were recurrent in the data. Identifying peculiar (or negative) cases that contrasted the majority of participant responses (Richards & Morse, 2007; Roper & Shapira, 2000) was important for understanding the range of perspectives surrounding guideline compliance. Atlas.ti (qualitative data analysis software) facilitated data organization. This software allowed "querying" the data (Friese, 2012) using the tools provided to question the characteristics of relationships of interest within the data. Saving records of these analytic processes using the software provided an audit trail that supported data interpretation (Cutfliffe & McKenna, 2004; Shenton, 2004). This enhanced the integrity and rigor of data analysis (Roper & Shapira, 2000) and provided clear linkage between interpretations and the data (Friese, 2012). This process advanced analysis from descriptive coding to more abstract concepts, by relating the data to the literature (Richards & Morse, 2007; Roper & Shapira, 2007) on malaria diagnosis and guideline implementation in resource-constrained settings.

Reflexivity

Reflexivity describes a researcher's continuous process of reflection on how his or her personal values, behavior, or interaction with the participants can affect the interpretation of participants' responses (Doyle, 2013; Parahoo, 2006). This study employed nonparticipant observations, interviews, and focus groups, all of which relay varying degrees of researcher interaction with participants in the setting (Bogdewic, 1999; Roberts, 2009). Reflexivity was essential to understand the potential influences of the researcher's biases and preconceptions on the processes of data collection and interpretation (Jootun, McGhee, & Marland, 2009) in this study. Continuous personal scrutiny and internal dialogue were key reflexive processes engaged in this study (Doyle, 2013). This led to greater clarification in data interpretation enabling the researcher to "prompt, probe, and encourage" participants' views (Hertz, 1997) particularly relating to areas of potential bias. Reflexive processes were practicalized through memoing, which documented inherent researcher biases held prior to conducting field investigations (Morse & Field, 1995;

Roper & Shapira, 2000). Memos were also important in identifying how these perceptions changed during the research process. This ensured the researcher's sense of self-awareness throughout the research process (Parahoo, 2006). Data collection and iterative analysis prompted further investigation and generated insider knowledge (Nicholls, 2009b, 2009c), which assisted in achieving data saturation (Walker, 2012). Memos allowed the researcher to compare previously held assumptions and even expected outcomes with the actual data that were generated in this study (Richards & Morse, 2007; Shenton, 2004). Maintaining careful documentation of background knowledge acquired prior to field investigations was also essential to ensure that this information did not interfere with the essence of learning from, and understanding participants' perspectives in, the field (Jootun et al., 2009; Parahoo, 2006).

Rigor

Rigor addresses measures of quality applied before, during, and after conducting a study, which determine the trustworthiness of its findings (Morse et al., 2002; Nicholls, 2009c). Lincoln and Guba (1985) document the criteria of confirmability, dependability, credibility, and transferability of findings as measures of rigor in qualitative research. This study employed various strategies to ensure rigor (Table 8.4). Methodological coherence involving a "good fit" between the underlying philosophical assumptions, the methodology of choice, and the prescribed method in this study (Nicholls, 2009c) established confirmability, credibility, and dependability of the information produced. Other strategies that ensured rigor included purposive sampling to support in-depth understanding (Higginbottom, 2004) of guideline compliance. Maximum phenomenal variation (within-sample variation) enabled full representation of the possible range of perspectives surrounding guideline compliance (Miles, Huberman, & Saldaña, 2013). Serial data collection using document analysis, observations, informal and in-depth interviews, and focus group interviews allowed data generated in earlier phases to be verified in later stages. Interview transcripts were carefully compared to the audio-recordings (verified) before analysis. Concurrent data collection and manual transcript analysis directed the inquiry toward more relevant investigation (Nicholls, 2009c). Key points from transcripts were summarized and discussed with participants for clarification, enhancing the authenticity, confirmability, and dependability of data interpretation (Lincoln & Guba, 2000; Richards & Morse, 2007). Regular memoing of guiding assumptions and rationale for decision making during data collection and analysis ensured a transparent process and provided audit trails (Shenton, 2004) that allow

Table 8.4 Data Collection Strategies in the FE Study on Guideline Compliance

Study Aspect	Data Collection Method				
	Field observation	Informal interviews (INFIs)	Individual, in-depth interviews (IDIs)	Focus group discussions (FGDs)	(Informal) Key informant interviews (KIIs)
Phase	1	2	3	4	5
Participants involved	Consenting frontline health care providers, laboratory personnel	Selected frontline health care providers, laboratory personnel	Heads of facility (HOFs), selected frontline health care providers, district health management (DHMT) representative	Selected frontline health care providers, laboratory personnel	District regional and national health policy officials
Data generated	First-hand information on provider practices involved in consultations with suspected malaria patients	Provider-reported challenges with RDT use and test result application in case management of febrile patients	Provider perspectives on guideline compliance, and attendant challenges in their settings	Provider agreement, disagreement, and consensus surrounding key elements of guideline compliance	Policy officials' perspectives on elements of provider-reported challenges with guideline compliance
Research questions (RQs) addressed	RQ 1 RQ 2	RQ 1 RQ 2	RQ 1 RQ 2	RQ 1 RQ 2 RQ 3	RQ 1 RQ 2 RQ 3
Element of rigor addressed	Credibility, dependability, transferability, confirmability				

readers to make informed decisions regarding transferability of the findings to other contexts. Continually negotiating consent from participants throughout the duration of the study ensured that no participants provided data under duress, coercion, or other undue influence (Roper & Shapira, 2000).

DISCUSSION AND CONCLUSION

Extensive background information on the research topic and the context facilitates meaningful investigation within the time boundaries of FE studies (Knoblauch, 2005). Background knowledge in this study was obtained through reviewing local policy and practice guideline documents, and from prior knowledge of the context as a Ghanaian citizen. Maintaining continual awareness of how this knowledge might influence the processes of data collection and analysis (Kingdon, 2005) was essential to ensure that the participants' perspectives were "re-presented" through their responses (Mayan, 2009). The researcher continually confirmed developing interpretations of the data across different participant categories in the setting.

Ethnographic studies involve close researcher–participant interactions. Early rapport and trust building can be delicate, requiring that the researcher clarify unrealistic or uninformed expectations among participants (Roper & Shapira, 2000). Tactful negotiation allowed the researcher to emphasize a "learner" role, and secured, rather than alienated, key informants (LeCompte & Schensul, 1999; Roper & Shapira, 2000). Gradually, tactful communication clarified erroneously held ideas that the researcher might facilitate RDT supply based on their responses.

Accommodating participants' schedules is common courtesy, in return for them accommodating the researcher's curiosity (Roper & Shapira, 2000). Frequent schedule changes were common among participating health care providers, based on heavy workloads and limited time availability. Employing methodological and data triangulation was beneficial in conducting data verification within the time frame of the study (Halcomb, 2005). Other considerations in this study included flexibly using various methods that appropriately elicited the required information (Cresswell, 2007). Informal interviews allowed policy and administrative officials to provide their valued opinions, which were critical to comprehensively describe guideline compliance in the setting. These perspectives would not have been secured in a timely manner if only formal interview processes were employed. Semi-structured interviews followed a topic guide (Gilchrist & Williams, 1999; Richards & Morse, 2007). This focused on the issues under investigation, while allowing participants to broadly share relevant information (Roper & Shapira, 2000). The inherent heterogeneity resulting from maximum variation sampling techniques ensured that the full extent and range (Higginbottom, 2004) of guideline compliance within the study setting was explored.

Limitations

This study investigated guideline compliance to elicit information to improve policy implementation for managing malaria in Ghana. RDT use is fundamental to guideline implementation and compliance in the setting. However, RDT availability was consistently limited during the study. This is likely to have influenced participants' perspectives regarding their use in case management of malaria. In this regard, it is also possible that participants' responses may be affected by recall of past rather than current RDT use. Congruent with sampling sizes in qualitative research studies, this study employed a sample size of 50 participants. Generalizability was not a guiding objective (Miles, Huberman, & Saldaña, 2013). Previous studies, particularly those relating to a health care provider's use of RDTs and guidelines in malaria management, have produced useful findings based on smaller sample sizes (Chandler, 2010; Tavrow, 2000). The study therefore documented data collection and analysis procedures to inform readers who can consequently make an informed decision regarding the transferability of the findings (Cutcliffe & McKenna, 2004), which may include policy or technology development for malaria diagnosis in other settings.

REFERENCES

Abdelgader, T. M., Ibrahim, A. M., Elmardi, K. A., Githinji, S., Zurovac, D., Snow, R., & Noor, A. M. (2012). Progress towards implementation of ACT malaria case-management in public health facilities in the Republic of Sudan: A cluster-sample survey. *BMC Public Health, 12*, 11.

Agar, M. (1996). *Professional stranger: An informal introduction to ethnography* (2nd ed.). New York, NY: Academic Press.

Ahorlu, C. K., Dunyo, S. K., Afari, E. A., Koram, K. A., & Nkrumah, F. K. (2007). Malaria-related beliefs and behaviour in southern Ghana: Implications for treatment, prevention and control. *Tropical Medicine and International Health, 2*, 488–499.

Amexo, M., Tolhurst, R., Barnish, G., & Bates, I. (2004). Malaria misdiagnosis: Effects on the poor and vulnerable. *Lancet, 364*, 1896–1898.

Ansah, E. K., Narh-Bana, S., Epokor, M., Akanpigbiam, S., Amu Quartey, A., Gyapong, J., & Whitty, J. M. (2010). Rapid testing for malaria in settings where microscopy is available and peripheral settings where only presumptive treatment is available: A randomized controlled trial in Ghana. *BMJ, 340*(c930). doi: 10.1136/bmj.c930

Asase, A., & Oppong-Mensah, G. (2009). Traditional antimalarial phytotherapy remedies in herbal markets in Southern Ghana. *Journal of Ethnopharmacology, 126*(3), 492–499.

Asiimwe, C., Kyabayinze, D. J., Kyalisiima, Z., Nabakooza, J., Bajabaite, M., Counihan, H., & Tiberandana, J. (2012). Early experiences on the feasibility, acceptability, and use of malaria rapid diagnostic tests at peripheral health centers in Uganda—Insights into some barriers and facilitators. *BMC Implementation Science, 7*, 5.

Baiden, F., Owusu-Agyei, S., Okyere, E., Tivura, M., Adjei, G., Chandramohan, D., & Webster, J. (2012a). Acceptability of rapid diagnostic test-based management of malaria among care-givers of under-five children in rural Ghana. *PLoS ONE, 7*(9), e45556. doi:10.1371/journal.p.one.0045556

Baiden, F., Owusu-Agyei, S., Webster, J., Owusu-Adjei, S., & Chandramohan, D. (2012b). Would rational use of antibiotics be compromised in the era of test-based malaria management? *Tropical Medicine and International Health, 16*(2), 142–144. doi:10.1111/j.1365/3156.2010.02692.x

Baiden, F., Webster, J., Tivura, M., Delimini, R., Berko, Y., Amenga-Etego, S., ... Chandramohan, D. (2012c). Accuracy of rapid diagnostic tests for malaria and treatment outcomes for malaria and non-malaria cases among under-five children in rural Ghana. *PLoS ONE, 7*(4), e34073. doi:10.1371/journal.p.one.0034073

Barbour, R. S. (2005). Making sense of focus groups. *Medical Education, 39*, 742–750.

Bell, D., & Perkins, M. (2008). Making malaria testing relevant: Beyond test purchase. *Transactions of the Royal Society of Tropical Medicine and Hygiene, 102*, 1064–1066.

Belzile, J., & Öberg, G. (2012). Where to begin? Grappling with how to use participant interaction in focus group design. *Qualitative Research, 12*(4), 459–472.

Bogdan, R. C., & Biklen, S. K. (1992). *Qualitative research for education: An introduction to theory and method* (2nd ed.). Boston, MA: Allyn & Bacon.

Bogdewic, S. P. (1999). Participant observation. In B. F. Crabtree & W. L. Miller (Eds.), *Doing qualitative research* (2nd ed.). Thousand Oaks, CA: Sage.

Brewer, J. D. (2000). *Ethnography*. Buckingham, UK: Open University Press.

Brink, P. J. (1982). Traditional birth attendants among the Annang of Nigeria. *Social Science and Medicine, 16*, 1883–1892.

Bryman, A. (2008). *Social research methods*. Oxford: Oxford University Press.

Carter, S. M., & Little, M. (2007). Justifying knowledge, justifying method, taking action: Epistemologies, methodologies, and methods in qualitative research. *Qualitative Health Research, 17*(10), 1316–1328.

Chandler, C. I. R., Mangham, L., Njei, A. N., Achonduh, O., Mbacham, W. F., & Wiseman, V. (2012). 'As a clinician, you are not managing lab results, you are managing the patient': How the enactment of malaria at health facilities in Cameroon compares with the new WHO guidelines for the use of malaria tests. *Social Science & Medicine, 74*, 1528–1535.

Chandler, C., Whitty, J. M., & Ansah, E. K. (2010). How can malaria rapid diagnostic tests achieve their potential? A qualitative study of a trial at health facilities in Ghana. *Malaria Journal, 9*(95). doi:10.1186/1475-2875-9-95

Charmaz, K. (2006). *Constructing grounded theory: A practical guide through qualitative analysis*. London, UK: Sage.

Cove, S., & Pelto, G. H. (1993). Focused ethnographical studies in the WHO programme for the control of acute respiratory infections. *Medical Anthropology: Cross-Cultural Studies in Health and Illness, 15*(4), 409–424.

Cresswell, J. W. (2003). *Research design: Qualitative, quantitative, and mixed methods approaches* (2nd ed.). Thousand Oaks, CA: Sage.

Creswell, J. W. (2007). *Qualitative inquiry and research design: Choosing among five approaches* (2nd ed.). Thousand Oaks, CA: Sage.

Crookes, P., & Davies, S. (Eds.). (2004). *Research into practice: Essential skills for interpreting and applying research in nursing and health care*. Edinburgh, UK: Bailliere Tindall.

Crotty, M. (1998). *The foundations of social research: Meaning and perspective in the research process*. London, UK: Sage.

Cruz, E. V., & Higginbottom, G. (2013). The use of focused ethnography in nursing research. *Nurse Researcher, 20*(4), 36–43.

Cutcliffe, J. R., & McKenna, H. P. (2004). Expert qualitative researchers and the use of Audit trails: hyperbole of the case for method or a path to enhanced credibility? *Journal of Advanced Nursing, 45*(2), 126–133.

Davies, M. B. (2007). *Doing a successful research project*. Basingstoke: Palgrave MacMillan.

Denscombe, M. (2003). *The good research guide*. Maidenhead, UK: Open University Press.

Denzin, N. K., & Lincoln, Y. S. (2005). Introduction: The discipline and practice of qualitative research. In N. K. Denzin & Y. S. Lincoln (Eds.), *The Sage handbook of qualitative research* (2nd ed.). Thousand Oaks, CA: Sage.

Dery, D.B., Brown, C., Asante, K.P., Adams, M., Dosoo, D., Amengo-Etego, S., ... Owusu-Agyei, S. (2010). Patterns and seasonality of malaria transmission in the forest-savannah transitional zones of Ghana. *Malaria Journal, 9*, 314.

Dew, K. (2007). A health researcher's guide to qualitative methodologies. *Australian and New Zealand Journal of Public Health, 31*(5), 433–437.

DiCicco-Bloom, B., & Crabtree, B. F. (2006). The qualitative research interview. *Medical Education, 40*, 314–321.

Doyle, S. (2013). Reflexivity and the capacity to think. *Qualitative Health Research, 23*(2), 248–255.

Drakely, C., & Reyburn, H. (2008). Out with the old, in with the new: The utility of rapid diagnostic tests for malaria diagnosis in Africa. *Transactions of the Royal Society of Tropical Medicine and Hygiene, 103*, 333–337.

English, M., Reyburn, H., Goodman, C., & Snow, R. (2009). Abandoning presumptive antimalarial treatment for febrile children aged less than five years—A case of running before we can walk? *PLoS ONE, 6*(1), e1000015.

Ezzy, D. (2002). *Qualitative analysis: Practice and innovation*. Crows Nest, NSW: Allen & Unwin.

Fetterman, D. M. (2010). *Ethnography: Step by step* (3rd ed.). Thousand Oaks, CA: Sage.

Friese S. (2012). *Qualitative data analysis with ATLAS.ti*. London, UK: Sage.

Ghana Health Service (GHS). (2007). *National health policy. Creating wealth through health*. Ministry of Health, Policy, Planning, Monitoring, and Evaluation. Accra: Ghana Health Service.

Ghana Health Service (GHS). (2009). *National Malaria Control Program*. Annual Report. Accra: Ghana Health Service.

Ghana Health Service (GHS), Atwima-Nwabiagya District Directorate. (2012). Annual Report. Kumasi: Ghana Health Service.

Ghana Statistical Service (GSS), Ghana Health Service (GHS). (2009). Ghana demographic and health survey (DHS) 2008. Accra: Ghana Statistical Service. Calverton, MD: ICF Macro.

Gilchrist, V. J., & Williams, R. L. (1999). Key informant interview. In B. F. Crabtree & W. L. Miller (Eds.), *Doing qualitative research* (2nd ed.). Thousand Oaks, CA: Sage.

Guba, E. G. (1990). The alternative paradigm dialog. In E. G. Guba (Ed.), *The paradigm dialog* (pp. 17–30). Newbury Park, CA: Sage.

Guba, E. G., & Lincoln, Y. S. (1988). *Qualitative approaches to evaluation in education* (pp. 89–115). New York, NY: Praeger.

Guba, E. G., & Lincoln, Y. S. (1994). Competing paradigms in qualitative research. In N. K. Denzin & Y. S. Lincoln (Eds.), *Handbook of qualitative research* (pp. 105–117). London, UK: Sage.

Grimberg, B. T., & Mehlotra, R. K. (2011). Expanding the antimalarial drug arsenal–Now, but how? *Pharmaceuticals, 4*, 681–712. doi:10.3390/ph4050681

Halcomb, E., & Andrew, S. (2005). Triangulation as a method for contemporary nursing research. *Nurse Res. 13*(2):71–82.

Hamlyn, D. W. (1995). *Epistemology, history of*. Oxford, UK: Oxford University Press.

Higginbottom, G. M. A. (2004). Sampling issues in qualitative research. *Nurse Researcher, 12*, 7–19.

Higginbottom, G. M. A. (2011). The transitioning experiences of internationally educated nurses into a Canadian health care system: A focused ethnography. *BMC Nursing, 10*, 1–13. doi:10.1186/1472-6955-10-14

Higginbottom, G. M. A., Pillay, J. J., & Boadu, N. Y. (2013). Guidance on performing focused ethnographies with an emphasis on healthcare research. *The Qualitative Report, 18*(Art. 17), 1–16. Retrieved from http://www.nova.edu/ssss/QR/QR18/higginbottom17.pdf

Hudelson, P. M. (1993). The management of acute respiratory infections in Honduras: A field test of the focused ethnographic study (FES). *Medical Anthropology: Cross-Cultural Studies in Health and Illness, 15*(4), 435–446.

Jootun, D., McGhee, G., & Marland, G. R. (2009). Reflexivity: Promoting rigour in qualitative research. *Nursing Standard, 23*(23), 42–46.

Kimchi, J., Polivka, B., & Stevenson, J. S. (1991). Triangulation: Operational definitions. *Nursing Research, 40*(6), 364–366.

Kingdon C. (2005). Reflexivity: Not just a qualitative methodological research tool. *British Journal of Midwifery, 13*(10), 622–627.

Knoblauch, H. (2005). Focused ethnography. *Forum: Qualitative Sozialforschung/Forum: Qualitative Social Research, 6*(3), Art. 44.

Kvale, S. (1996). *Interviews: An introduction to qualitative research interviewing.* London, UK: Sage.

Kyabayinze, D., J., Asiimwe, C., Nakanjako, D., Nabakooza, J.,Bajabaite, M., Strachan, C., . . . Van Geetruyden, J. P. (2010). Programme level implementation of malaria rapid diagnostic tests (RDTs) use: Outcomes and cost of training health workers at lower level health care facilities in Uganda. *BMC Public Health, 12,* 291.

LeCompte, M. D., & Schensul, J. J. (1999). *Designing and conducting ethnographic research* (Ethnographer's toolkit, Vol. 1). Walnut Creek, CA: AltaMira.

Leininger, M. M. (1985). *Qualitative research methods in nursing.* Orlando, FL: Grune and Stratton.

Lincoln, Y. S., & Guba, E. G. (1985). *Naturalistic inquiry.* Beverly Hills, CA: Sage.

Lincoln, Y. S., & Guba, E. G. (2000). Paradigmatic controversies, contradictions, and emerging confluences. In N. K. Denzin & Y. S. Lincoln (Eds.), *Handbook of qualitative research* (2nd ed., pp. 333–355). Thousand Oaks, CA: Sage.

Lubell, Y., Reyburn, H. M., Mbakilwa, H., Mwangi, R., Chonya, S., & Whitty, C. J. M. (2008). The impact of response to the results of diagnostic tests for malaria: Cost benefit analysis. *BMJ, 336*(7637), 202–205.

Magilvy, J. K., McMahon, M., Backman, M., Roark, S., & Evenson, C. (1987). The health of teenagers: A focused ethnography. *Public Health Nursing, 4*(1), 35–42.

Malinowski, B. (1922). *Argonauts of the Western Pacific.* London, UK: Routledge.

Mayan, M. J. (2009). *Essentials of qualitative inquiry.* Walnut Creek, CA: Left Coast Press.

Maynard, M. (1994). *Methods, practice and epistemology: The debate about feminism and research.* London, UK: Taylor & Francis.

Mays, N., & Pope, C. (2000). Assessing quality in qualitative research. *BMJ, 320* (7226), 50–52.

McElroy, T. A., Davis, A., Hunt, C., Dadul, J, Stanba, T., & Larson, C. (2011). Navigating a way forward: Using focused ethnography and community readiness to study disability issues in Ladakh, India. *Disability and Rehabilitation, 33*(1), 17–27.

Mertens, D. M. (2005). *Research methods in education and psychology: Integrating diversity with quantitative and qualitative approaches* (2nd ed.). Thousand Oaks, CA: Sage.

Miles, M. B., Huberman, A. M., & Saldaña, J. (2014). *Qualitative data analysis: A methods sourcebook* (3rd ed.). Thousand Oaks, CA: Sage.

Moonasar, D., Goga, A.E., Frean, J., Kruger, P., & Chandramohan, D. (2007). An exploratory study of factors that affect performance and usage of rapid diagnostic tests for malaria in the Limpopo Province, South Africa. *BMC Central, 6,* 74.

Morgan, D. L. (1988). *Focus groups as qualitative research.* London, UK: Sage.

Morse, J. M. (1987). Qualitative nursing research: A free-for-all? In J. M. Morse (Ed.), *Qualitative nursing research: A contemporary dialogue* (pp. 14–22). Newbury Park, CA: Sage.

Morse, J. M. (2010). How different is qualitative health research from qualitative research? Do we have a subdiscipline? *Qualitative Health Research, 14*(10), 1459–1468.

Morse, J. M., & Field, P. A. (1995). *Qualitative research methods for health professionals* (2nd ed.). Thousand Oaks, CA: Sage.

Msellem, M. I., Mårtensson, A., Rotllant, G., Bhattarai, A., Strömberg, J., Kahigwa, E., . . . Björkman, A. (2009, April). Influence of rapid malaria diagnostic tests on treatment and health outcome in fever patients, Zanzibar—A crossover validation study. *PLoS Med, 6*(4), e1000070. doi:10.1371/journal.pmed.1000070

Muecke, M. A. (1994). On the evaluation of ethnographies. In J. M. Morse (Ed.), *Critical issues in qualitative research methods* (pp. 187–209). Thousand Oaks, CA: Sage.

Nicholls, D. (2009a). Qualitative research: Part one—philosophies. *International Journal of Therapy and Rehabilitation, 16*(10), 526–533.

Nicholls, D. (2009b). Qualitative research: Part two—methodologies. *International Journal of Therapy and Rehabilitation, 16*(10), 586–592.

Nicholls, D. (2009c). Qualitative research: Part three—methods. *International Journal of Therapy and Rehabilitation, 16*(10), 638–647.

Onwujekwe, O., Uzochukwu, B., Dike, N., Uguru, N., Nwobi, E., & Shu E. (2009). Malaria treatment perceptions, practices and influences on provider behaviour: Comparing hospitals and non-hospitals in south-east Nigeria. *Malar J, 8*, 246. doi:10.1186/1475-2875-8-246

Parahoo K. (2006). *Nursing research: principles, process and issues* (2nd edition), Basingstoke: Palgrave Macmillan.

Patton, M. Q. (2002). *Qualitative research and evaluation methods* (3rd ed.). Thousand Oaks, CA: Sage.

Pope, C., & Mays, N. (1995) Qualitative research: reaching the parts other methods cannot reach: An introduction to qualitative methods in health and health services research. *British Medical Journal, 311*, 42–45.

Reyburn, H., Mbatia, R., Drakely, C., Carneiro, I., Mwakasungula, E., Mwerinde, O., . . . Whitty, J. M. C. (2004). Overdiagnosis of malaria in patients with severe febrile illness in Tanzania: A prospective study. *BMJ, 329*, 1212.

Reyburn, H., Mbakilwa, H., Mwangi, R,, Mwerinde, O., Olomi, R., Drakeley, C., & Whitty, J. M. C. (2007, February 24). Rapid diagnostic tests compared with malaria microscopy for guiding outpatient treatment of febrile illness in Tanzania: randomised trial. *BMJ, 334*(7590), 403. doi:10.1136/bmj.39073.496829.AE

Richards, L., & Morse, J. M. (2007) *Readme first for a user's guide to qualitative methods* (2nd ed). Thousand Oaks, CA: Sage.

Roberts, T. (2009). Understanding ethnography. *British Journal of Midwifery, 17*(5), 291–294.

Roper, J. M., & Shapira, J. (2000). *Ethnography in nursing research. Methods in nursing research* (Vol. 1). Thousand Oaks, CA: Sage.

Schwandt, T. A. (2001). *Dictionary of qualitative inquiry* (2nd ed.). London, UK: Sage Publications.

Shenton, K. (2004). Strategies for ensuring trustworthiness in qualitative research projects. *Education for Information, 22*, 63–75.

Spradley, J. P. (1980). *Participant observation.* New York, NY: Holt, Rinehart & Winston.

Stewart, M. K., Parker, B. J., Chakraborty, J., & Begum, H. (1993). Acute respiratory infections (ARI) in rural Bangaldesh: Perceptions and practices. *Medical Anthropology: Cross-Cultural Studies in Health and Illness, 15*(4), 377–394.

Tavrow, P., Knebel, E., Cogswell, L. (2000). Using Quality Design To Improve Malaria Rapid Diagnostic Tests in Malawi. In: USAID (Ed.), *Operations research results*. Bethesda, MD: Quality Assurance Project.

Thomson, D. (2011). Ethnography: A suitable approach for providing an inside perspective on the everyday lives of health professionals. *International Journal of Therapy and Rehabilitation, 18*, 10–16.

Thurmond, A. V. (2001). The point of triangulation. *Journal of Nursing Scholarship, 33*(3), 253–258.

Tavrow, P., Knebel, E., Cogswell, L. (2000). Using quality design to improve malaria rapid diagnostic tests in Malawi. In: USAID (Ed.), *Operations research results*. Bethesda, MD: Quality Assurance Project.

Tuckett, A. (2004). Qualitative research sampling: The very real complexities. *Nurse Researcher, 12*(1), 47–61.

Uzochukwu, B. S. C., Onwujekwe, E., Ezuma, N. N., Ezeoke, O. P., Ajuba, M. O., & Sibeudu, F. T. (2012). Improving rational treatment of malaria: Perceptions and influence of RDTs on prescribing behavior of health workers in southeast Nigeria. *PLoS ONE, 6*(1), e14627.

Walker, J. L. (2012). The use of saturation in qualitative research. *Canadian Journal of Cardiovascular Nursing, 22*(2), 37–41.

Wells, T. N. C. (2011). Natural products as starting points for new anti-malarials: Going back to our roots? *Malaria Journal, 10*(Suppl 1), S3. doi:10.1186/1475-2875 -10-S1-S3

Williams, H. A., Causer, L., Metta, E., Malila, A., O'Reilly, T., Abdulla, S., Kachur, S., … Bloland, P. (2008). *Malaria Journal, 7*, 239.

World Health Organization (WHO). (2003). Malaria rapid dagnosis. Making it work. *Meeting Report, January 20–23, 2003*. Regional Office for the Western Pacific. Geneva: World Health Organization.

World Health Organzation (WHO)/United Nations International Children's Emergency Fund (UNICEF). (2005). *Handbook IMCI. Integrated management of childhood illnesses*. Geneva: World Health Organization, United Nations Children's Fund.

World Health Organization (WHO). (2006). *Guidelines for the treatment of malaria*. Geneva: World Health Organization.

World Health Organization (WHO). The Roll Back Malaria Partnership (RBM). (2008). *The global malaria action plan*. Geneva: WHO, RBM Secretariat.

World Health Organization (WHO). (2010a). *Guidelines for the treatment of malaria* (2nd ed.). Geneva: World Health Organization.

World Health Organization (WHO). (2010b). *World malaria report*. Geneva: World Health Organization.

World Health Organization (WHO). (2012). *World malaria report*. Geneva: World Health Organization.

CHAPTER NINE

META-ETHNOGRAPHY

Mikki Meadows-Oliver

Qualitative research is a method of inquiry that allows researchers to gather in-depth data on a topic of interest. Such in-depth data collection allows qualitative researchers to gain a deeper understanding of participant experiences regarding a phenomenon of interest. Qualitative research is often used when only a few studies are available on a particular topic or when researchers want to obtain an alternative view of an issue (Meadows-Oliver, 2009). It may employ research questions not easily answered by quantitative research. Qualitative research employs different traditions to research a topic, including ethnography, phenomenology, and grounded theory—to name a few. Qualitative research is oftentimes exploratory—researching topics that have been scarcely studied; there have been an increasing number of qualitative studies published within the past decade. Researchers have long since noted that although individual qualitative studies are informative, "like pieces of a jigsaw puzzle," the isolated, individual studies do not always contribute to the fullest understanding of the experience under study (Jensen & Allen, 1996, p. 553). Sandelowski, Docherty, and Emden (1997) noted that more research from individual studies is not necessary to gain a more complete understanding of the topic of interest. They recommended that qualitative synthesis projects be undertaken to enhance the development of knowledge (Sandelowski et al., 1997). Such syntheses of qualitative research findings may result in a comprehensive analysis of the phenomenon of interest (Finfgeld, 2003).

For individual qualitative findings to have more of an effect, they need to be placed in a larger interpretive context. Metasynthesis is one such method that can be used to situate findings within a larger context. It can transform several individual studies into a unified, powerful body of knowledge (Beck, 2003). Noblit and Hare (1988), in their seminal work on integrating and synthesizing qualitative research, coined the term, "meta-ethnography" to describe their method of integrating qualitative research findings. Since then, the majority of researchers have used the term metasynthesis to describe the process of integrating qualitative research findings. Because most publications use the term metasynthesis, I use the term here. The scholar conducting the metasynthesis is referred to as the synthesist. This chapter describes my process of conducting a metasynthesis and the challenges faced.

THE STUDY

In the course of doing background work for a qualitative study on homeless mothers caring for their children in shelters, I began to accumulate published literature on the topic. I noted there were an increasing number of qualitative studies focusing on homeless families, in particular on homeless women with children. The single study provided a glimpse into the lives of homeless mothers and their children. As I began reading the articles, it became clear that to advance knowledge on the topic of nursing the findings needed to be synthesized. My search of the literature revealed no previous metasynthesis on the topic. Therefore, I conducted a metasynthesis of 18 qualitative studies on homeless mothers.

What Is Metasynthesis?

Metasynthesis is research of research and is often considered to be a study unto itself. Synthesists do not return to the original data but use findings presented by the original researcher. The findings from previous research publications are the primary data for a metasynthesis (Bondas & Hall, 2007). A metasynthesis compares and analyzes text of research publications and creates, in the process, a new and enhanced interpretation. The process of conducting a metasynthesis enlarges the interpretive possibilities of the data when compared to individual studies, and the findings further knowledge that develops and advances the discipline. The aim of the metasynthesis is to generate a novel, integrated, and more complete interpretation of findings that offers greater understanding in depth and breadth than those from individual studies. The outcome will be a common understanding of the nature of a phenomenon.

How Was the Metasynthesis Conducted?

Whereas the term metasynthesis is used most commonly in published articles, the meta-ethnographic synthesis method proposed by Noblit and Hare (1988) is the most common methodological choice cited in nursing science to synthesize qualitative research articles (Bondas & Hall, 2007). Similar to many other researchers, I used Noblit and Hare's (1988) approach when I conducted my qualitative metasynthesis that focused on homeless mothers caring for their children while living in shelters. Noblit and Hare's (1988) approach involved the systematic comparison of studies in which they are translated into one another—a process that entails going beyond a single account to reveal analyses between accounts. The comparison and translation are accomplished by following these seven steps.

The first step in this process is for the synthesist to identify a topic of interest. When considering an area of study for the metasynthesis, the topic being considered must be comprehensive enough to encompass the phenomenon of interest but adequately focused to guarantee that the findings are meaningful to health care providers, researchers, and policy makers. Many researchers have done preliminary studies in their metasynthesis area of research, and their own progression of work appears to have guided their topic selections. Metasynthesis is often used by seasoned qualitative researchers to move their work forward rather than continuing to conduct serialized investigations (Finfgeld, 2003). I had done preliminary work in the area of homeless mothers. When conducting the search for articles for the metasynthesis, I was developing a study in this area which would later be further refined and the population narrowed to homeless adolescent mothers.

The second step is deciding what is relevant to the initial interest. The synthesist should assemble a list of studies that might be included in the metasynthesis. Although I did not report the databases used or provide a full accounting of my search history in my published metasynthesis (Meadows-Oliver, 2003), synthesists are encouraged to disclose criteria they have used in the selection of studies for the metasynthesis (Finfgeld, 2003). Synthesists should keep track of databases searched as well as any search terms used to locate studies. When conducting the literature search, I used electronic databases and also performed ancestry searches of articles that I had already obtained. The electronic databases that I searched included Medline, CINAHL, ERIC, Psycinfo, and dissertation abstracts. I used the search terms homeless families, homeless mothers, homeless parents alone, and in combination to accumulate citations and abstracts.

To properly conduct the metasynthesis, the synthesist requires sufficient research reports that meet inclusion criteria. The criteria for exclusion and inclusion should be stated, recorded, and applied. The inclusion criteria, procedures for data handling and collection, description of the sample, and rules for data analysis and interpretation have to be explicit (Bondas & Hall, 2007). Having rigid elimination criteria may lead to the risk of losing relevant data. Developing broad inclusion criteria may allow the most comprehensive understanding of the phenomenon of interest (Jensen & Allen, 1996).

For my metasynthesis, my first inclusion criteria set was that I wanted research articles using only a qualitative design. I did not differentiate between studies that were phenomenological, grounded theory, or ethnographic. Although some scholars recommend limitations when determining inclusion criteria regarding different qualitative traditions (Estabrooks, Field, & Morse, 1994), others state that the goal is to retrieve all of the relevant studies in a field—not simply a sample. They encourage that synthesists undertake a robust search on the topic area (Walsh & Downe, 2005). Because I set my inclusion criteria to studies published in only English, relevant non-English research may have been overlooked. Synthesists can choose to set a year limitation for publications that they will include in the metasynthesis. I chose not to limit the publication years of the articles included in my synthesis because I wanted to include as many articles as possible in my metasynthesis.

Although there are differences of opinion on using unpublished or gray literature such as master's theses and dissertations, I chose to include dissertations in metasynthesis. Beck (2002) recommends including unpublished literature in metasyntheses to avoid publication bias. Similarly other researchers note that to gain a fuller, more in-depth understanding of the phenomenon under study, synthesists may require access to full research reports, such as dissertations or unpublished theses (Walsh & Downe, 2005). Whereas some researchers object to including dissertations and master's theses because they have not been peer-reviewed and the quality of the findings cannot be ensured, others note few grounds exist for the exclusion of qualitative data from metasyntheses because of the lack of methodological quality (Bondas & Hall, 2007; Sandelowski et al., 1997).

When conducting the literature search and reviewing the abstracts of the selected articles, it is important for the synthesist to decide which of the studies are really about the same phenomenon or experience (Sandelowski et al., 1997). It is essential for the synthesist to review the stated research purpose of the article, the research questions posed, and findings produced to ensure that the article is relevant to the phenomenon of interest.

Scholars are divided on the issue of appropriate sample size for the metasynthesis. Because large analyses of data are thought to hinder deep analysis, some researchers recommend not including more than 10 studies in the synthesis. To prevent having an overly large sample, it is recommended that the synthesist have a clearly defined aim and use purposive and theoretical sampling to set tighter boundaries for the metasynthesis. In contrast,

Finfgeld (2003) states that the type of metasynthesis should determine the sample size needed. The sample size may need to be maximized in an effort to offer the broadest and most comprehensive analysis and interpretations possible. As opposed to having too much data, the opposite problem of having too few studies may be encountered. The greater the number of studies there are to work with, the more saturated and transferable is the product of the analysis (Bondas & Hall, 2007).

After obtaining the abstracts and determining which studies met inclusion criteria, 18 studies using different qualitative research traditions were included in my metasynthesis of homeless mothers caring for their children in shelters. I used purposive sampling to ensure a fair representation of study findings. I included studies conducted across professional disciplines. For example, my metasynthesis contained studies from nursing, medicine, public health, psychology, social work, and education.

In addition to determining the study sample size, the synthesist must decide whether or not differing qualitative methods will be included in the metasynthesis. Jensen and Allen (1996) state that multiple qualitative approaches should not be combined in a metasynthesis because the differing views of reality that underpin the varying approaches may lead to the generation of substantively different kinds of knowledge. Conversely, Walsh and Downe (2005) state that because the qualitative paradigm sees truths as multiple, it is acceptable and valid to include a variety of qualitative approaches in a metasynthesis. Beck (2003) concurs, writing that a metasynthesis profits from the assortment of methodological and theoretical contexts within various studies included in it. Similarly, Noblit and Hare (1988) do not limit the inclusion of multiple types of qualitative research in qualitative synthesis projects. They described meta-ethnography as a rigorous procedure for deriving substantive interpretations about "any set of ethnographic or interpretive studies" (p. 9). Blending studies from diverse approaches may counterbalance the limitations inherent in using only one qualitative method (McCormick, Rodney, & Varcoe, 2003).

I did not want to omit any relevant data related to or limit my understanding of the experiences of homeless mothers caring for their children in shelters, so I included studies from differing qualitative traditions. My metasynthesis used studies labeled as phenomenological, descriptive qualitative, interpretive qualitative, grounded theory, ethnographic, naturalistic inquiry, and feminist inquiry. After establishing inclusion criteria, conducting the literature search of nursing and related literature, and reviewing abstracts on homeless women with children living in shelters, I uncovered 18 qualitative studies on this phenomenon.

The third step in the metasynthesis process is for the synthesist to read the studies obtained from step 2. The selected studies are read and reread with close attention paid to the details of the studies. Jensen and Allen (1996) caution synthesists to pay careful attention to the details in the individual accounts included in the synthesis to ensure inclusion of all pertinent findings. The findings should be supported by raw data such as the participants' quotes (Finfgeld, 2003).

The fourth step in the metasynthesis process is for the synthesist to determine how the studies are related. The accounts may (a) be directly comparable (reciprocal), (b) stand in opposition to each other (refutational), or (c) represent a line of argument. When the studies concern similar topics and the findings are directly comparable, as in my case, the metasynthesis takes the form of reciprocal translations.

Translating the studies into one another is the fifth step in the metasynthesis project. Translations are comparisons of the concepts of one study with the concepts of the other studies involved in the metasynthesis. The translation of study findings makes metasynthesis distinct from traditional literature reviews. Literature reviews are typically undertaken to provide background on a topic being researched and are defined as analytical summation of research focused on a particular area of interest. Metasynthesis should also be differentiated from a secondary analysis, which is defined as a form of research in which the raw data collected by researchers are reanalyzed to answer a new question. When combining the qualitative data on homeless mothers, I was not looking to conduct a secondary analysis of data or to perform a traditional literature review. I was looking to view the experiences of homeless mothers from a new perspective. I wanted the results of the synthesis of the qualitative findings to be more interpretive, to develop new knowledge and to deepen the understanding of the experiences of homeless mothers caring for their children in shelters.

It is important to note that every study within the metasynthesis does not have to relate to the concept being translated. However, representation of the concept must be frequent enough and salient enough that the author feels that it demonstrates the essence of the experience. When analyzing the data from the studies, synthesists should ensure that both principal and contrasting findings of the primary studies are identified (Beck, 2003).

Looking at the original concepts of several studies, the concepts were compared with one another and translated into each other. Although these concepts did not occur in all 18 studies, the concepts were salient enough that I believed that it showed the essence of the experiences of homeless mothers caring for their children in shelters. For example, concepts from nine studies that were translated into each other include *web of stress, experience of distress, self-blaming and depression, feelings, frustration, initial reactions, feeling down, living under pressure,* and *feelings of helplessness and hopelessness.*

Synthesizing the translations is the sixth step in the metasynthesis process. Synthesizing the translations refers to developing overarching themes and metaphors from the concepts of the original studies. Synthesis is achieved by maintaining the central metaphors and/or concepts of each account and comparing them to the other key metaphors or concepts in that account (Bondas & Hall, 2007).

The concepts of *web of stress, experience of distress, self-blaming and depression, feelings, frustration, initial reactions, feeling down, living under pressure,* and *feelings of helplessness and hopelessness* were translated and synthesized to come up with the metaphor "Stressed and Depressed." The metaphor of "Protective Mothering" was derived when the concepts of *for the sake of the children, concerns about the welfare of the children, safety, parental concern, heightened awareness, guarding, guarding from harm, children as motivators,* and *concerned for the safety of the children* were translated and synthesized.

Six reciprocal translations of homeless mothers caring for their children in shelters emerged from the translation of the themes and concepts from the 18 included studies *on becoming homeless, protective mothering, loss, stressed and depressed, survival strategies,* and *strategies for resolution.*

The seventh and final step of Noblit and Hare's (1988) process is expressing the synthesis. In this final phase, the findings of the synthesis are communicated to the researcher's audience. Before expressing the synthesis, the synthesist needs to ensure that rigor was maintained (Jensen & Allen, 1996). The findings of the metasynthesis are deemed to be credible if the people who have had that experience would identify as their own from the descriptions or interpretations depicted. Credibility is aided if the original studies provide exemplars and/or evidentiary quotes (Finfgeld, 2003). Synthesists should share as much of their sampling and data analysis procedures as possible to support the credibility of their work. The criterion of fittingness is satisfied when the findings can fit into varying contexts and when the findings are grounded in the life experiences of the participants, reflecting both typical and atypical elements (Jensen & Allen, 1996).

Provided the same data, metasynthesis findings are auditable when similar findings can be attained. Internal validation is achieved through study participant quotes and the metaphors used to describe the experiences. External validation is accomplished through comparisons with theoretical literature. Confirmability of the metasynthesis findings occurs when auditability and truth value are achieved. Truth value is defined as the "discovery of human phenomena or experiences as they are lived and perceived by subjects, rather than in the verification of a priori conceptions of those experiences" (Jensen & Allen, 1996, p. 556).

Thorne and colleagues (2002) suggest returning to the original researchers and asking them if the integrity of their original research is intact following the metasynthesis. However, this task is easier to accomplish if researchers are synthesizing data based on their own studies (Walsh & Downe, 2005). Paterson, Thorne, and Dewis (1998) state that trustworthiness can be established by having other researchers independently check the metasynthesis process at each step. Limitations of using previously published data should be noted. After ensuring rigor in the metasynthesis, to express the synthesis, I presented the findings at an international conference and published the metasynthesis in a peer-reviewed nursing journal.

CAVEATS OF CONDUCTING A METASYNTHESIS

Sandelowski (2006) cautions those conducting metasynthesis to realize that metasyntheses of qualitative research findings are far removed from the lives of those persons participating in the original qualitative research projects. It is only through interpretation of researchers that synthesists have access to research participants. Qualitative metasyntheses are interpretations that are at least three times removed from the experiences that were originally studied. Metasyntheses are created from the synthesists transformations of primary research findings. The primary research findings are themselves compilations of the original researcher's transformations of the data they collected from research participants. The participants' words are, in turn, transformations of their experiences in an unrepeatable "remembering moment." Large differences can exist between the actual lived experiences and the participants' retold lives (Sandelowski, 2006).

CONCLUSION

Metasyntheses should reveal the essence of the phenomenon under study by generating novel interpretations of findings. Qualitative synthesis projects may lead to a more holistic understanding of patient experiences. Metasyntheses can help strengthen evidence-based practice, and care to patients may be improved when grounded more firmly in the evidence. Such evidence can positively affect decision making in health care policies. Rigorously conducted metasyntheses can drive research, practice, and policies forward.

REFERENCES

Beck, C. (2002). Postpartum depression: A metasynthesis. *Qualitative Health Research, 12,* 453–472.

Beck, C. (2003). Seeing the forest for the trees: A qualitative synthesis project. *Journal of Nursing Education, 42,* 318–323.

Bondas, T., & Hall, E. (2007). Challenges in approaching metasynthesis research. *Qualitative Health Research, 17,* 113–121.

Estabrooks, C., Field, P., & Morse, J. (1994). Aggregating qualitative findings: An approach to theory development. *Qualitative Health Research, 4,* 503–511.

Finfgeld, D. (2003). Metasynthesis: The state of the art—so far. *Qualitative Health Research, 13,* 893–904.

Jensen, L., & Allen, M. (1996). Meta-synthesis of qualitative findings. *Qualitative Health Research, 6,* 553–560.

McCormick, J., Rodney, P., & Varcoe, C. (2003). Reinterpretations across studies: An approach to meta-analysis. *Qualitative Health Research, 13,* 933–944.

Meadows-Oliver, M. (2003). Mothering in public: A meta-synthesis of homeless women with children living in shelters. *Journal for Specialists in Pediatric Nursing, 8,* 130–136.

Meadows-Oliver, M. (2009). Does qualitative research have a place in evidence-based nursing? *Journal of Pediatric Health Care, 23,* 352–354.

Noblit, G., & Hare, R. (1988). *Meta-ethnography: Synthesizing qualitative studies.* Newbury Park, CA: Sage.

Paterson, B., Thorne, S., & Dewis, M. (1998). Adapting to and managing diabetes. *Image Journal of Nursing Scholarship, 30,* 57–62.

Sandelowski, M. (2006). "Meta-Jeopardy": The crisis of representation in qualitative metasynthesis. *Nursing Outlook, 54,* 10–16.

Sandelowski, M., Docherty, S., & Emden, C. (1997). Qualitative metasynthesis: Issues and techniques. *Research in Nursing & Health, 20,* 365–371.

Thorne, S., Paterson, B., Acorn, S., Canam, C., Joachim, G., & Jillings, C. (2002). Chronic illness experience: Insights from a meta-study. *Qualitative Health Research, 12,* 437–452.

Walsh, D., & Downe, S. (2005). Meta-synthesis method for qualitative research: A literature review. *Journal of Advanced Nursing, 50,* 204–211.

CHAPTER TEN

APPLICATION OF LEININGER'S ETHNOGRAPHY/ETHNONURSING RESEARCH METHODOLOGY IN STUDYING THE ZAPOTEC INDIANS OF OAXACA, MEXICO

Carol Holtz

I saw a need for a theory related to culture and care which had to be developed and used in nursing in order to establish a field of transcultural nursing.... to guide nursing's new and imperative future. ... Moreover nurses needed to overcome cultural ignorance, ethnocentrism, and racism in their practices.... (Leininger, 1997, p. 32)

This chapter gives an overview of Dr. Madeleine Leininger's transcultural nursing theory, the cultural research enabler, with a focus on the sunrise model; and an overview of ethnography and ethnographic nursing research methodology. The chapter also describes, with anecdotal comments, the author's personal journey in establishing a relationship with Dr. Leininger. The chapter includes a review of the culture of the indigenous Zapotec Indians of Oaxaca, Mexico, and the application of Leininger's theory and the sunrise model for obtaining transcultural knowledge, contributing to a culturally congruent plan of care for this population.

DR. MADELEINE LEININGER

Madeleine Leininger is the founder of the transcultural nursing theory, a leader in care theory, and the first professional nurse to hold bachelor's and master's degrees in nursing and a doctorate in cultural and social anthropology. During her employment at the College of Nursing at the University of Cincinnati, she began the first graduate program in psychiatric nursing at that institution. While working at the child guidance home in Cincinnati, she became concerned about the lack of understanding of cultural factors that influenced the children's behaviors. During Dr. Leininger's time at the University of Cincinnati, Dr. Margaret Mead was a visiting professor in the Department of Psychiatry at the same university. Leininger and Mead became friends and discussed the potential relationship between nursing and anthropology. Leininger later studied for a PhD in anthropology and during this time worked with the Gadsup people of New Guinea. While researching this culture, she used ethnographical and ethnonursing research methodology. Later she continued to develop her culture care theory of diversity and universality (culture care theory) and ethnonursing research methodology (Leininger, 1991, pp. 14, 18).

Leininger's Theory

Leininger's theory is based on a belief that *care* is the essence of nursing, and values, meanings, and expressions of care are important to establish and compare. This knowledge is influenced by worldviews (paradigms), meanings, patterned expressions, and structured forms of care knowledge that influence health, well-being, or illness knowledge. Transcultural nursing is the study and practice of comparative cultural care including the values, beliefs, and practices of people of different cultures. *The goal* of this theory is to *provide culturally congruent care to patients*. This care includes sensitive, creative, and meaningful practices to fit with the values, beliefs, and practices of clients (Leininger, 1991, 1997, 2006).

Leininger defines nursing as a learned, scientific, and humanistic profession and discipline focused on human care and caring activities to assist, support, facilitate, or enable individuals or groups to maintain or regain their health or well-being in culturally meaningful and beneficial ways, or to help individuals face handicaps or death. Leininger proposes three modes for guiding nursing care judgments, decisions, or actions to provide appropriate, beneficial, and meaningful care: (a) preservation and/or maintenance; (b) accommodation and/or negotiation; and (c) repatterning and/or restructuring. She states that the modes substantively influence nurses' ability to provide culturally congruent nursing care and foster the development of culturally competent nurses (Leininger & McFarland, 2002).

The immediate purpose of Leininger's theory is to discover, document, interpret, and explain the predicted and multiple factors influencing and explaining care from a cultural holistic perspective. The ultimate goal of her theory is to provide culturally congruent care. Her theory is used within the qualitative research paradigm, and the ethnonursing method is used for naturalistic and open discovery (Leininger, 1997).

Assumptions and orientation definitions within Leininger's cultural care theory include the following:

1. Care is the essence of nursing and a distinct, dominant, and unifying focus.
2. Care (caring) is essential for well-being, health, healing, growth, survival, and facing handicaps or death.
3. Culture care is the broadest holistic means to know, explain, interpret, and predict nursing care phenomena to guide nursing care practices.
4. Nursing is a transcultural, humanistic, and scientific care discipline and profession with the central purpose of serving human beings worldwide.
5. Care (caring) is essential to curing and healing; there can be no curing without caring.
6. Culture care concepts, meanings, expressions, patterns, processes, and structural forms of care are different (diversity) and similar (toward commonalities or universalities) among all cultures of the world.
7. Every human culture has lay (generic, folk, or indigenous) care knowledge and practices and usually some professional care knowledge and practices that vary transculturally.
8. Cultural care values, beliefs, and practices are influenced by and tend to be embedded in the worldview of a culture and in its linguistic, religious (or spiritual), kinship (social), political (or legal), educational, economic, technological, ethnohistorical, and environmental context.
9. Beneficial, healthy, and satisfying culturally based nursing care contributes to the well-being of individuals, families, groups, and communities within their environmental context.
10. Culturally congruent or beneficial nursing care can only occur when the individual, group, community, or culture care values, expressions, or patterns are known and used appropriately and in meaningful ways by the nurse.
11. Culture care differences and similarities between professional caregiver(s) and client (generic) care receiver(s) exist in any human culture worldwide.
12. Clients who experience nursing care that is not reasonably congruent with their beliefs, values, and caring lifeways show signs of cultural conflicts, noncompliance, stresses, and ethical or moral concerns.
13. The qualitative paradigm provides new ways of knowing and different ways of discovering the epistemic and ontological dimensions of human care (Leininger, 1991).

Leininger's Cultural Enablers

Leininger uses her coined term *enablers* to tease out data relating to cultural care, which include:

1. **Observation-participation reflection (OPR) enabler**—The researcher is an active observer, listener, and participant, to identify what occurs naturally in the environment. This consists of (a) primary observation and active listening; (b) primary observation with limited participation; (c) primary participation with continued observations; and (d) primary reflection and reconfirmation of findings with informants.
2. **Stranger to trusted friend (STF) enabler**—This enabler describes the stranger (researcher) who is initially distrusted by informants, who avoid sharing their cultural stories and secrets. The informants later share their cultural knowledge (secrets) so that they will be understood more accurately. The goal is to obtain honest, credible, and in-depth data from the informants. Plowden and Wenger (2001) described the research that they conducted with African American participants demonstrating this enabler model. The investigator moved from a stranger within the community to a trusted friend and began to collect rich and valuable data as given from the informants' perspective.
3. **Acculturation health care assessment enabler**—This enabler identifies formal and nonformal values, beliefs, and general lifeways of the informants.
4. **Sunrise model, a cultural enabler**—Leininger provides a visual aid to her theory as shown by her model of 2002, originally developed in 1970 with numerous later revisions. The ultimate outcome is culturally congruent care for health or well-being of people or culturally congruent care for the dying (Leininger & McFarland, 2002).

The components of Leininger's cultural assessment as shown in her sunrise model (Leininger & McFarland, 2002) consist of the elements of:

- communication and language
- gender considerations
- sexual orientation
- ability/disability
- occupation
- age
- socioeconomic status

- interpersonal relationships
- appearance
- dress
- use of space
- foods
- meal preparation and related lifeways

Culture and Cultural Concepts

Leininger's concept of culture states that culture is the complex whole that includes knowledge, beliefs, art, morals, law, customs, and any other capabilities and habits acquired by a society. It consists of shared ideas, concepts, rules, and meanings, having explicit guidelines that members of a society learn and which guide them in viewing their world experiences. Among her beliefs is the concept that one must be careful to not overgeneralize or stereotype members of a society because not all members of a group share the same worldviews. There are different levels of culture which consist of (a) the tertiary level, which creates a public appearance given to outsiders; (b) the secondary level, which includes rules and assumptions known to inside members, rarely shared with outsiders; and (c) the primary level, which is the deepest level known to each individual member but hidden from outsiders, and which is stable and resistant to change (Andrews & Boyle, 2008; Purnell & Paulanka, 2008).

The concept of a worldview or paradigm is necessary to understand culture. It consists of a perspective shared by individuals or a group, which explains the universe and life events. One perspective originally noted in the works of Purnell and Paulanka (2008) is that health and illness are related to harmony, unity, and a balance between humans and the universe. Cultures often have their own lens or perspective for viewing the world as well as categorizing their members.

Ethnography as a Research Methodology

Ethnography is the description of culture using a process to learn *about* people by learning *from* them (Spradley, 1979). The researchers reside in natural settings to gain an in-depth perspective. Historically, nursing professionals have applied ethnography in diverse settings to enhance and understand nursing practice by understanding patients' life experiences, which cannot be studied using the scientific method (Cruz & Higginbottom, 2013).

Leininger's Ethnonursing Research Methodology

To use her theory for a cultural investigation for nursing research, Leininger developed the *ethnonursing* research methodology based on ethnographic research methodology, previously used mainly by anthropologists and sociologists. She developed the ethnonursing research methodology to help with the discovery of data related to her transcultural nursing theory. Leininger (1997) defines this method as a qualitative research method focused on naturalistic, open discoveries and largely inductive modes to document, describe, explain, and interpret the informant's worldview, meanings, symbols, and life experiences as they bear on actual or potential nursing phenomena. The purpose of this method is to (a) mainly discover unknown or vaguely known nursing phenomena bearing on nursing knowledge; (b) to enter the people's world with an open mind and learn from them about their insiders' or emic life worlds, experiences, and current or past perspectives about human care and health; (c) to study how the outsiders or etic view contrasted with the local culture and areas of conflict; (d) to gain in-depth knowledge about the meanings, expressions, symbols, metaphors, and practices related to care, human life conditions, and experiences; (e) to tease out nursing knowledge related to the theory of culture care using the dimensions within the sunrise model; (f) to discover ways to obtain meaningful data; and (g) to identify knowledge about human care and health that is similar or diverse.

Leininger uses Lincoln and Guba's (1985) criteria for qualitative studies, which are:

1. Credibility—direct evidence from the people and the environment
2. Confirmability—documented verbatim evidence from people who can confirm the data or findings
3. Meaning-in-context—meaningful or understandable findings that are known and relevant to the people within their familiar and natural environment
4. Recurrent patterning—documented evidence of repeated patterns, themes, and acts over time reflecting consistency
5. Saturation—in-depth evidence of taking in all that can be known or understood about the phenomena or a domain of inquiry under study
6. Transferability—whether findings from one study have similar but not identical meanings and relevance in another situation or context (Leininger, 1997)

Leininger lived for more than 1 year in the East-Highlands of New Guinea where she studied the Gadsup Akuna people and hoped to learn more about their ways of caring from an emic or insider perspective. She would ultimately contrast this knowledge with that of the Western cultures, which included Americans. This research guided her development of her culture care theory, unifying the disciplines of nursing and anthropology. She believed that health care providers could provide more individualized care (culturally congruent care) when they had knowledge of the patient's background (Leininger, 1997).

Leininger (1985) notes that the origins of ethnography, as a qualitative research methodology, have been used in anthropology for more than a century. Ethnography consists of a process of observing, detailing, describing, documenting, and analyzing lifestyles or particular patterns of culture to understand people within a particular environment. It is an older research methodology, often conducted by anthropologists such as Franz Boas, Malinowski, and Margaret Mead. The studies consist of observations and active participation within the culture to document, describe, and analyze the cultural lifeways of a group of individuals including social, economic, kinship, language, values, art, education, customs, beliefs, practices, religion, and other factors, which are needed to explore the culture of a group of people. Health and illness behaviors are within the context of culture and no part is entirely separate from other parts. Political, social, and economic factors also influence health. In their article, "Ethnography: Contributions to Nursing Research," Robertson and Boyle (1984) state that health and illness behaviors occur within the context of culture. Ethnographic research methodology facilitates the investigation of a patient's beliefs of health and illness and helps to identify the cultural components.

Leininger states that ethnographic research methodology, when applied to nursing, is called *ethnonursing* (Leininger, 1985). It is designed to relate culture care theory to obtain meaningful data. Ethnonursing is a qualitative methodology that can be used to investigate those of different cultural backgrounds, geographic locations, and time. It can be used to document, describe, and understand the experiences, meanings, and symbols involved in nursing care, which is related to their values, beliefs, health practices, and culture. The researcher maintains open discovery, active listening, demonstrates respect, and tries to avoid an ethnocentric bias (McFarland, Mixer, Webhe-Alamah, & Burk, 2012). Higginbottom, Pillay, and Boadu (2013) state that ethnographies can have meaningful and useful applications for primary care nursing and often improve care. The authors justify ethnography as a methodology useful to many disciplines when there is a need for learning about cultural subgroups.

Depending on the scope and nature of the research, ethnonursing methodology can be described as *mini-ethnography*, which is confined to a small-scale focus or narrow area of inquiry, or a *maxi-ethnography*, defined as a large and comprehensive study of a particular culture necessitating a broader investigation and requiring details about the culture. Data can be used to obtain insight into health beliefs, practices, and care, and further understanding of a particular culture, which can bring much needed insight to health care providers. Nurses and other health care providers can incorporate this knowledge to plan more precise patient care. Leininger states that giving more culture-specific care reflects a strong element of caring. In addition, this knowledge can be used to generate new nursing and health care theories. Leininger founded this methodology in the mid-1960s (Leininger, 1985).

The ethnonursing methodology primarily focuses on *emic* knowledge (insider's perspective) as compared to *etic* (outside observer's) perspective. Leininger developed the sunrise model in 1965, modified numerous times to be used as a guide or domain of inquiry. The ethnonursing research data analysis process includes four steps: (a) collecting and reviewing all data including interviews, observations, recordings, transcriptions, participatory activities, and field notes; (b) recording and classifying data; (c) identifying and categorizing data, reviewing for saturation, which consists of looking for similarities and differences, including pattern and contextual analysis (additional codes may be added or deleted); and (d) interpreting and synthesizing of findings. This process leads to the development of major themes, research findings, recommendations, and/or theoretical findings. Ultimately, the researcher creates themes with confirmation with the original informants (McFarland et al., 2012).

Leininger describes three different types of research interviews within the ethnonursing methodology. The first is the open-ended interview in which the researcher does not ask questions that lead to fixed or predetermined answers, but the participant is encouraged to talk, clarify, and/or give examples. The second type is a structured or closed interview, in which questions are phrased to elicit specific responses. The third type is the semi-structured interview which is a combination of the open and closed types of interviews. For ethnographic methodology, it is often helpful if the researcher has some limited background before the interview. Another essential element is to allow the participants to have an opportunity to interpret, clarify, verify, or confirm what they have stated. Leininger also suggests the phrases "tell me," "I am interested to hear," or "I would like to learn more about that" to encourage people to talk about themselves, which she calls "lead in" questions (Leininger, 1985).

Data analysis is focused on the use of *emic* (data obtained directly from the participants by observation and participation). It also includes *etic* information from the researcher's general observations while studying people over time. Particularly for ethnonursing, data analysis focuses on studying areas related to health, care, prevention of illness, illness, and other aspects of nursing. Data from several key informants, as well as the observations made by the researcher, are reviewed. The researcher also includes all the influences such as social structure, politics, worldview, and health care environment (Leininger, 1985).

Author's Personal Journey to Meet Madeleine Leininger (Leading to the Use of Her Theory)

I studied at the University of Cincinnati College of Nursing in the late 1960s; the university had a School of Anthropology. Dr. Margaret Mead, a world-famous anthropologist, and a visiting professor within the University of Cincinnati's Medical School Department of Psychiatry, gave a lecture to our nursing student body in a large auditorium on campus one afternoon. All the students had read her book, *Coming of Age in Samoa* as required reading for the sociology class. I was inspired by her lecture and thought that someday I would like to travel, learn, and perhaps even work with people of other cultures in the world. Little did I know that Madeleine Leininger was also on our University of Cincinnati campus at some point in her career. I also did not know then that many years later in my career I would meet Dr. Leininger and understand the focus of her nursing theory, the connection relating nursing with anthropology. Years later, in Atlanta, Georgia, I began studying for my master's degree in nursing. With little background in nursing theory, I took a nursing theory course and was assigned to review and present the works of Dr. Leininger, as an example of a famous nursing theorist. After reading several of her books, I was so inspired that I wanted to locate her and talk with her.

I traced her to Tuscaloosa, Alabama, at that time. I was successful in reaching her on the phone and getting the opportunity to tell her that she had written in her books everything I believed about nursing, yet she had also stated it far better than I ever could have. Dr. Leininger was interested in my desire to use her theory as a framework for my master's thesis entitled, "What do Jewish clients wish their nurses to know to better meet their health care needs?" Leininger and I corresponded with lengthy handwritten letters, and she encouraged me to attend a Transcultural Nursing Conference and meet her. I eventually did, and I also became more active in the organization, becoming friendly with Leininger. She encouraged me to come to Detroit for my doctoral program, but I stayed in Atlanta and received my PhD in nursing there. Her work again guided me to write my dissertation inspired by her theoretical framework. This thesis is titled, "A study of poor African American women who received no prenatal care." After completing my doctorate degree I had an opportunity for a podium presentation at one of the Transcultural Nursing Conferences, and Dr. Leininger was in the audience, sitting in the center of the front row, as I nervously gave my presentation. Many years later as a faculty member of an Atlanta nursing program, I started a study abroad program in Oaxaca, Mexico. That was my 19th annual event, taking students there for a 2-week, 3-credit-hour course. I was able to conduct research with my dean, using both qualitative and quantitative research methodologies with the indigenous Zapotec Indians, some of whom were HIV positive. With the desire to explore the culture of these Indians, I began to re-examine Leininger's sunrise model, and her transcultural nursing theory, to use an ethnonursing research methodological investigation of the culture and health needs of the community. The following is a summary of my research experiences with the Zapotec Indians. As Leininger suggests, one must investigate the culture first, before beginning a research project. I began by examining the cultural background of the Zapotec Indians of Oaxaca, Mexico.

I have had numerous experiences working with indigenous Zapotec Indians in my study abroad program in Oaxaca, Mexico, and conducting cultural investigations with my dean, using qualitative research methodology (and quantitative in some studies) with HIV-positive men and women at the HIV/AIDS clinic (COESIDA), a part of the Health Department of the State of Oaxaca, Mexico. The need for greater HIV/AIDS health education and for care for depression were found. To give the COESIDA agency data to use in requesting more Mexican federal government funding for psychological services for the patients, my dean and I were requested by the Health Department of the State of Oaxaca to conduct the research investigations at COESIDA. Listed here are some of the publications based on investigations into the needs of Zapotec Indians conducted by Dr. Richard Sowell, dean of the College of Health and Human Services at Kennesaw State University; Dr. Gabriela Velasquez, the medical director of the COESIDA clinics in Oaxaca; Dr. Lewis VanBrackle, chair of the Department of Statistics at Kennesaw State University; and myself. Much of the information about the Zapotecs was gathered firsthand by in-depth qualitative interviews in Spanish, which were conducted over many years.

Cultural Background of the Zapotec Indians of Oaxaca, Mexico

The Zapotec Indians of Oaxaca, Mexico, are indigenous people who are native, original inhabitants of a land. They have a history of having been conquered by the Spanish who later colonized parts of their land, which resulted in a new culture that retained some aspects of the original pre-Hispanic Zapotec culture. The current Zapotecs have a culture with a distinct language (containing numerous dialects), beliefs, dress, and societal norms, as well as a blend of Spanish culture, which includes Catholicism (or some modification of this religion) and the Spanish language. The Spanish conquistadors used their strength and (culturally) imperialistic force to conquer the Zapotecs and create a Spanish influence on the pre-Hispanic Zapotec culture. According to Purnell and Paulanka (2008), *cultural imperialism* is defined as the practice of promoting, distinguishing, separating, or injecting the culture or language of one culture into another culture. This often results in overt racism, classism, or prejudice by the dominant culture. Much of the history as told by the Zapotecs, who currently live within Mexican governmental laws, reflects those experiences. Zapotec Indians often believe that they are victims of discrimination, which frequently results in unequal local and federal governmental treatment in regard to federal laws, health care, education, employment opportunities, housing, and other government services. To gain a greater understanding of the Zapotec culture, and more specifically, the health and health care values, beliefs, customs, and practices of the people and their society, one can use Leininger's cultural assessment with the guidance of Leininger's sunrise model, which is part of her transcultural nursing theory.

Background of the Indigenous Zapotec Indians of Oaxaca, Mexico

The Zapotecs (Didxazon), are an indigenous people of Mexico, descended from an Indian society that existed in Central America and Mexico from 500 BCE until 1500 CE. The name *Zapotec* comes from *Nahuatl*, which means inhabitant of the place of *sapte*. The people are indigenous Indians descended from the pre-Columbian Indians who inhabited the Americas prior to the arrival of the Spanish conquistadors. Oaxaca, Mexico, today has a population of 3.5 million people, containing an indigenous Indian population of more than 1 million. There are 16 different groups each speaking its own language and many speaking different dialects of those languages. Zapotec Indians have over 60 language dialects and many also speak Spanish. This area is one of the most ethnically, culturally, and linguistically diverse areas in the Western Hemisphere. Of the indigenous Indians of Oaxaca, 500,000 speak no Spanish at all. The Zapotecs live in small remote villages, of usually less than 500 people, and are often difficult to access. Oaxaca is a very diverse area located in the southwest part of Mexico on the Pacific coast. The Sierra Madre, Oriental, and Sur mountains emerge in this location. Included in this region are deserts, rainforests, high mountain cloud forests, and coastal areas. Historically, the Zapotecs possessed a highly developed communication and technology system for their time. They were talented craftsmen, providing nearly all the high-quality clothing in pre-Hispanic Mesoamerica and have continued that tradition. Now they mainly reside in the State of Oaxaca de Juarez, at an altitude of 5,034 ft. The population of Zapotecs, at present, is approximately 800,000 to 1 million people. There are four basic groups of Zapotecs: the *istmenos*, who live in the southern Isthmus of Tehuantepec, the *serranos*, who live in the northern mountains of the Sierra madre de Oaxaca, the *southern Zapotecs*, who live in the southern mountains of Sierra Sur, and the *Central Valley Zapotecs*, who live in and around the valley of Oaxaca (Zapotecs, n.d.) The language group is composed of over 60 variations or dialects. Analysis of the speech of the people living in the village of Santa Maria Lachixio indicates that high voice tones are used to show respect toward others. Kinship, age, and authority are important determiners of high pitch. Children are taught at 6 to 12 years of age how to speak and behave respectfully (Chinas, 1973; Joyce, 2010; Persons, 1997; Stephen, 2005).

Most Zapotecs are Catholic, yet some of their ancient beliefs and practices, such as burial of the dead with their valuables, still exist today. Zapotec women's roles are in the context of marriage, childbearing, and work. Today there are strong hierarchical gender roles that value males and masculinity more than females and femininity. Many of the Zapotecs' lives reflect the strongly separated gender roles. Women are concerned about their sexual reputations and young girls, by 10 or 11 years, are not allowed to walk the streets alone. People are free to choose their marriage partners, and monogamy is valued. Men are freer to have sexual relations with others. Women's activities are often more controlled by their husbands, fathers, or brother(s). Women are sometimes the victims of violence within the marriage. There are specific gender roles for men and women. Women are expected to take care of the children and the home and also work outside the home if needed. Within their mostly agrarian society, females help with weeding and harvesting but rarely plant or plow, except when no males are available. Many men and women are weavers and make clothing, rugs, pottery, and woodcarvings (Chinas, 1973; Joyce, 2010; Persons, 1997; Stephen, 2005).

Cultural Assessment of the Zapotec Indians of Oaxaca, Mexico, Using Leininger's Sunrise Model Enabler

By using parts of Leininger's sunrise model one can examine various aspects of the cultural knowledge of the Zapotecs. This knowledge is extremely valuable for planning culturally congruent health care interventions and also for gaining trust and engaging in ethnonursing research methodology.

Influences

1. **Worldview**—Zapotecs are very proud of their heritage, do not want to assimilate, and wish to maintain their culture in a private manner, being respected by the federal and local governments.
2. **Technological factors**—Zapotecs have a history of exceptionally high levels of achievement in astronomy and mathematics; today they continue to live in an agrarian society, using manual labor, and also engaging in labor-intensive crafts.
3. **Religion**—The majority is Catholic, yet some are Protestant followers. They originally had their own religion, as shown by archeological evidence. Many are resentful of the Spaniards' destruction of their original places of worship and continue to distrust outsiders.
4. **Kinship and social factors**—The Zapotec culture is a male-dominant society with specific gender roles. They believe that males should protect females, and they support the traditional roles of females. Women are homemakers with childbearing and childrearing as a high priority. Women also assist in farm labor or crafts. Males mainly work in farming or crafts. The majority live in small isolated areas, with village members acting as extended family. There are strong traditional family and friend relationships.
5. **Cultural values, beliefs, and lifeways**—The culture is male dominant, with some male family violence. People are somewhat religious, have traditional gender roles, and a belief in natural foods and traditional medicines.
6. **Political and legal factors**—Some people refuse to cooperate with the local, state, and/or federal government because they resent the lack of recognition and acceptance of their specific cultural lifeways. Many participate in demonstrations against the local government in the hope of receiving greater respect, tolerance, and assistance.

7. **Economic factors**—Because of low education levels and subsistence farming with low wages, most Zapotecs have extremely low incomes, necessitating that all family members pool resources to generate an adequate family income.

8. **Educational factors**—Most Zapotecs have less than a third grade education; many speak a mainly non-Spanish indigenous language, creating a very low socioeconomic household level and a low health literacy level with little employment options. Health literature and health care are given by Spanish-speaking health care providers who seldom speak the indigenous languages. (Health context in Oaxaca, 2012; Zapotec culture, n.d.)

Use of Leininger's Cultural Assessment Data: Knowledge Needed to Create Culturally Congruent Care Interventions for Zapotec Indians of Oaxaca, Mexico

Ethnographic and ethnonursing research methodology requires cultural knowledge to build trust among community leaders and members, respect for outsiders, and an emic comprehension to assist the community. The following is cultural information needed for conducting ethnonursing research and planning culturally congruent nursing interventions related to the Zapotec cultural background.

1. **Health literacy**—Because of the low literacy resulting from low income, living in isolated rural areas, and low education levels, there is minimal or no medical care or health education among Zapotecs. Their health education needs to be more visual rather than written. Use of posters rather than written materials and translators would be beneficial.

2. **Traditional healers and medicines**—Most Zapotecs, especially in isolated rural areas, use natural medicine and traditional healers (curanderos(as) and partas). Their traditional health interventions need to be incorporated into their health education programs. Professional health educators need to respect traditional health practitioners and increase the health knowledge and practices of lay health providers in a nonthreatening manner (Health context in Oaxaca, 2012; Lowenberg, 2010; Zapotec culture, n.d.)

3. **Nutritional education**—Education addressing nutritional needs should include cultural likes and dislikes, and food readily available. Because there is low consumption of fruits, vegetables, dairy, and high-protein

products, there are high rates of malnutrition, anemia, poor longevity rates, extremely high maternal and infant mortality rates, and high rates of congenital anomalies. Health education needs to address nutritional needs as well as the consumption of iron, folic acid, and prenatal vitamins during pregnancy (Holtz & Sowell, 2010, 2012; Joyce, 2010; Sowell, Holtz, Vanbrackle, Velasquez, & Hernandez-Alonso, 2013; Stephen, 2005; Zapotec culture, n.d.)

4. **Politics and community trust/distrust for outsiders**—The community members are very sensitive to outsiders criticizing their socioeconomic status and cultural lifeways. Great care needs to be taken to gain trust within the community to allow outsiders to participate in health-related activities.

   There is general frustration with government policies, which do not support the sustainment of indigenous cultures including values, beliefs, language, customs, and practices, which may result in lack of government health services in the remote and isolated areas. There is also a lack of employment and educational opportunities, perpetuating poverty. Zapotecs strongly want to maintain their ancient culture in spite of government wishes to incorporate them into mainstream society. This situation often results in community members' isolation from large cities and government benefits, which ultimately results in less government services and lowering of quality education and health care. Generally, the local priest or other community leader needs to give positive sanction for outsiders to be received by the community and for community members to give serious consideration to the importance of their health education (Stephen, 2005; Zapotec culture, n.d.)

5. **Geographic area**—Zapotecs generally live in rural isolated communities in mountainous regions with poor or no paved roads, making access to health care more challenging, resulting in delays or absence of health care, particularly needed for emergencies (Holtz & Sowell, 2010, 2012; Sowell et al., 2013; Stephen, 2005; Zapotec culture, n.d.).

6. **Family beliefs and values**—There is a strong focus on family members, with concern about elders and children and their health. The community is group-oriented rather than individual oriented. Women sometimes feel less powerful in family decision making, and economics. They adhere to traditional gender roles and family expectations. There is an obligation to care for family elders by providing financial support, housing, and health care within their home when needed. The entire extended family is united in supporting one member's illness, often traveling together for numerous miles and hours to receive

health care and support seriously ill family members (Health context in Oaxaca, 2012; Lowenberg, 2010; Zapotec culture, n.d.).

7. **Language**—Zapotecs have a unique language with a variety of dialects within it, which is maintained to promote the culture, but which, without knowledge of the Spanish language, also inhibits education potential, thereby limiting health education and family income. The people may need translators for health care and social worker consults to access and use medical knowledge and care. There is great difficulty in learning new information, requiring many educational picture posters (more visual than written) (Holtz & Sowell, 2010, 2012; Sowell et al., 2013; Stephen, 2005; Zapotec culture, n.d.).

8. **Family violence**—Excessive use of alcohol causes many women and children to be abused. Victims need great support from family and friends, and could also use professional psychological support, if available (O'Nell, 1981).

9. **Occupational hazards**—The community members are often employed in high risk occupations, requiring low education levels. As a consequence, there are many occupational injuries and lack of or nonadherence to occupational rules such as the use of hard hats, eye protective shields, and heavy gloves. Occupational injuries often result in chemical contamination, burns, and head injuries (lack of hard hats), or broken bones. Men may need to leave the region or the country for long periods of time to look for and obtain work. This may result in men having greater exposure to HIV/AIDS and sexually transmitted diseases (STDs), which are given to their wives and girlfriends, and passed on in pregnancy to babies (vertical HIV transmission; Chinas, 1973; Holtz & Sowell, 2010, 2012; Sowell et al., 2013; Stephen, 2005; Zapotec culture, n.d.).

SUMMARY

This chapter addressed the historical journey of Dr. Madeleine Leininger's development of the transcultural nursing care theory. Leininger's theory and her ethnographic research methodology are described. The author also gave a personal anecdote of her relationship with Dr. Leininger. Leininger's sunrise model was used as a guide to obtain cultural knowledge of the Zapotec Indians of Oaxaca, Mexico, allowing for planning and evaluation of culturally congruent care for this population.

REFERENCES

Andrews, M. M., & Boyle, J. S. (2008). *Transcultural concepts in nursing care* (5th ed). New York, NY: Lippincott, Williams & Wilkins.

Chinas, B. (1973). *The Isthmus Zapotecs: Women's roles in cultural context* (pp. 119–122). New York, NY: Rinehart and Winston. Social life and customs; Indian women-Mexico.

Cruz, E. V, & Higginbottom, G. (2013). The use of ethnography in nursing research. *Nurse Researcher, 20*(4), 36–43.

Health context in Oaxaca. (2012). Retrieved from http://www.clinicadelpueblo .org.mx/index.php?option=com_content&view=article&id=72&Itemid=197& lang=en

Higginbottom, G., Pillay, J., & Boadu, N. (2013). Guidance on performing ethnographies with an emphasis on healthcare research. *The Qualitative Report, 18*(17), 1–16.

Holtz, C., & Sowell, R. (2010). Study abroad as a strategy for nursing education. In M. Bradshaw & A. Lowenstein (Eds.), *Innovative teaching strategies in nursing and related health professions*. Boston, MA: Jones and Bartlett.

Holtz, C., & Sowell, R. (2012). Oaxacan women with HIV/AIDS: Resiliency in the face of poverty, stigma, and social isolation. *Women and Health, 52*(6), 517–535. doi: 10.1080/03630242.690839

Joyce, A. (2010). *Mixtecs, Zapotecs, and Chatinos* (pp. 1–42). West Sussex, UK: Wiley-Blackwell.

Leininger, M. (1985). *Qualitative research methods in nursing* (pp. 33–69). Orlando, FL: Grune & Stratton.

Leininger, M. (Ed.). (1991). *The theory of culture care diversity and universality* (pp. 44–45). New York, NY: National League for Nursing.

Leininger, M. (1997). Overview of the theory of culture care with the ethnonursing research method. *Journal of Transcultural Nursing, 8*(32), 52.

Leininger, M. (Ed.). (2006). *Culture care diversity and universality* (2nd ed.). Sudbury, MA: Jones and Bartlett.

Leininger, M., & McFarland, M. (2002). *Transcultural nursing: Concepts, theories, research and practice* (p. 46). New York, NY: McGraw Hill.

Lincoln, Y. S., & Guba, E. G. (1985). *Naturalistic inquiry*. Newbury Park, NY: Sage.

Lowenberg, S. (2010). The plight of Mexico's indigenous women. *The Lancet, 375*(9727), 1680–1682.

McFarland, M., Mixer, S., Weble-Alamah, H., & Burk, R. (2012). Ethnonursing: A qualitative research method for studying culturally competent care across disciplines. *International Journal of Qualitative Methods, 11*(3), 260–263.

O'Nell, C. (1981). Hostility management and the control of aggression in a Zapotec community. *Aggressive Behavior, 7*, 351–366.

Persons, J. (1997). *High pitch as a mark of respect in Lachizio Zapotec*. Retrieved from http://www.und.nodak.edu/dept/linguistics/wp/1997Persons.pdf

Plowden, K., & Wenger, F. (2001). Stranger to friend enabler: Creating a community of caring in African American research using ethnonursing methods. *Journal of Transcultural Nursing, 12*(1), 34–39.

Purnell, L., & Paulanka, B. (2008). *Transcultural health care.* Philadelphia, PA: F.A. Davis.

Robertson, M., & Boyle, J. (1984). Ethnography: Contributions to nursing research. *Journal of Advanced Nursing, 9,* 43–49.

Sowell, R., Holtz, C., Vanbrackle, L., Velasquez, G., & Hernandez-Alonso, V. (2013). Depression in HIV positive Oaxacan women: Implications for mental health services. *Online Journal of Medicine and Medical Science Research, 2*(1), 6–12.

Sowell, R., Holtz, C., & Velasquez, G. (2008). HIV infection returning to Mexico with migrant workers: An exploratory study. *Journal of the Association of Nurses in AIDS Care, 19*(4), 267–282.

Spradley, J. (1979). *The ethnographic interview.* Belmont, CA: Wadsworth.

Stephen, L. (2005). *Zapotec women: Gender, class and ethnicity in globalized Oaxaca* (2nd ed.). Durham, NC: Duke University Press.

Zapotec culture. (n.d.). http://zapotec.agron.iastate.edu/cultura.html

CHAPTER ELEVEN

ETHNOGRAPHY IN A
BLACK STOREFRONT CHURCH:
THE WOMEN, THE RESEARCH, AND ME

Mary E. Abrums

*T*his chapter is taken from an ethnographic study done with a small group of poor and working-class African American women who live in Seattle, Washington, and are sustained by their storefront church—Morning Sun Missionary Baptist (a pseudonym; Abrums, 2010). Ethnographic description and life history narratives explore the day-to-day realities and challenges that the women face, as well as the long-term impact of poverty and racism on the women and their families.

The research that forms the basis for this chapter took place in Seattle in the 1990s. Although Seattle is seen as a progressive city, the poor, for the most part, are invisible. Little has been done to examine the lives of the relatively small African American population in this city. With only 47,541 African Americans (registered in the U.S. census as black or African American) in Seattle (City of Seattle, 2004), it is assumed that blacks have necessarily assimilated, but this is not really true. The majority of African Americans currently live in South and Central Seattle, but they have, like the families in this research, traditionally lived in the Central District ("the CD"). Small storefront churches dot the landscape—churches that maintain communities and traditions from an earlier Southern black lifestyle, and that support their members as they go to work in a White world or send their children to schools, sometimes to schools across town, that have predominantly White populations, where teachers, nurses, and social workers are primarily White, college-educated, and middle class.

By sharing their narratives and their lives, the women in this study hoped that they could make things better for poor black women. (The women self-identified as black and the terms *black* and *African American* have been used interchangeably.) Throughout the research, they demonstrated the interconnections of family, kinship, faith, and values within a small church community. The purpose of this chapter is to share my experiences of working as a researcher and highlighting the differences in race and class between the women who were constant companions in the research process and myself.

BEGINNINGS

The first day of my research project was a gray Sunday morning in February. Driving to Morning Sun Church, I passed south of the Montlake Cut on 23rd Avenue. As I went deeper into the CD I gradually began to see more black than White people on the street. At a busy intersection, an old black man was selling newspapers to motorists and pedestrians. There were several men standing with him, casually dressed, visiting on a Sunday morning, and I locked my car doors. I recognized this as a racist reaction, and I was not proud of myself. But I was worried about driving through the CD—my perception was that it was not a safe part of town.

As I drove, I was nervous about being accepted in a black church. How would I fit in? I knew that the women dressed up for Sunday, but I did not want to overdo it and look too well off. I finally chose a nice dress and high heels, but covered the dress with a casual sweater instead of my red wool coat. I selected earrings that my older daughter had made for me and took off my mother's diamond wedding ring. I tried to be early, but not too early, and parked around the corner and waited for 10 minutes before entering so as not to appear too eager.

Learning to Follow

This chapter is about my growth and development in the process of doing this research study. I originally wanted to understand more about African American women, health, and health care. In health care research, black women, particularly poor and working-class women, are routinely represented as having poor health statistics. As a nurse, I was appalled at the statistics, particularly the pregnancy complication and infant mortality rates, but accepted them as factual. However, I was puzzled by the usual reasons given to explain the data—high-risk behaviors such as smoking, drinking, drugs, adolescent motherhood, poor nutrition, poor prenatal care, and so on.

The focus was always on how black women contributed to their own and their children's health problems.

I recognized this "blaming the victim" attitude, and I questioned it as I started my research. I believed that the women from Morning Sun Church had probably come to some questions and conclusions of their own and wanted to hear what they had to say. Nevertheless, it was hard for me to get around my educational socialization, and I quickly discovered that my "routine" questions created brick walls over and over again as I asked them about health issues. My basic and most inaccurate assumption was that the women saw themselves as I had been trained to see them and as they were presented in the dominant discourse—as an "at risk" and vulnerable group. Through trial and error and much painful experience, it gradually became apparent to me that this assumption was puzzling and insulting to the women, as well as subtly, blatantly, and pervasively racist. The women clearly and adamantly rejected the scientific and cultural stereotyping and the racial and gender objectification of African American women seen in the majority of research studies. Framing their lives within "poor health status" was not relevant to their worldview or to how they defined themselves (Abrums, 2000a).

I do not claim to have completely or even partially overcome the problems that are inherent in research done by a member of the dominant social group who studies poor people of color. All I can say is that the women led me in a particular direction, and I had to follow them to learn what they wanted me to learn. I tried to leave my assumptions behind and step away from the dominant ideology, and I started to pay close attention to the women's experiences and stories, as well as to the meticulous details of the everyday life. It was only then that I began to move into the space that they wanted me to occupy to better hear and portray their life histories. It was only then that I began to look beyond the stereotypes and statistics to see how the women understood and influenced the world around them.

In our conversations, the women were willing to discuss their personal health, but more often, they wanted to talk about other interests: gospel music, spirituality, men, work, discrimination, teaching, family, cooking dinner, motherhood, loving Jesus, and surviving. It took me awhile to learn that this *meant* something.

Later, when I asked the women to review their stories, they told me that what I had written was "just fine," "funny," "all right," and that they did not want to change anything. To me, these comments meant that I had presented, at least in part, the stories that they wanted to be told.

A Question of Entry

As in Stack's (1974) landmark study of poor black women, I believed that the question of how to enter the research setting was an important one. I wanted to join a small group in an environment where the women were comfortably at home and traditionally "held the cards" and I did not—I wanted to be where the women held the power. I also wanted a setting where I had some level of familiarity and where I felt safe. I recognized that this issue of safety was based on stereotypes I held, but I could not entirely get around the fact that the CD had a high crime rate. When the opportunity arose to visit a small storefront church where another nurse anthropologist had studied, I seized the chance.

In retrospect, my reasoning was sound from a "power" perspective. I consistently felt that the church members had the power in our relationship. They could choose to reject or accept me as they wished, and they did so. The women were not dependent on me for social services or good health care or kindness to their children in a school setting. They did not have to invite me into their homes nor did they have to agree to be interviewed (and several refused). All they had to do was tolerate my presence in church and be courteous to me between services. Even as I gradually developed relationships with some of the women, they were not under any pressure or obligation to forge these friendships.

There were drawbacks to this setting as well. As women meeting in church, we had certain roles to fulfill. No matter how they truly felt about me or I about them, we generally were on our best behavior with one another. Charity, tolerance, kindness, and courtesy were the order of the day. This role of "Christian women" may have precluded some measure of our truly knowing one another. For instance, one woman hesitated to tell me that she loved to play the horses. If the women partied, I never knew about it (and maybe they didn't). But being in a setting that essentially demanded thoughtfulness was good for all of us as we tried to know one another, especially because fears, stereotypes, and prior negative experiences all played a part in our interactions.

FEARS AND STEREOTYPES

Unlearning racism or becoming anti-racist was a process of "two steps forward, one step back" for me during the entire research experience. I found that I grappled with racism within myself as much as I did with the societal racism that affected the lives of the women of Morning Sun (Abrums, 2000b). This struggle and resulting growth will undoubtedly continue all of my life. There has been progress: I now recognize many of the hidden dimensions of racism and I "own" what Sister Kent [the pastor's wife] taught me—that we are all "unique" and yet are "all of one blood." I will never be able to see, feel, or hear the world as the women of Morning Sun do, but I have come a little bit closer to their angle of vision.

This process of learning a new way to see the world required constant and vigilant monitoring of my words, thoughts, and questions. For example, I felt reassured and safe when I saw a police car in my neighborhood. But the women of Morning Sun were nervous around policemen: If there was an incident on the street, they sympathized with the person in trouble; If they saw a problem at night outside of their homes, they did not call the police because they feared someone might get hurt. Reverend Kent [the pastor] often said that police had a hard job and that "there are some good ones," but the underlying and occasionally spoken feeling in the church was that police were "mean." When I drove into the CD on a Friday or Saturday night to pick up a church member, I was shocked at the differences between the CD and my north-end White middle-class neighborhood. Police cars were on every other block, and black adolescent girls and boys were spread-eagled against police cars by 10 p.m. I began to understand that the CD was more dangerous than my neighborhood, especially for teenagers. But the danger came from both criminal activity and from the ever-watchful surveillance of the police.

I worried that racist thinking motivated me to lock my car doors as I drove into the CD, but the women of Morning Sun consistently locked their own car doors and locked me in when I dropped them off at home. Safety was an issue for all of us, and they had a realistic assessment of the dangers of living in a poor neighborhood.

I also found that the churchwomen saw danger where I did not. I felt uneasy when I saw groups of young black men, and they were anxious when they saw groups of young White men, whether they were "skinheads" or athletes playing basketball. As we drove through White business districts near the university or on Broadway, they carefully checked their car doors and stared straight ahead. We often made different decision about who and what situations were safe or unsafe; and these judgments related to our personal stereotypes, experiences, and histories.

Stereotypical and racist thinking clouded my view in other ways. One time when I was driving downtown with several of the women, I spotted a row of six White men and women in their twenties, sitting on the sidewalk, obviously homeless or traveling, looking grubby but healthy with sleeping bags and backpacks. An old black man walked by and reached into his pocket to give each young person some money. His passing kindness startled me. The whole picture was out of focus, and I was ashamed that I had trouble accepting this image.

I found that I was often distinctly uncomfortable as the only White woman in a black church, especially when the church overflowed and yet no one joined me in my empty pew. I became exhausted from going week after week into a community where I was unsure of my place and my welcome—even though the churchwomen were friendly and tried to include me. I had to take breaks from the strain of facing a black world and from constantly watching my thoughts, words, and actions. From these stressful, albeit illuminating experiences, I learned how the many small discriminatory actions that black people face daily at work and school create the constant stress that causes serious health problems.

GATHERING DATA

The research study took 18 months to complete. I have remained in close contact with some of the women; however, the data represents only the experiences and conversations that occurred during the official research period. I began my research initially by meeting with Missionary Mahalia Lake, the church member responsible for outreach activities. She and I agreed on three approaches: I would explain my study to and obtain permission from the pastor of the church, meet with Missionary Lake every week to discuss church-related questions, and attend Morning Sun Church "to watch and see."

When I told Missionary Lake that I would like to interview church members, she said, "We'll see about that. We're a small church." So I patiently pursued traditional ethnographic methods, hoping that once the women knew me better, they would agree to do life history interviews. Meanwhile, I found that using participant–observation methods at church generated rich data as Reverend Kent interpreted life experiences and gave his congregation "rules to live by" from the Bible. The music and songs offered concrete lessons about how to make it in this world and eventually enter heaven.

Each week before church services I attended Sunday school with several of the older women and learned how they applied the church lessons in their daily lives. In between the morning and the afternoon Sunday services I joined the women for lunch and informal conversations. I often participated in additional services with neighboring congregations on Friday evenings or Sunday afternoons when Morning Sun members were invited to "fellow-ship." Outside of church I visited with Missionary Lake on a weekly basis at the housing project office, in her home, or out on errands. Gradually I became more involved with other members of the Lake family. We did errands and ate out and went to doctor's appointments. I provided the transportation and sometimes lunch; in exchange they tolerated my barrage of questions, sometimes willingly, sometimes impatiently.

The Interviews

In addition to using participant–observation methods, I interviewed eight of the women to learn their life histories. I spent 15 months in the church prior to being granted the majority of the interviews that took place in the final 3 months of the study. In structuring the life history interviews I hoped to use a collaborative approach, so I asked Sister Kent and Missionary Lake to help me formulate the questions. But they said that it was my project, not theirs and that I was the one who wanted "to know," so I should just ask what I wanted to know.

At last Sister Kent endorsed my credibility and "good heart" and encouraged some of the women to participate in the interviews. I finalized my questions and scheduled lunch and an interview at my home with Mahalia Lake. Mahalia dressed up and brought her photo album. She seemed to enjoy lunch, but the interview process was tense and uncomfortable. I learned quickly from this interview that I needed to let go of any ideas I had about controlling the interaction. I left my questions and all ideas about chronolog-ical order behind, and I let the women choose the meeting place—this was always in the women's homes with the exception of Betty Jones, who asked to meet at her daughter Joann's house.

At the beginning of each interview, I simply told the woman that I was trying to understand more about black women and that I wanted to hear her life story as if she were writing it herself. I told her that she could start anywhere that she wanted. I assured her of anonymity and told her that she could change or delete any part of the story. Each woman chose her own name for her life history. Using Minister's (1991) method, I referred to a sin-gle sheet of paper that highlighted topics of interest. All of the interviews were taped and professionally transcribed. They lasted anywhere from 2 to 6 hours over the course of 2 days. During each interview, I acted as a "witness" to the woman's testimony through honest response, expressions of empa-thy and laughter, and by sharing my own experiences, beliefs, and values. I never left behind the idea of "making meeting," and I always took a gift of food, sometimes lunch, but more often snacks of cookies and fruit for the children (Banks-Wallace & Saran, 1992).

With these approaches to the interviews, the process was successful and enjoyable for all of us. The stories were told through conversations about context, historical forces, opinions, beliefs, and spiritual searches. In short, they were dialogues of meaning.

On Forging Relationships

During the interview process, I found that my own stereotypes sometimes got in the way of accuracy. For example, I misheard Marie Jones Smith when she told me that she was 19 when she had her first baby, and I noted that she was 17. When I listened to the interview tape I realized my error. I became wary of the subjective influence of my preconceived ideas on the research data. If this error occurred in my interview with Marie, a clear-speaking, well-educated woman, how many more errors did I make when class and education, as well as race, were barriers? I learned to strongly value tape recorders and meticulous transcription.

Sometimes the women seemed evasive or guarded about their information, and at first this frustrated me. Things were left unsaid, and they focused on the positive parts of their lives and on how they overcame challenges. I finally realized that each woman deserved the right to share her history, her memories, in the way that she saw fit. In trying to ferret out information that was not readily offered, I was often looking for content that fit my preconceptions. I learned to critique my questions and examine how I had led the interview. I learned that privacy was a valued space that needed to be respected.

Forging relationships, both during the interviews and in everyday life, took time and persistence. I had always depended on my ability to read people, accommodating my style accordingly to help smooth the rough edges of an encounter, but I found that I could not judge my interactions with the women accurately—I was at a loss as I tried to understand them and how to fit into their world.

I had originally wanted to model my research relationships on Stack's (1974) work, but I found I could not do this. I learned that I had to be myself. Unlike Stack, I was not willing to give up the convenience of my car and found it was more of an asset than a liability in that I traded transportation for the women's time and stories about themselves.

Marie Jones Smith, Joann Jones Newton, and I were similar ages and closer in terms of social class and educational level than were the other participants. These were important variables that helped overcome some racial barriers. I was comfortable visiting their homes, and they were comfortable having me. Mutual concerns about our children's health, safety, and education were commonalities that allowed us to communicate on many levels. Mable Jackson loved entertaining me in her home. In spite of the poverty of her surroundings, she always made each visit an occasion by dressing up and graciously welcoming me into her life.

In contrast, my most successful encounters with the Lakes were on "neutral territory." We went to their usual stores and fast food restaurants, to church and health clinics; we took "field trips" to places that Mahalia selected. In these settings, I did not have to struggle with the poverty of their homes, and they (and I) did not have to be reminded of the privilege in my world.

My relationship with the Lake family was a complicated one. Over the months, Molly and I became friends, but it was an unequal friendship because of the differences in our resources. Although Molly and I were close and her children sat with me at church, we did not trade childcare arrangements as did Stack (1974) and the women in her study. My children were older than Stack's were at the time of the study; they recognized and felt uncomfortable with the abject poverty of the project apartments, and I did not leave them there for any extended period of time.

I was frustrated with my inability to develop more trusting relationships with the Lakes, especially with Mahalia, but it was hard to gain the intimacy I hoped for. The Lakes knew and I knew that I could escape from their world into my nice house, safe neighborhood, healthy children, and employed husband; they had no such escape. As much as I wanted to be a part of their lives, their intimacy was based on shared problems and mutual need as well as on love, affection, and trust. I was not, nor could I ever be, part of that context. I felt compassion for them and admiration for their pride and ability to sustain. I learned that it takes courage to face the lives they lead every single day. Courage just to keep going is an important virtue, and it is one that Molly and Mahalia have and that Caren is rapidly learning. I admire them for this, but I do not want to go through what they have had to go through to have it. I am not trying to idealize them—the women are simply doing what they need to do. In the eyes of the church community, Mahalia and Molly are neither better nor worse off than any other members. They are poorer, but they are required and expected to do their best.

I struggled and still struggle with the idea that when someone enters your field of vision, you have an obligation. However, each time I left Molly and Mahalia's homes, I "counted my blessings." And when I finished my fieldwork, I felt a sense of relief that I no longer had to face their pain and my own ambivalence about how involved I wanted to be with that pain on a daily basis. It was only later that I was able to try again.

On Social Context

My relationship with each woman taught me something important about the meaning of being black and/or a black woman in our society. From the Lake family members, the poorest women in the congregation, I learned the most about the confluence of class, gender, and race. Unlike the Jones family with inherited property and Mable Jackson with a working husband, the Lakes never had a break in any way. The Jones family could trace property and family through several generations, but the Lakes' knowledge of previous generations was sketchy, a legacy of slavery in some black families. In addition, for the past three generations, the Lakes had been female-headed households. Although husbands, partners, and brothers/sons lived with and supported the women and children emotionally and even financially when they could, the lack of steadily employed men was a serious problem for the Lakes. With barely enough for day-to-day survival, family members were unable to accumulate any money for savings or a safety net.

In spite of these challenges, with each generation, Lake family members obtained a little more education—Mahalia's mother finished sixth grade, Mahalia finished tenth, Molly and her brothers earned their GEDs, and Roberta was the first in all the generations to graduate from high school. The Lake women were intelligent and articulate, but their educational history was variable: Mahalia, raised in the South and in Chicago, read and wrote fluently; but Molly, educated in Seattle public schools, struggled with these skills and could barely do math. Her daughter Roberta labored over English and language courses when she began to attend community college.

Because of their poverty, the Lakes faced ongoing health problems related to stress, poor nutrition, and possibly environmental exposure. Molly had two miscarriages, a stillborn baby, another baby born with leukemia, and her daughter Shani had a kidney problem. Mahalia cared for her grandson who had behavioral problems probably related to prenatal drug and alcohol exposure. Molly had asthma and hypertension, and Mahalia was pre-diabetic and also had hypertension. Caren suffered placenta previa with one of her births. These health problems took a continual toll on the entire family unit, depleting emotional resources and physical energy that might have been used to improve life for the family as a whole.

Giving Gifts

There were difficulties in maintaining equality in relationships given the vast discrepancies in resources between the women and myself, and I grappled with the idea of gift giving or of paying the women for their help with my research project. I often questioned my own intentions—did I give them gifts or food in the hope of manipulating further revelations or were these gifts freely given? When they confided in me, was this a "payback" on their part for perceived favors from me or was this information generously shared? Probably all were true to some extent. In anthropological research, giving gifts for knowledge is a legitimate form of exchange, but I never felt "right" about it. I wondered whether it destroyed honest exchange from the outset.

However, in spite of my misgivings, gradually a pattern emerged. I provided transportation for the women's errands, and they answered questions during the drive. I often bought meals and gifts for the women who were struggling. In time they came to expect this system of payment; however, we also became closer, and gifts and lunches were part of sharing friendship as well. Although I wanted our friendships to be equal, I never allowed the women to pay for me because I knew that they did not have the resources. They gave me small gifts when they could and sent cards and thank-you notes when I did something for them. The women were not hesitant to let me know if I transgressed privacy boundaries; thus, if I was manipulating them (which I'm not sure I was), it did not work too well. In fact, I often felt quite powerless.

Although Mable Jackson and the Lakes welcomed gifts and lunches, the Jones family members were clear that they would be insulted if I paid for their help in any way. When I interviewed them I brought snacks, so we could have something to eat while we visited or so the family could eat while they waited for a delayed meal. I drew up a formal kinship chart for the Jones family for Betty's birthday, and the family happily accepted it and had the chart framed for Betty.

Gift giving probably had a different meaning to each of us because of differences in social class. Molly seemed to accept this exchange system of sharing information for small resources most easily. She talked freely to me about her beliefs and her life, and she took advantage of the meals, my babysitting offers, the gifts, and the handed-down clothes for her children. At times her mother Mahalia, or Sister Kent, chastised her for "using" me. But Molly was pragmatic and, unlike her mother and Sister Kent, she did not feel she could afford to refuse favors, especially when she needed things for her children. She often said, "You're here, and I need and you have."

WRITING

I had one primary rule that I tried to follow in my writing. This rule was taped above my desk: "Write this story for the people at Morning Sun Church to read and you won't have any trouble." Thus, I tried to write so that all readers could readily understand and use the material. In addition, as I wrote the women's stories, I tried to maintain the primacy of the women as subjects and agents. I kept in mind that whatever I wrote could be used for political purposes, both to help black women and to harm them. Thus, I attempted to examine my words from every possible angle to see whether they might be used to support efforts for liberation or employed to maintain oppression. In the end, I was not sure that I had any control over how a reader might choose to interpret and use this content.

In writing the women's stories and my interpretations, I tried to keep judgment out of the discussion. Hancock (1989) suggests that continually asking the question "How?" instead of "Why?" assists this process. Knowing that the stories were to be returned to the women for reading helped in this regard—I never wanted to say anything that might hurt someone.

Other minor issues of writing style needed to be resolved in the presentation of this research. In writing my research study, I used the term *black* interchangeably with *African American* because *black* was the preferred term of the people of Morning Sun Church. In the research literature *black* has been alternately capitalized and not capitalized, depending on the writer, and I have not used capitals for any terms referring to specific groups unless they are proper names.

Interpretation and Analysis

I began my analysis by studying the women's life stories to firmly orient my interpretation in the women's voices. Their spoken life histories were not neat and tidy stories: They flowed quickly between past and present and future and back again. Scattered throughout the women's stories were the theories, principles, or belief systems by which they lived their lives.

In presenting these life histories, I tried to refrain from discussing and analyzing material, preferring as much as possible to let the women speak for themselves. In general I organized each woman's story into a readable form, and I sometimes summarized lengthy episodes without sacrificing essential content. In addition to the interviews, some of the story content evolved from my written records of day-to-day interactions with the women. Each woman read and approved her story.

Interviewing members of the same family at different stages in their lives vastly enriched the stories. It became possible to see how beliefs and values were passed from generation to generation through historical, environmental, and social changes. Different vantage points regarding the same experiences lent depth to particular stories and demonstrated how family members developed separately and together, and how they influenced one another's growth.

A World of Contrast

Moving between my world and theirs on a daily basis forced me to continually juxtapose the two, comparing and contrasting. However, I found that the most traumatic times of encounter occurred not in the black world of the women of Morning Sun, but in my own White world. In my relationships with the women, while I struggled to build a bridge, I was suspended over a chasm. I was surprised and angry to find that I was no longer comfortable and sure of finding a landing place in my own world. hooks (2004) notes that:

> The meaning of "home" changes with . . . radicalization. At times, home is nowhere . . . Home is that place which enables and promotes varied and ever changing perspectives, a place where one discovers new ways of seeing reality . . . reveals where we are, who we can become, an order that does not demand forgetting (p. 155).

It took me some time after completing the research to redefine and reclaim the meaning of "home," but now, several years later, I move easily between both worlds. I am very cognizant of the fact that, sadly, there are two separate worlds—one for poor women/people of color and one for primarily White middle-class people. The churchwomen, other women of color, and some White professors in academia are allies as I continue to work on these issues through my teaching and writing.

Social and health statistics and the women's stories help students to understand both the macro picture and the everyday impact of poverty. Stories especially help students to see the unique individuals who share some, but not all, experiences related to race, class, and gender. Each portrait removes a brick in the wall of stereotypes and generalizations, and students begin to understand the extraordinary depth and breadth of the wall. As students grapple with questions of difference and sameness, they find hope in the promise of these words—"We are all of one blood." Some students take this promise to heart, become motivated to help others to understand what they have learned, and begin to tackle the problems of oppression in their personal and health care work environments. In this and in other small ways, I know that I am "moving the rock."[1]

There is one more important lesson that I learned from the members of Morning Sun Church. It would be an injustice to them and to myself if I failed to mention it. From the churchmen and women, I learned how to pray.

NOTE

1. This chapter was originally published in the book, *Moving the Rock: Poverty and Faith in a black Storefront Church*. The title of the book comes from the following story:

> A group of Catholic sisters met with a diverse group of women from their community. The panel was scheduled from 9:00 a.m. until 3:15 p.m. The lone Black participant said that she did not know much about Catholic sisters and would just listen. She did so until 3:00 p.m. when she said:
>
> > Well, I don't know if I can say it too good, 'cause you know I didn't go to school much. But in my heart I know. I'll just tell you a little story. Now all you nice ladies imagine that you lived in a house by a road on the top of a mountain. And there's a big rockslide and a big boulder came down right around the corner on this mountain. And every car that came round that corner hit that boulder and smashed up. Now I can understand what all you'd do. I heard you. You'd run right out and you'd take those people out of that car. You'd bandage them up, and you'd bring them in you house and feed them, and you'd pray with them. And when they got well, you'd send them home. Well, sister, what I think you ought to do is send somebody out to move the rock. (Gifted with Hope, 1985, p. 16)

REFERENCES

Abrums, M. E. (2000a). "Jesus will fix it afterwhile": Meanings and health. *Social Science and Medicine, 50*, 89–105.

Abrums, M. E. (2000b). The meaning of racism when the "field" is the other side of town. *Journal of Cultural Diversity, 7*(4), 99–107.

Abrums, M. E. (2010). *Moving the rock: Poverty and faith in a black storefront church.* Lanham, MD: Alta Mira Press.

Banks-Wallace, J., & Saran, A. (1992). *Sisters in session.* Paper presented at the Women's Health Research Group. Seattle, WA: University of Washington.

City of Seattle. (2004). Population by race and neighborhood district. *Census 2000 (Summary file 1).* Prepared by Department of Neighborhoods, Department of Planning and Development. Seattle. Retrieved from http://www.seattle.gov/dpd/cms /groups/pan/@pan/documents/web_informational/dpds_007745.pdf

Gifted with Hope (1985, April). Five religious women talk about their changing roles. An interview with Majorie Tuite, Melinda, Roper, Luanne Schinzel, Joan Chittister, and Rosemary Radford Ruether by the editors. *Sojourners: Faith, Politics, Culture*, 12–22.

Hancock, E. (1989). *The girl within*. New York, NY: Faucett Columbine.

hooks, b. (2004). Choosing the margin as a space of radical openness. In S. Harding (Ed.), *The feminist standpoint theory reader: Intellectual & political controversies* (pp. 153–159). New York, NY: Routledge.

Minister, K. (1991). A feminist frame for the oral history interview. In S. Berger & D. Patai (Eds.), *Women's words: The feminist practice of oral history* (pp. 27–41). New York, NY: Routledge.

Stack, C. B. (1974). *All our kin*. New York, NY: Harper and Row.

CHAPTER TWELVE

QUALITATIVE INQUIRY: ONCE A DOUBTING THOMAS, NOW A PROPHET

Joanne K. Singleton

Once upon a time, I did not know the value, courageousness, and creativity of qualitative inquiry. Today I am a nurse scientist who answers questions using the most appropriate methods. When I did my first qualitative study, I was a doctoral student—a doctoral student grounded in the love of statistics, and cause and effect, and a believer in the power of prediction. I now understand humans better—how unpredictable they are and why questions that involve the human experience may need to be answered qualitatively.

My research interest was directed toward helping people to care for themselves. There were theories for me to extend or test, and tools to use. What more could a developing scientist have wanted? Then it all started to fall apart as I critiqued the said theories and grappled with the validity and reliability of tools through my experience with pilot studies.

Yikes! What was a frustrated doctoral student to do when after all of this, the questions that needed to be answered became clearer, only to suggest a different direction for the inquiry? Listening to this doctoral student's questions, as her understanding of her area of inquiry increased, the student's doctoral committee convened and said, "You are asking qualitative questions!"

Oh no! The dreaded words had been uttered. The warnings of doctoral students who had gone before played like tracks of music in my head: "You will never get done if you go qualitative! Even if you get done, it will be hard to publish; it is impossible to get qualitative studies down to a 20-page article!"

Challenged, but not defeated, I knew I had a lot to learn on many levels. For example, qualitative research was considered by some to be nonobjective. How would that work for someone such as me who was grounded in the notion that research must be objective? Could I tolerate that? In qualitative research, the researcher is said to be the instrument. Would I be able to be the "research instrument"? At the end of it, assuming I finished, would I be able to believe the findings from my own study? It seemed daunting. Not having traveled in this territory, I knew I needed a roadmap to guide me. As a "Doubting Thomas," I needed to find my true way.

There are always many ways to shape the questions that guide scientific inquiry, just as there are many ways to look at a phenomenon of interest. Role models in nursing, such as Madeleine Leininger and Janice Morse, who forged this path, provided excellent examples. Reading their work, and that of others across disciplines, was the first and very valuable step toward thinking deeply to better understand the direction the inquiry would take.

THE STUDY

How do nurses help patients to care for themselves? This remains an important area of inquiry, harking back to Florence Nightingale's first reference to self-care when she declared, "Whatever a patient can do for himself, it is better" (1969, p. 38). Contemporary nursing theories and models also support this perspective (Henderson 1966; Orem, 1980; Rogers, 1970), as does the American Nurses Association in its definition of professional nursing practice (1980). In addition, taking care of one's own health continues to strengthen as a value in the United States and will continue to be recognized and shaped by the Affordable Care Act, as individuals will increasingly be required to engage in and take responsibility for their own health.

On a personal level, encouraging others to help them care for themselves is something I learned about as a teenager. I was working in a program for teens in a New York City medical center, in which we were introduced to nursing and we learned to provide care to patients. Although at the time I was not interested in becoming a nurse, it was during my first summer in that program that I learned how I could help someone to care for himself or herself. I call it my Nightingale experience, as it became clear to me how as a nurse I would be able to help others in this way. My direction became clear that day (Singleton, 2000a).

While self-care is valued by the nursing profession, historically, it has been identified that this value may be challenged in actual nursing practice in long-term care. Kane and Kane (1986) said that "Nursing home residents' self-care efforts are circumscribed by the rules and customs of the institution" (p. 262). Further, in protected living environments, such as long-term care, residents may lose some control over their day-to-day personal schedules, which may result in a feeling of powerlessness. This can be compounded by caregivers' perceptions of the residents as being sick and dependent, and result in a focus on behavioral interventions that promote dependence and discourage self-care.

Having practiced for a short time in long-term care, and with many colleagues in this area of practice, this indictment did not sit well with me. Further, as mentioned before, I had piloted some tools used to measure practitioners' beliefs about patients engaging in self-care, and I was shocked that the nurses in my pilot study scored very low, which suggested that they were not supportive of patients engaging in self-care. My pilot study experience led me to question the validity of the tools. What I did then was to ask nurses who practiced in a variety of settings to complete the tool and then to have an interview with me to discuss their score. It was most interesting to find that while the nurses may have had a low score, suggesting they did not support patients in self-care, what they said during their interviews showed a very different perspective. While talking to the nurses about supporting patients in self-care, it was very clear that they did support it and that it was part of their practice.

Self-care in nursing has primarily been understood through Orem's self-care deficit theory. While it is not within the scope of this chapter to provide an in-depth discussion of the limitations of Orem's theory, an important limitation, relevant to this study, is the significance of how culture may influence self-care. Although Orem spoke of culture, this concept was not developed, leaving the context in which nursing practice occurs unaccounted for in the development and testing of Orem's theory. In addition, the theory does not account for the influence of the nurse–practitioner relationship on outcomes of care, and self-care has a biologic focus and may direct inquiry based on that focus. It is this author's belief that in the case of Orem's theory, determining what nursing self-care interventions are and developing tools to measure them is premature. First, there must be an understanding of nurses' values, assumptions, and beliefs of self-care and self-care interventions as reflected in nursing practice.

Description of the Study

Culture refers to "a set of shared assumptions, values, beliefs, and behaviors of interacting individuals ... acquired by experience through the process of enculturation" (Tripp-Reimer, 1985, p. 91). The profession of nursing can be defined as a culture, as it is shaped by the American Nursing Association (ANA) Code of Ethics, Scope and Standards of Practice, state definitions of practice and practice acts, history, and rituals. Within the culture of nursing, there are many subcultures, as nurses who practice together develop, over time, norms of behavior and patterns of interaction, for example, nurses who work in a particular specialty, or nurses who work together on the same shift, to name a few. The aim of this study was to explore and describe nurses' perspectives of encouraging patients/residents in long-term care to care for themselves. To gain this understanding, the researcher sought to study the actual practice of nurses, over time, in the context in which it occurs. Qualitative research methods offer a way to study human experience and behavior in this context, and ethnography is a qualitative method through which the world of a particular cultural group can be described.

Leininger introduced nursing to ethnography through her work in the 1960s. Leininger (1985) identified the value of this anthropologic method when little was known about the phenomenon. Ethnography allows the researcher to learn about a person's perspective and obtain data on meaning in the context of the individual or group environment. This is accomplished through identifying patterns and rich descriptions of significant events and daily situations of the cultural group. According to Aamodt (1991, p. 4), ethnography offers a way of "collecting, describing, and analyzing the way in which human beings categorize the meaning of their world."

Questions that guided this study were framed accordingly and included:

- What is the nurses' perspective of self-care interventions?
- What knowledge of self-care interventions is shared by this culture of nurses and informs their practice?
- What cultural behavior or actions describe how these self-care interventions inform their practice?
- In relation to the self-care interventions described by this culture of nurses, do the nurses make and/or use things that can be considered cultural artifacts?

CONCEPTUAL ISSUES

How Was the Study Framed, and What Was the Approach to a Review of the Literature?

A review of the literature was conducted to determine whether the research questions proposed may have already been addressed. This is important to develop and justify the significance of the study. The results at the time showed no studies that described nurses' self-care interventions in nursing homes or nursing practice. Based on this outcome, the review of the literature focused on the conceptual framework for the study, including culture and symbolic interactionism; self-care and nursing practice; and the use of ethnography in the study of nursing.

The conceptual framework established culture as the "acquired knowledge people use to interpret experience and generate behavior" (Spradley, 1980, p. 6). Humans use cultural knowledge to interpret and evaluate situations, and have both explicit and tacit cultural knowledge. Explicit cultural knowledge is what can be easily communicated, while tacit cultural knowledge is outside of our immediate awareness and not easily communicated. Culture is an interpretative process, a cognitive map that guides human actions and interpretation of our experiences (Spradley, 1979).

To study humans in a cultural group requires understanding of how humans derive meaning from, and make meaning with, others. This is understood through symbolic interactionism first described by Margaret Mead in 1934; however, the actual term was coined by Blumer in 1969. The three principles of symbolic interactionism are extremely valuable for a deeper understanding of ethnographic methods. According to Blumer (1969, p. 2):

> Human beings act toward things on the basis of the meanings that the things have for them ... the meaning of such things is derived from, or arises out of, the social interaction that one has with one's fellows ... these meanings are handled in, and modified throughout, an interpretive process used by the person in dealing with the things he encounters.

Meaning frames human experience, and humans organize their lives based on what things mean to them. Humans are constantly interpreting and defining meaning as they move from situation to situation. How one interprets and assigns meaning is influenced by roles, norms, values, and goals, which in turn influence, but do not determine, what one will actually do. All situations include an actor, others and their actions, and objects. It is the actor who determines the action through the process of interpretation, which is based on meaning. Cultural meaning is created through symbols, which involve three elements: the symbol itself, one or more referents to the symbol, and the relationship between the symbol and referent. Symbolic meaning is understood through this triad (Spradley, 1979).

At the most basic level of explanation from a symbolic interactionist perspective, humans move toward what has meaning for them. Therefore, through observing the practice of nurses within the same cultural group, in this case long-term care, and talking with these nurses, their perspectives, both explicit and tacit, on nursing interventions to encourage residents' self-care can be understood. Including this as part of the review of the literature was extremely important to show how the ethnographic method selected to guide the actual study process, Spradley's developmental research sequence, was appropriate to answering the study questions within a cultural context. Further, it provided a necessary and truly valuable map for a new qualitative researcher.

METHODOLOGY

What Did I Do, and Why?

Nursing care is delivered in a variety of settings, over shifts, and across a plethora of specialties. In each of these situations, nurses interact together and share values, assumptions, and beliefs about the care of their patients. Nursing is a culture, and each of the situations described can be considered a subculture of nursing. To gain an understanding of nursing interventions to encourage residents' self-care in long-term care, nurses in this setting were identified as a cultural group supporting an ethnographic approach to the inquiry.

Sample

The sample was a function of the subculture of nurses to be studied. In consultation with the director of nursing, three units were selected by the director of nursing for consideration. The researcher had the opportunity to meet with the head nurse from each unit to learn about the nurses, staff, and self-care interventions used by the nurses as identified by the head nurse. In addition, it was identified that the overall philosophy of the long-term-care facility focused on rehabilitation, and that two of the possible study units were designated as short-term rehab units with up to a 3-month length of stay. Because of the overall rehab philosophy, the short-term designation of two of the three units was determined to be a noncontributing factor in unit selection. Unit selection was made from observation/assessment of the day shift in three units based on the following criteria:

- During the observation, as identified by the head nurse, how many kinds of nursing interventions to encourage patients' self-care were distinguished and how frequently were they observed?

- Comfort of interaction between the researcher and the nurses
- Nurse staffing
- How often are the RNs scheduled to work together?

Observation of the nurses in all three units showed four self-care interventions; however, one unit—unit 2—had the highest observation frequency of these interventions; the comfort level of the researcher's interactions was high for all three units; nurse staffing in two units was identical—units 2 and 3—with each having a head nurse, two RNs, and one licensed practical nurse (LPN). However, in unit 2, the RNs were almost always scheduled to work together, versus unit 3 in which this was not as regular. In addition, in unit 2, the LPN was educated and practiced as an RN in another country and was awaiting her New York State RN licensure; effectively, this increased the number of RNs in unit 2 to 4. The unit with the most nurses assigned to the day shift at the same time and selected to be the study unit, based on the above criteria, was unit 2. Selection of unit 2 to be the study unit reinforced the importance of challenging what had been said about nurses in long-term care as probably not encouraging self-care among their patients/residents.

It is important to note that while there were four nurses assigned to the study unit, data collection included multiple formal individual (two with each of the four nurses) and group interviews (four with all four nurses), participant observation (with ongoing informal interviews over 6 months), event and record analysis, and member checks. Unlike a quantitative study in which the analysis is based on the number of participants (N) to determine statistical significance, in qualitative research, each interview, observation, event, and record provided data for analysis.

Institutional Review Board (Any Challenges, Privacy of Participants, Data Storage?)

When the long-term care facility was approached to present and discuss the possibilities of sponsoring the research, it was identified that they did not have an institutional review board (IRB). The first step for them was to set up their IRB, which they did very quickly, and the study was the first to be reviewed and approved by their IRB. In addition, and as is the usual practice, the study was reviewed and approved by the IRB at the university where I was a doctoral student. The value of ethnography is that it offers a close look into the lives of the subjects studied. Ethical guidelines for this study included the Federal Policy for the Protection of Human Subjects and the Principles of Professional Responsibility of the American Anthropologic

Society (1971). The data collection plan included observation of the nurses during their shift, which included observing their interactions with patients/ residents. It was agreed that the researcher would wear a name tag that identified her as a nurse researcher, and how to respond to the patients/residents' questions about the actual study was left to my discretion. Because of the "close look" offered by this method, some additional challenges had to be addressed. Participant observation can disclose information that may confirm or, conversely, violate the rights of participants. Participants, therefore, were afforded the protection of speaking "off the record." At any time, participants could confirm that they were speaking "off the record," and they were assured that the information would not be included in the researcher's field notes. A process was also established with the participants and the institution for the researcher to report any situations observed that in the researcher's professional opinion identified a patient/resident to be in imminent danger.

It was agreed that the sponsor institution and the participants would not be identified by name to ensure confidentiality, and that any research reports made available to the institution would also be available to the participants and the general public. In this study, full anonymity could not be provided as the researcher knew the participants and interacted with them regularly. Confidentiality and anonymity of the data were ensured through the use of pseudonyms. The nurse participants selected the name they were identified by in the study. All research reports were made available to the nurse participants who determined what they wished to read. Further, it was agreed that the researcher had access to collection of data during the day shift on weekdays, weekends, and holidays, and this access included patient, unit, and organizational information as appropriate to the study.

DATA COLLECTION METHODS

How Were Interviews and Observations Conducted and How Was Rigor Established?

Data collection methods in this study included formal and informal individual and group interviews, participant observation, event analysis, record analysis, and the researcher's journal. In addition, a demographic profile of the nurse participants was generated.

The development of the roles of researcher and participant takes time, and according to Spradley (1979), has the predictable stages of apprehension, exploration, cooperation, and participation. Indeed, these predictable stages were experienced, and milestones were identified in the data collection process. As expected, there was an initial apprehension in both the researcher and the participants at the start of data collection. Following the first formal group interview, the apprehension gave way to exploration, which was characterized as a several-week period of time during which the researcher and the participants came to understand each other's roles. Then, following a period of descriptive observations and the first formal individual interviews, a profound change in interaction toward the cooperative stage occurred. This was quickly followed by the researcher and participant roles developing into full participation. The quick progression from cooperation to participation coincided with one of the participants returning from a leave of absence and may have been encouraged by the researcher consulting with the nurses already participating, seeking their advice and recommendations to determine whether the returning nurse should be invited into the study. Individually and collectively, the recommendation was to invite the returning nurse into the study. This reinforced the fact that the nurses assigned to the day shift of this unit saw themselves as a group or team interacting together in practice. The nurse returning from leave was invited by the researcher and her fellow nurses to join the study, and she accepted the invitation. This strengthened the researcher's and the participants' collaboration, which was aimed at producing an accurate description of the nurses' perspective of their interventions to encourage residents' self-care.

Data Collection Procedures

Spradley's (1979) developmental research sequence (DRS) was used as a guide for data collection and analysis. The DRS is a cyclical process and the phases within the DRS helped to guide the researcher. Following data collection, the researcher transcribed interviews, reviewed condensed accounts and expanded them in great detail, and analyzed the data to direct the next step of inquiry aimed at addressing the research questions. The DRS progresses from descriptive observation, to focused, and then selected observations. Each phase in this study began with a formal group interview to direct observation and inquiry. A final formal group interview was conducted at the end of the study to share the final study findings, terminate the study, and leave the field. A formal interview can be with an individual or a group; it is purposefully scheduled by the researcher and has a clear direction. The purpose of the formal interviews in this study was to tap into the nurses' cultural knowledge of self-care interventions. Nursing administration agreed to provide coverage for the formal group interviews, which took place in the unit in a private room and were tape recorded. The formal group interviews were scheduled for 30 minutes. An interview guide was used to direct the discussion, and the purpose of each interview was identified. The first formal group interview, for example, was to have the nurses identify their self-care interventions. Questions that the nurses were asked to respond to included:

- Will you please share with me the kinds of things you do in your practice in this setting to encourage residents to be independent and to care for themselves in whatever way they possibly can?
- What does independence mean to your patients?
- Whom do you involve in these interventions?
- How do you communicate these interventions?

Each of the nurses also participated in two formal individual interviews. The formal individual interviews allowed for the collection of demographic data, and also provided a private opportunity to each of the nurses to speak to the researcher about the self-care interventions they had identified. An interview guide was used. Formal individual interviews were scheduled for up to 60 minutes, took place in a private room in the unit, and were tape recorded. Questions the nurses were asked to respond to included demographic data about themselves and their practice, and the following information:

- If there was one thing they could tell the researcher about nurses' interventions to encourage residents' self-care, what would that be?
- What is the point of the interventions they have told the researcher about?

During the formal interviews, descriptive, focused, and contrast questions were asked to tap into the nurses' cultural knowledge of their self-care interventions. Descriptive questions helped to identify their self-care interventions; focused questions helped to organized self-care interventions into categories and also to determine any discreet interventions that did not fit into a named category; and contrast questions helped to identify differences within similarities or categories of their self-care interventions.

Participant observation was an essential data collection strategy for this study and included descriptive, focused, and selected observations throughout the study. Descriptive observation begins with the broad question: "What is going on here?" From the answers to this broad question, major aspects of the cultural system are identified, and they in turn lead to more detailed questions and observations that become more selective.

Conducting fieldwork in one's own culture has been identified as potentially beneficial for facilitating entry. It was ethically important, however, for this study to be clear that while the researcher was a nurse, she was acting as a researcher, not a nurse. This was publicly identified at the start of the study. The role of observer-as-participant was maintained, the focus being on observation and participation taking place with the researcher being present in this cultural group over a 6-month period of time.

Informal interviews took place throughout the study and were recorded in the researcher's field journal. Informal interviews helped to clarify what the researcher was observing across the study. Event and record analysis were also important data collection strategies. Event analysis included observation of change in shift report, night-to-day and day-to-night. This took place twice for each shift change to understand how the nurse participants communicated their self-care interventions to other nurses. Record analysis was conducted to gain an understanding of how self-care interventions were communicated and included organizational and nursing department documents related to resident care, resident charts, nursing orders, general institutional correspondence to staff, and communications between and among the participants related to resident care (informal notes they shared with each other).

Critically important is the researcher's field journal, which is where field notes and observations are recorded. Three sections were established and included condensed notes that were recorded in the field; the researcher's personal feelings, reactions, and insights; and expanded accounts that fleshed out the condensed notes after the researcher left the field.

DATA ANALYSIS

Within Spradley's DRS, there are four types of data analysis: domain, taxonomic, componential, and cultural theme analysis. Data collection and analysis are cyclical with one informing the other, and through this process, cultural themes are identified. Domain analysis is the first step. A domain represents a unit of cultural knowledge and as such can be considered a category of cultural meaning. There are three basic elements of a domain: the name for the cultural term, also known as the cover term; the included terms—the names for smaller or subcategories within a domain; and semantic relationships, which link the cover term and included terms within a domain. In this study, domains represented the nurses' knowledge of their self-care interventions.

Once the domains were identified, a taxonomic analysis was completed to show relationships among the included terms within the domain, which helped to show how the domains were organized. Taxonomies helped to show the cultural knowledge of participants through the observed cultural patterns. The taxonomic analysis then directed selected observations and componential analyses of those domains. A componential analysis is a systematic search for components of meaning, also known as attributes that are associated with cultural categories. At this point, a cultural theme analysis was able to be conducted. The data were then searched for "any principle recurrent in a number of domains, tacit or explicit, and serving as a relationship among subsystems of cultural meaning" (Spradley, 1979, p. 141).

Multiple data collection methods, including interviews, observations, events, records, and field notes were analyzed using the procedures previously discussed, guided by Spradley's DRS. Trustworthiness of data was ensured through information cross-checking one source with one or more other sources. Review and confirmation of the levels of the data analysis that led to the subsequent theme identification were confirmed by methods experts. In addition, findings were shared with the nurse participants throughout the study to ensure accurate representation of their cultural knowledge of their self-care interventions. At the completion of the study, when the final study results were shared with the nurse participants, their consensus was that the findings offered a true representation of their explicit and tacit knowledge of their self-care interventions to encourage residents' self-care in their practice setting.

As previously reported, "Through ongoing observations and formal and informal interviews with the nurses, broad categories of the nurses' explicit knowledge of encouraging patients/residents in caring for themselves were identified, named, refined, collapsed, and organized. This resulted in five categories that represented the way the nurses encouraged patient/residents in caring for themselves. Within each category, the specific actions of the nurses, their interactions with their patients/residents, and contrasts were identified" (Singleton 2000b, p. 25).

The five categories included:

- Coordinating and involving others in carrying out the patient's/resident's plan of care
- Talking and communicating with patients/residents
- Assessing patients/residents
- Teaching patients/residents, staff, and families
- Reinforcing the plan of care with patients/residents.

Themes were then identified to help explain the relationship between the categories. Within this practice setting, it was noted that all other professional staff—physical therapy, occupational therapy, and social workers—were assigned to patients/residents. Nurses, however, were assigned to tasks, and the nursing assistants whom the nurses oversaw had patients/residents assigned to them. Nursing practice in this setting at the time of this study was based on a hierarchical medical model. While the nurses spoke of the importance of collaboration with the other disciplines and interdisciplinary practice, in reality, this broke down as they began to "see" and make explicit their tacit knowledge. Acknowledging the task-oriented hierarchical medical model presented a *Conundrum of Collaborative*, which was identified as an overarching theme. How the nurses managed this conundrum was seen in three themes, *Taking time, Engaging dialogue of presence*, and *Day trips toward restoration*. These three themes were seen as mediating themes and allowed the nurses, despite the task-oriented hierarchical medical model, to find ways to develop and maintain patient/resident–nurse relationships. Encouraging patients/residents to care for themselves occurred within the patient/resident–nurse relationship. What was illustrated through the themes was the nurses, through the tasks they completed, taking time to engage with the patients/residents by being fully present with them in these interactions, and by accompanying the patients/residents, supporting them daily in caring for themselves. From this study, a new term, *care-of-self* was identified. Care-of-self includes the physical needs of the patients/residents, which has been the major focus of the self-care theory, and goes beyond to include the bio-psycho-social-spiritual self.

DISSEMINATION

Following a successful dissertation defense, this study, in its entirety, was published through University Microfilms International (Singleton, 1993). Numerous aspects of this study were presented as papers at national conferences. The goal of this publication, first and foremost, was to bring out data-based publication. That was when the warnings of doctoral students who had gone before, as mentioned at the beginning of this chapter, began to play again like tracks of music in my head. In particular, the following lines played over and over, "If you get done, it will be hard to publish; it is impossible to get qualitative studies down to a 20-page article!"

The challenge faced in pursuing publication, staying focused, and translating the outcomes of the study so that they can be applied to practice is not uncommon. Sounds easy? I have come to learn that writing is an art form. Writing requires clarity of purpose, skill, ego-integrity, strategy to find the right journal fit, and persistence. It took many different manuscripts, rejections, and suggestions to find the right fit for article and journal. What became clear and really helped to find the focus was determining who the findings would best serve in practice. Eventually, it became clear that the findings might be most useful to nurses practicing in rehabilitation settings, as the study unit was a short rehab unit in a long-term care facility. Focusing in this way, the data-based article was published in *Rehabilitation Nursing* in January 2000.

In addition, this study was the foundation for developing and submit-ting a paper for a National Institutes of Health (NIH)-, National Institute of Nursing Research (NINR)-mentored research award to further develop my expertise in qualitative methods while continuing to develop the care-of-self concept coined in the study. Although the mentored research award was not granted funding twice, it did allow me to establish a mentorship, with sup-port from my university and with internationally renowned nurse scientists, to support my continuing work on developing qualitative methods, mixed methods, and triangulation of study results. This study has been the founda-tion for continuing research, presentations, and publications on care-of-self.

SUMMARY

When I came to understand that the questions I needed to ask for this inquiry were qualitative, I did not realize how important this "challenge" was going to prove to my development as a scientist. Throughout the inquiry, I expe-rienced, from the inside, the rigor of qualitative methods. As I mentioned at the beginning of the chapter, I was a Doubting Thomas. There were many things that I learned through this experience about qualitative research in particular, and research in general. Things I learned:

- A systematic process is essential to any type of inquiry.
- The method of inquiry is directed by the question or questions asked.
- One is not a qualitative or quantitative researcher per se; if one is truly directed by the research question, one will use the appropriate method.
- Qualitative research is flexible within the structure/process defined; it must be flexible for one to be able to talk to the people who know best about what one is studying, as well as for one to be able to see, through observation, what one is studying; sometimes, until one gets into the field, one does not know if the data collection plan one has outlined will result in the data one is looking for; sometimes, the data collection plan will need to be revised.

- All research is subjective, as the researcher determines what he or she will study.
- Qualitative researchers are good listeners, and courageous and deep thinkers.

REFERENCES

Aamodt, A. M. (1991). Ethnography and epistemology: Generation nursing knowledge. In J. Morse (Ed.), *Qualitative nursing research* (pp. 4–53). Newbury Park, CA: Sage.

American Nurses' Association. (1980). *Nursing: A social policy statement.* Kansas City, MO: Author.

Blumer, H. (1969). *Symbolic interactionism: Perspective and method.* Englewood Cliffs, NJ: Prentice Hall.

Henderson, V. (1966). *The nature of nursing: Reflections after 25 years.* New York, NY: National League for Nursing.

Kane, R. A., & Kane, R. L. (1986). Self-care and health care: Inseparable but equal for the well-being of the old. In K. Dean, T. Hickey, and B. Holsetin (Eds.), *Self-care and health in old age: Health behavior implication for policy and practice.* London, UK: Croom Helm.

Leininger, M. M. (Ed.). (1985). *Qualitative research methods in nursing.* New York, NY: Harcourt Brace Jovanovich.

Nightingale, F. (1969). *Notes on nursing: What it is and what it is not* (unabridged republication of the 1st American edition as published in 1860 by D. Appleton & Co.). New York, NY: Dover.

Orem, D. (1980). *Nursing: Concepts of practice* (2nd Ed.). New York, NY: McGraw-Hill.

Rogers, M. (1970). *An introduction to the theoretical basis of nursing.* Philadelphia, PA: F.A. Davis.

Singleton, J. K. (1993). *Nursing interventions to encourage residents' self care in long term care: An ethnography.* UMI Dissertation Services (UMI Order PUZ 9401935).

Singleton, J. K. (2000a). Nurses' perspectives of encouraging clients' care-of-self in a short-term rehabilitation unit within a long term care facility. *Rehabilitation Nursing, 25*(1), 23–30, 35.

Singleton, J. K. (2000b, December). Reflecting on reflections. *American Journal of Nursing, 100*(12), 53–54.

Spradley, J. P. (1979). *The ethnographic interview.* Fort Worth, TX: Holt, Rinehart and Winston.

Spradley, J. P. (1980). *Participant observation.* Fort Worth, TX: Holt, Rinehart and Winston.

Tripp-Reimer, T. (1985). Expanding four essential concepts in nursing theory: The contribution of anthropology. In J. McCloskey & H. Grace (Eds.), *Current issues in nursing* (2nd ed., pp. 91–103). Boston, MA: Blackwell.

CHAPTER THIRTEEN

A FOCUSED ETHNOGRAPHIC STUDY OF WOMEN IN RECOVERY FROM ALCOHOL ABUSE

Leslie K. Robbins

*A*lcohol abuse and its related problems are among the most pervasive health and social concerns in the United States today. Women are especially vulnerable to the physical and social devastation of alcohol abuse. Yet, although there is extensive research on alcohol drinking patterns, treatment strategies, and early recovery, there is little information about the factors that facilitate successful, sustained abstinence in women.

The purpose of this study was to examine and describe the common factors in successful recovery from alcohol abuse among women and to place these factors within the context of both their social networks and the larger social environment. This study draws from the population of New Mexico, where alcohol-related deaths are the highest of any state in the United States and the leading cause of death among individuals under the age of 65 years. The study was a focused ethnography of women who had successfully maintained long-term recovery from alcohol abuse. As an ethnographic study, data collection included participant observation, in-depth interviews with 21 women, and the collection of historical and current, culturally relevant data. A purposive sampling plan was used to maximize the selection of participants who had used traditional and nontraditional approaches to recovery. As such, the analysis of the success narratives revealed two distinct findings. The first was that women used several different trajectories to achieve longterm recovery. Three trajectory typologies were identified from the success narratives and labeled Alcoholics Anonymous (AA) as ceremony, AA as grounding, and recovery as self-management. However, within each of these trajectories, variations in successful recovery were seen.

The second major finding was that all women articulated an overarching theme of connections as an indispensable aspect of sustained recovery.

The success narratives demonstrated the powerful role that connections played in their long-term recovery, and the analysis distinguished two unifying concepts of connections—those that focused beyond self (spirituality, social support, and pets) and those that focused toward self (self-nurturance, agency, and identity). This discussion focuses on the implications for clinical practice related to both women who are still actively abusing alcohol and those who are successfully maintaining long-term recovery.

The specific aims of the research were:

1. Describing the factors common to women who have achieved long-term recovery (abstinence) from alcohol abuse.
2. Describing the situations that have contributed to sustained/long-term recovery.
3. Describing how recovery has affected their perceptions of themselves.

Ethnography was selected as the research methodology for the study, and an ecological, ethnographic approach was used to guide the theoretical structure of the study. This approach situates the analysis at the level of the individual within the micro- and macro-cultures (McElroy & Jezewski, 2003). This approach located illness narratives within the individual analytic level and supported the use of observational data collection as well as individual interviews. A pilot study, to explore recruitment of study participants and evaluate different participant interview schedules, was conducted over a 2-month period after institutional review board (IRB) approval was obtained. The pilot study included four women aged 21 or older with greater than 24 months of recovery from alcohol abuse.

During a pilot study varying schedules of participant interviews were evaluated. Participants were interviewed either once, twice, or three times, with the goal of identifying the schedule that yielded the richest information collection. This information led to the use of one to two interviews per participant in the larger study. Themes identified in the pilot study were used to refine the probes utilized in the larger study.

A purposive sampling plan was used in the larger study to maximize the selection of participants who had utilized traditional and nontraditional approaches to recovery. This plan enhanced the diversity of participants' ethnicity, their years of recovery, and their approaches to recovery itself. Several different nodes of participants were identified using this method. The analysis of success narratives obtained from the 21 study participants revealed two distinct findings: (a) that women used different trajectories to achieve long-term recovery and (b) that all women articulated an overarching theme of connections as being indispensable to sustained recovery. Within the different trajectories, three typologies were identified and labeled: "AA as ceremony," "AA as grounding," and "recovery as self-management."

Within each of these three typologies, additional variations to successful recovery were identified. The theme of connections included two unifying concepts identified as important to sustaining long-term recovery—those that focused "beyond self" (spirituality, social support, and pets) and those that focused "toward self" (self-nurturance, agency, and identity). The emergent theoretical framework and supporting ethnographic evidence are described in the manuscript, *Women's Ways of Recovery: An Ethnography of Sustained Sobriety* (Robbins, 2004).

BACKGROUND AND SIGNIFICANCE

Addiction, as a phenomenon, constitutes one of the most significant social and public health problems in North America (Suissa, 2003). Alcohol is the most commonly accepted psychoactive substance in use today (Becker & Walton-Moss, 2001). Nearly 14 million Americans (1 in every 13 adults) exhibit severe problems with alcohol, such as dependence or abuse, and millions more engage in risky drinking (Callahan, 2001). Risky drinking is defined as "drinking that increases the chances of adverse consequences; drinking more than guidelines on moderate drinking suggest" (Callahan, 2001, p. 34). The moderate drinking guidelines are two drinks per day for men and one drink per day for women (Callahan, 2001).

Alcohol use disorders are often seen as chronic and relapsing behavioral conditions that involve multiple biological, psychological, and sociological causes (Helman, 2001; Kadden, 2001; Snow & Anderson, 2000), and its related problems are among society's most pervasive health and social concerns (U.S. Department of Health and Human Services [USDHHS], 2000). Conservative estimates place the annual dollar cost at over $185 billion for alcohol abuse, which makes this the most expensive of all drug-related problems except for tobacco (Gordis, 2001). The social cost of alcohol abuse is staggering; among the calculable economic costs are those resulting from lost productivity, resources expended on health care and alcohol abuse treatment, and death resulting from chronic liver disease and cirrhosis (Gordis, 2001; Madden, Montoya, & Richard, 1995; Rice, Miller, & Dunmeyer, 1990).

Alcohol abuse also appears to play a major role in violent crimes and domestic assaults. Callahan's (2001) research showed that up to 86% of murderers, 60% of sex offenders, and 37% of assault offenders, along with

57% of men and 27% of women who committed domestic violence, had been drinking when they committed the crime. In addition, studies reported that 36% to 50% of suicides involved alcohol (Chassin & DeLucia, 1996; Kendall, 1983). It has also been suggested that alcohol tends to be related to suicides that are impulsive and that death is more likely to have resulted from gunshot wounds (Welte, Abel, & Wieczorek, 1988).

Alcohol abuse is one of New Mexico's most serious problems. New Mexico has the highest rate of alcohol-related deaths in the country, and alcohol is the leading cause of death among New Mexicans under the age of 65 and a contributor to deaths from cirrhosis, motor vehicle crashes, homicide, suicide, and some cancers (New Mexico Department of Health, 2002b). Drinking and driving (at least one time during the previous month) was reported by 70% of adults in New Mexico. This reflects not only an overall increase but also, for the first time, an increase in the percentage of women drinking and driving (National Institute on Alcohol Abuse and Alcoholism [NIAAA], 2000). The statewide rate of alcohol-involved traffic deaths at 18/100,000 is one of the highest among the states and is more than twice the national rate of 6/100,000 (New Mexico Department of Health, 2002a). New Mexico's rate of deaths from illness in which the primary cause was alcohol use is more than double the national rate, even excluding traffic deaths, suicides, and homicides (New Mexico Department of Health, 2002a). In 1998, alcohol was involved in 47% of suicides and 55% of homicides (New Mexico Department of Health, 2002a).

Although New Mexico's alcohol problems apply generally to men and women, some problems are specific to women. Nearly 44% of New Mexican women drank alcohol in the 3 months before pregnancy and 4% continued to drink in late pregnancy. There has been an increase in the incidence rate of fetal alcohol syndrome over the past 10 years. Almost one infant in a hundred has an alcohol-related health problem, and one in one thousand has fetal alcohol syndrome (FAS; New Mexico Vital Records and Health Statistics Public Health Division, 2002).

Although women have lower overall rates of alcohol abuse than their male counterparts, the number of young women with serious alcohol problems has steadily increased over the past decade (Callahan, 2001). According to the National Women's Health Information Center (2000) there are about 4.5 million women in the United States who abuse alcohol. Differences in the development and nature of alcohol problems between men and women have been identified. These differences can be attributed to biological (Copeland & Hall, 1995), psychological (O'Connor, Esherick, & Vieten, 2002), and social factors (Amaro & Hardy-Fanta, 1995).

The increasing rate of alcohol abuse among women is especially problematic in that long-term abuse of alcohol has more severe medical consequences in women than in men (Becker & Walton-Moss, 2001; Weiss, Kung, & Pearson, 2003). Women who drink may find themselves with health-related problems after fewer years of problem drinking and may become disabled for longer periods of time; they also have a 50% to 100% higher alcohol-related death rate than men (Becker & Walton-Moss, 2001; Snow & Anderson, 2000). In general, women who drink consume less alcohol and have fewer alcohol-related health problems and dependence symptoms than men (Wilsnack, Vogeltanz, Wilsnack, & Harris, 2000). However, among the heaviest drinkers, women at least equal—and, in some cases, surpass—men in the number of problems that result from their drinking (Wilsnack & Cheloha, 1987; Wilsnack & Wilsnack, 1990).

Nixon (1994) reported that neurocognitive functioning was adversely affected in women after a shorter period of drinking smaller amounts of alcohol compared to men. Moderate alcohol consumption in postmenopausal women taking estrogen replacement therapy increased the circulating estrogen levels by 300%, which can potentiate alcohol-related hepatic injury (van der Walde, Urgenson, Weltz, & Hanna, 2002; Zilberman, Tavares, Blume, & el-Guebaly, 2002). As a result of research findings such as these, Brady and Randall (1999) suggested that the course of alcohol use disorder seems to be different in women, with them progressing through the trajectory of physical and psychosocial consequences of sustained abuse over a much shorter period of time. This accelerated progression has been called "telescoping" and indicates that there is a much smaller window of opportunity for intervention before serious progression (Cook, 2004).

In the United States, more than 700,000 people are being treated for alcohol dependence on any given day; 13.5% receive inpatient care whereas 86.5% receive care in an outpatient setting (NIAAA, 2000). Treatment approaches encompass self-help programs, psychotherapy, and medications, as well as both outpatient and inpatient rehabilitation programs. However, after the initial treatment period of abstinence (not drinking alcohol), rates of relapse range from 50% to 60% within the first year and rise to 90% within 4 years of initial treatment (Connors, Maisto, & Donovan, 1996; Donovan & Chaney, 1985; Doweiko, 1990; Marlatt & Gordon, 1985; Suissa, 2003). This indicates that there is more to the recovery process than simply not drinking alcohol and that a limited focus on only "not drinking" erroneously implies that the process of recovery might be completed within a certain period of time. In contrast to this narrow view, alcohol use disorders are more often seen as chronic, with relapse behaviors involving complex biological, psychological, and sociological interactions (Helman, 2001; Kadden, 2001; Snow & Anderson, 2000).

Although the ultimate goal of recovery from alcohol abuse is to achieve a balanced lifestyle and prevent the development of unhealthy consequences (Marlatt & Gordon, 1985; Tonigan, 2001), the definition of recovery differs according to the theoretical framework being applied (Tomko, 1988). For instance, in the addiction literature, recovery is viewed as an outcome in some theories and as a process in others. In contrast, in the alcohol abuse literature, recovery includes the absence of symptoms, along with behavioral, cultural, and social changes, which creates a new lifestyle and identity (DiClemente, 2003; Marcus, 1998; Marlatt & Tapert, 1993; Marlatt & VandenBos, 1997; Morgan, 1995; Tucker, Donovan, & Marlatt, 1999). Recovery from alcohol abuse has been defined as beginning with the last drink and progressing as long as abstinence (not drinking) is maintained. When drinking behaviors begin again, a relapse is said to occur (DiClemente, 2003).

Women in recovery have higher rates of anxiety, loss of self-esteem, feelings of shame and guilt, posttraumatic stress disorder (PTSD), and depression than the general population (Anderson, Stevens, & Post, 2001; Covington, 2000; Snow, Prochaska, & Rossi, 1994). In studies of women recovering from substance abuse, findings indicate that an important component of recovery involved aspects of healing from guilt and shame, the importance of social support, and a redefinition of self-identity (Bowden, 1998; Ehrmin, 2001; Hall, 2000; Koski-Jannes, 1999; Millar & Stermac, 2000; Rush, 2002). In addition, researchers have shown that substance abuse is always a part of a bigger picture that includes individual history, socioeconomic interactions, and cultural influences that combine into an individual identity (Brown, Melchior, Panter, Slaughter, & Huba, 2000; Covington, 2002; Kearney, 1997; Rubin, Stout, & Longabaugh, 1996).

Unfortunately, much of the research on alcohol abuse treatment and recovery has a male-as-norm bias and has not adequately dealt with factors that facilitate or hinder recovery in women (Becker & Walton-Moss, 2001; Nelson-Zlupko, Dore, Kauffman, & Kaltenbach, 1995; Walton, Blow, & Booth, 2001; Wilke, 1994). In addition, research on women has tended to focus on specific populations of pregnant, postpartum, or lesbian women (Hall, 2000; Kearney, 1998). Moreover, although women continue to experience psychosocial difficulties 5 years into recovery (Weaver, Turner, & O'Dell, 2000), most recovery research has concentrated only on early recovery (less than 2 years). Though it is clear that women often relapse for different reasons than men, it is still common for women in recovery to be offered the same resources as their male counterparts (Becker & Walton-Moss, 2001; Nelson-Zlupko et al., 1995; Walton et al., 2001; Wilke, 1994).

Accordingly, research studies are needed to explore women's experiences of successful long-term recovery. Research studies focusing on the constraints and facilitating factors to successful long-term recovery in ordinary women (versus specific populations) will provide information to better inform treatment and aftercare in clinical practice.

RESEARCH DESIGN AND METHODS

This study is a focused ethnography of 21 women who have maintained long-term recovery from alcohol abuse. A focused ethnography is used to evaluate or elicit information on a special topic or shared experience (Morse & Richards, 2002). The topic is specific and is conducted with a subculture group made up of participants who share some features (Muecke, 1994). In a focused ethnography, the participants may not know each other, but the researcher focuses on common behaviors and experiences. This enables the researcher to apply the assumptions from a shared culture (Morse & Richards, 2002). This type of study is highly descriptive, and is congruent with the ideas of naturalistic inquiry, or the qualitative research orientation of studying a phenomenon in its natural state (Sandelowski, 2000).

The focus of this study was to describe, examine, and illuminate the experience of women residing along the southern New Mexico border, who have been successful in maintaining long-term recovery (greater than 24 months) from alcohol abuse. The specific aims of the study were to describe (a) the factors common to women who have achieved long-term recovery (abstinence) from alcohol abuse, (b) the situations that have contributed to sustained long-term recovery in women, and (c) the ways in which recovery has affected women's perception of themselves. The study was reviewed and approved by the IRB (CPHS) of the University of Texas Health Science Center at Houston.

Ethnographic focused interviews are used primarily to evaluate or to elicit information on a special topic or shared experience. Although descriptive studies and ethnography are generally considered atheoretical, this study used an ecological ethnographic approach as a theoretical structure. This approach situated the analysis at the level of the individual within the micro- and macro-cultures (McElroy & Jezewski, 2003). These analytical levels are defined as (a) the individual (personal identity; biogenetic/ontogenetic traits), (b) the micro-cultural (interpersonal roles and interactions; household and group traditions), and (c) the macro-cultural (cultural and transcultural systems; McElroy & Jezewski, 2003). Illness narratives are located within the individual analytic level, and support the use of observational data collection, as well as individual interviews.

Setting and Population

The setting for this study was a large geographic area of southern New Mexico, generally known as the "border area." This geographic area covers approximately 3,804 square miles, and includes a total population of approximately 256,000 individuals aggregated into many smaller communities. The ethnic makeup of the "border area" is 63% Hispanic, 32% Caucasian, 2% African American, 2% Native American, and 1% Asian (U.S. Bureau of the Census, 2000). Within this geographic area, there are three inpatient and nine outpatient treatment facilities, specifically for the treatment of alcohol abuse. In addition, each geographic community within the "border area" has at least one AA group actively meeting. One community also has a non-AA group, which meets as a support network for women in recovery from alcohol abuse. The population of interest, women in long-term recovery from alcohol abuse, was drawn from communities in New Mexico that inhabited the geographical area known as the "border area."

Sampling

Community-based purposive sampling was used to maximize the selection of participants who have experienced the phenomenon of long-term recovery. The choice was appropriate to access this hidden population of participants. Recruitment of potential participants into the study utilized two community-based key informants or "gatekeepers" who had become familiar to the principal investigator (PI) through years of professional association with the local recovering community and AA (Hammersley & Atkinson, 1995). One key informant/gatekeeper was an individual who was involved in the recovery community and provided the initial entrée for recruitment. Another key informant/gatekeeper participated in the study and shared information regarding the study among her social or interactional networks. In addition, other informants were encountered by word of mouth through the context of everyday social exchanges. These informants were identified as chance informants to differentiate them from key informants/ gatekeepers. As the study progressed, participants were specifically asked about women they knew who had not used AA in their recovery. Network sampling involves group members identifying additional members to be included in the sample (Maxwell, 1992). This allows cases of interest to be identified that are information-rich (Miles & Huberman, 1994).

Through both chance and key informants, any interested individual was given the name and contact information of the PI. Women who were over 21 years of age, with a self-reported history of alcohol abuse, and had maintained successful recovery for at least 24 months were recruited for the study. The sample of 21 participants ranged in age from 37 to 67 years and included 15 women who self-identified as White and 6 women who self-identified as Hispanic. Two of the participants were single, 14 were married, and 5 were separated or divorced. All had graduated from high school, 9 participants had some college education, and 10 participants were college graduates. Of the 10 college graduates, 4 held graduate degrees.

Data Collection

Data collection included ethnographic, focused interviews, demographic information, field notes, participant observation and a demographic survey. Fieldwork included attendance at open AA meetings, accessing articles related to state and national news about treatment and recovery, and conversations with professional contacts from the addiction field. A qualitative interview is a guided conversation, with emphasis placed on the researcher asking questions and listening carefully to the respondent's answers. In qualitative interviewing, participants are likely to be viewed as "meaning makers," rather than as passive conduits of information (Warren, 2002). Ethnographic conversational interviews are intended to elicit information and allow participants to tell stories that arise from their experiences of situations important to the study. Survey questions in an ethnographic study are intended to be "grand design" questions that elicit narratives representative of the participants' world. Experts in ethnographic research design suggest no more than three to five of these grand survey questions (Creswell, 1998; Fetterman, 1998). These questions lead to information that can then be explored through more-detailed questions. The intention is to discover new information and expand existing understanding. The ethnographic interview is informal and general but is not nondirective. The objective is to allow the PI to maintain the focus of the interview, with the participants bringing forth the dimensions they find important within the focus area (Kvale, 1996).

After written informed consent was obtained, semi-structured interviews were conducted either in the home of the participant or in the home of the PI to maintain confidentiality. The interview sites were selected by the participants. These interviews typically lasted between 1 and 2 hours and were audiotaped. Each interview began by asking participants the first grand question: Describe what it is like to be in recovery from alcohol abuse. Interviews were allowed to flow in a conversational style, with conversational probes ("Could you say something more about … ?") used to assist participants to expand or clarify ideas. The other grand questions asked were as follows: (a) What has helped you to maintain your recovery? (b) How has recovery worked for you? and (c) What does it mean to be a member of the recovering community? The interview was refocused on the specific areas of research interest as necessary.

Follow-up interviews were conducted with nine participants to further explore, saturate, or verify emerging themes. Audiotapes were reviewed by the PI for any identifying information prior to submission to a professional transcriber. Tape recordings were transcribed verbatim and validated by the PI for accuracy. Data collection concluded after 21 interviews when it became apparent that a point of redundancy had been reached and saturation of major categories established.

The PI was a psychiatric-/mental-health nurse practitioner and clinical nurse specialist, and her professional history included involvement with different aspects of the addiction and recovery community since 1987. In this capacity, she had attended many addiction conferences, provided individual and family counseling, was instrumental in facilitating inpatient treatment programs for addictions along with aftercare and partial hospitalization programs, and had facilitated support groups related to aspects of addiction and recovery. For the purposes of this study, she investigated more macro-level influences related to the social context of alcohol and alcohol abuse in New Mexico by accessing public documents and professional contacts in the addiction field to flesh out the current state of affairs in clinical and policy arenas. Furthermore, field notes were used to record aspects of the interview encounter, the immediate surroundings, and any thoughts of the PI related to analytic reflections. The field notes were recorded, categorized, and compared to the initial data for the analysis.

Data Analysis and Interpretation

Data collection and analysis occurred simultaneously. Interview data were read and analyzed for content similarities and variations. As each individual success story was read, the text was initially coded for content (e.g., social support, spirituality), and a descriptive summary was developed of the success trajectory. As specific content areas were identified within individual stories, they were grouped and regrouped using visual displays and matrices to facilitate the recognition of patterns or themes. Likewise, as patterns of trajectories became apparent in the success narratives, they provided the basis for further exploration and participant selection. Peer debriefing sessions occurred with peers experienced in qualitative research. These sessions occurred at various points throughout the data collection and analysis process, with the peers providing another level of analytical perspective and facilitating the identification of themes and synthesis of an explanatory framework. These analytic processes followed the general procedures described by Miles and Huberman for use with qualitative data (1994).

The purpose of this study was to examine and describe the common factors in successful recovery from alcohol abuse among women and to place these factors within the context of both their social networks and the larger social environment. As an ethnographic study, the focus of the analysis was on the culturally influenced norms of social relations that either constrained or facilitated successful long-term recovery from alcohol abuse. As such, the analysis of the success narratives revealed two distinct findings: (a) that women used distinct typology trajectories to achieve long-term recovery and (b) that all women articulated an overarching theme of connections as an indispensable aspect of sustained recovery.

Prior to the study, there had been concerns regarding the ability to access this hidden population on which little research had been conducted (Bowser, 1990; Braunstein, 1993). However, in reality, the women were eager to talk about their successful recovery stories. More women agreed to participate in the study than could participate, and at the end of the individual interviews, many women wanted to refer friends to be part of the study because the experience of discussing their recovery had been so important. In addition, the PI was able to access women who were not connected to the formal recovery community. The use of this sampling strategy allowed the PI to interview six Hispanic women in successful long-term recovery who were recruited into the study through a variety of informants. This was a surprising finding because the local biomedical community had many stereotyped Hispanic women as nondrinkers. In all, the 21 women who participated in this study had been in recovery from alcohol abuse over periods ranging from 2 to 28 years and had a total of 294 years of collective recovery.

In the study, 17 of the women reported a history of childhood abuse including sexual, physical, or emotional abuse; 15 of the women also reported having been in abusive adult relationships. At the beginning of the interview, women were asked to describe their successful recovery and told they could start the story wherever they wanted. Most of the women chose to tell their story in a chronological fashion. Those who did start with successful recovery later returned to the beginning of the drinking story. Although several women became tearful, all expressed feeling much better at the end of the interview. Several women later recounted the interview experience to key or chance informants, stating that they felt much better after telling their recovery success story. The interview had given them the opportunity to stop and reflect on the entire journey of successful recovery.

Recovery Typologies

Although there were distinct variations in successful achievement of long-term recovery, these variations clustered into three recovery typologies. Whereas the majority of participants (15 out of 21) used the traditional 12-step program of AA, the social significance and meaning of AA varied widely for individual women after the initial early recovery period. AA remains a pivotal focus in the lives of many women in recovery. However, for some women, AA was not a meaningful approach to successful recovery. For these women, other avenues provided the necessary therapeutic support systems that are essential to long-term abstinence.

AA is a worldwide organization that accepts new members into a culture of sobriety and socializes them into the tenets of the 12-step program. This 12-step program is promoted as a necessary component of successful recovery from alcohol abuse and is usually recommended as an adjunct to traditional treatment. Membership in the organization is voluntary and free; the only requirement is a history of alcohol abuse and the desire to stop drinking. The basic tenets are presented in the "Big Book" and the "12 Traditions," and AA members have immediate access to other members both nationally and internationally, by the use of code words, in any public setting. Members can be active at all levels of the organization or not participate any further than local meetings. The international organizational structure is sustained by voluntary contributions from its members at various levels of the hierarchical structure.

The AA 12-step program is a structured approach to abstinence and every meeting includes time for introductions, sharing stories of "hitting bottom," and finding a "lifeline" in AA The 12-step program is based on the recognition that the individual is powerless over the disease, on an acknowledged belief in a higher power, and on making amends to others for past transgressions. The need to participate in fellowship with others in recovery is a pivotal point for success. New recruits are encouraged to attend "90 meetings in 90 days," which is an intense time of socialization into the new culture of sobriety. New members must find a "sponsor" within the organization,

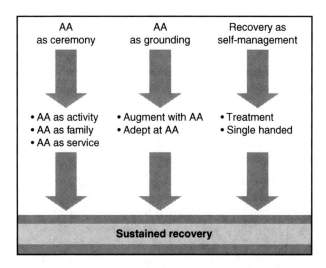

Figure 13.1 *Recovery typology and trajectories model.*

and these relationships are considered very important to successful long-term recovery.

The three typologies that were identified from the success narratives were (a) "AA as ceremony," (b) "AA as grounding," and (c) "recovery as self-management." However, within each of these typologies, variations in successful recovery were seen. These variable typologies and their trajectories (Figure 13.1) are discussed and illustrated with exemplars from the data (Table 13.1).

Table 13.1 *Exemplars From the Data Showing How a Matrix Was Used to Identify Patterns and Themes*

Condition	AA	Non-AA
Family support	#202—This is my family of choice #207—Husband in AA and knows how to help me	#216—Significant other is always there for me #218—My family just engulfed me with love
Social support	#207—All my friends are in AA #211—Need to feel connected to others	#216—Having friends is very important to recovery #218—Church is social support for me not spiritual
Spiritual support	#202—God important #202—Spiritual connection very important	#203—Spirituality helped me gain self-respect

AA as Ceremony

For the women in the AA as ceremony recovery typology, the AA meeting itself is the cornerstone of successful long-term sobriety. Coming together in the meeting with "others like me" reinforces the decision and desire not to drink. It is the attendance at the meeting that is essential to maintaining recovery in the early years, and all the women in this study who used AA had begun their success journey in this manner. Although the majority of women in this study had maintained an active involvement in the AA throughout their recovery (11 out of 21), for many of these women, the meaning of attendance and the social roles adopted in relation to the organization varied from this initial orientation. For all the women who utilized AA, the early years (1–2 years) had provided a traditional engagement in the AA environment of recovery, sometimes called "the white knuckle" time; however, differences in using AA developed as recovery progressed beyond this initial period. After the initial recovery period, the classification, AA as ceremony, branched into three different trajectories: (a) AA as activity, (b) AA as family, and (c) AA as service.

For some women, attendance at the ceremonial meeting remained the necessary ritual for maintaining sobriety and continued to be a pivotal component of their life. This trajectory was labeled AA as activity, and described someone who found it necessary to be physically present at a structured meeting for successfully maintaining long-term recovery. For these women, the agency to abstain from drinking was embodied in being physically present at the AA meeting itself. For instance, one participant attended an AA meeting at least daily as an essential factor for her long-term recovery, even after 18 years of sobriety. The AA meeting appeared to provide her an opportunity to receive daily, positive reinforcement for her decision to abstain from alcohol. For other women in the AA as ceremony typology, as they moved out of the early years of recovery, the pathway and the meaning of AA meetings shifted.

The second trajectory identified in the AA as ceremony classification was labeled AA as family, and described an individual who had shifted the meaning of attendance from a restorative focus to a meaning focus, with the focal point on the supportive network of social relations, such as those typically found within families or at church. For these women, the socialization function of the AA organization extended to dating and marrying from within the boundaries of this AA culture.

Except for occupational associations, all social relationships revolve around activities with other members of AA. For example, one woman in the study said, "AA is my family of choice." By this, she meant that she had substituted the AA community for a relationship with her family of origin. Another woman in this trajectory said, "AA is my church now," indicating that for her, AA represented both the spiritual and fellowship needs that she had previously found in attending church. For the women in this trajectory, the agency to sustain long-term recovery resided in the external support system.

The third trajectory in the AA as ceremony typology is labeled AA as service. Like the other women in this category, each woman spent her early years as a typical participant in the 12-step program. However, for these women, there was a shift: The meaning of the meeting with the focus on being a service recipient shifted to the meaning of the meeting as an opportunity for service to others. After the initial period of sobriety, women in this trajectory maintained the focus on service to others within the AA community as an integral part of their sustained recovery. This service role is reinforced as part of the 12-step program.

The AA organization provides an opportunity for service roles at the local level through sponsorship of new recruits, opening meetings, or holding a local office such as treasurer. Five of the women in this study clustered into this trajectory. Some of these women participated in service roles at higher levels of the organizational hierarchy. For instance, one woman in the study was active in writing for the national magazine. Another woman did volunteer work for both regional and national conventions. However, similar to the other trajectories, in this AA as ceremony typology, the women restricted their social networks to individuals who were part of the AA culture. The agency to sustain long-term recovery continues to reside in the organization as an external support system.

AA as Grounding

A second typology described women who were initially part of the traditional AA 12-step program for several years but then moved away from the organization, which was a significant part of their daily lives. After internalizing the philosophy and practices of the program, these women were able to move away from meeting attendance and still continue successful long-term abstinence on their own. However, these women were explicit in expressing that they still "worked" the program as part of their continued recovery. A defining feature of women in this classification, labeled AA as grounding, was that they were able to enlarge their social networks to include others outside of the AA culture. However, the social network that involved members of the AA community remained an important part of these women's lives. Women in this typology described returning to a more normal lifestyle than that of life as a "recovering" alcoholic. Within this typology, there were two different trajectories identified: (a) women who augment with AA and (b) women who become adept at AA.

The women in the first trajectory, those who augment with AA, internalized the 12-step program and eventually stopped attending AA meetings on any type of regular basis. However, these women discussed returning occasionally for "tune-ups" when they felt vulnerable to temptation. In this way, they were able to re-energize their commitment and grounding in the 12-step principles, and continued to maintain successful long-term recovery. As one of the participants described, "Returning to AA meetings when I feel vulnerable or under a lot of stress is important to me, it helps me stay sober, it allows me to see where I started, and reinforces why I don't want to drink again."

Women in this trajectory were able to integrate their social networks to include both members of the AA community and individuals who were not part of the recovery community. For instance, one woman maintained a close connection with her sponsor, but this relationship shifted to more of a reciprocal friendship than an exclusively mentor–protégé relationship. Some of these women married men from the AA community, but now neither of the spouses attended meetings. Another defining feature of these women was the ability to return to social settings where alcohol was served without jeopardizing their sobriety. As one woman explained, "I love to dance and usually there is drinking at the places where I go, but I am able to be there and not be tempted to drink, I am having such a good time dancing." For women in this trajectory, the agency to maintain long-term recovery resides to a lesser degree in the external support systems of the AA community and to a greater degree in the internalized power of individual agency.

In contrast to the women who augment with AA trajectory, women who become adept at AA trajectory were originally part of the AA community, internalized the principles and practices of the 12-step program, and then moved away from the AA community. Although the two women in this trajectory still maintained social friendships within the AA network, their day-to-day social interactions shifted to encompass a much wider circle of social relationships. For instance, one participant explained how she was now very involved with her church and had friends who now made up a larger component of her social network.

Friendships that developed from many different areas of life, including both drinkers and nondrinkers, were common to the women in this trajectory. Similar to the women in the augment with AA trajectory, being in social settings where alcohol was served was not a problem for these women. However, after the initial recovery period, these women had never felt the need to return to the AA community for any type of reinforcement. As one woman described, "Early on I picked up the good habits of AA and now they are a part of who I am." For these women, the agency to maintain long-term recovery had completely shifted from an external influence to an internalized discipline.

Recovery as Self-Management
A third typology identified women who had never used the traditional AA approach to sobriety; this classification was labeled recovery as self-management. Women in this classification either had never attended an AA meeting or had attended a few AA meetings and determined that this was not a meaningful approach for them. These women were able to maintain long-term recovery using the existing support systems in their families or larger community. Women in this classification explained that they did not feel the need to be constantly reminded of how alcohol dependency had impacted their lives. These women successfully moved back into the social roles and relationships they had had before they developed an alcohol problem. These women were also able to maintain larger social networks that included both drinkers and nondrinkers. Women in this classification did not feel that they were part of the "recovery" community—they just did not drink anymore. Within this classification, there were two different trajectories: (a) those who utilized treatment, and (b) those who achieved sobriety single-handedly.

Among the women in the treatment pathway, two used some type of inpatient treatment facility at the beginning of their recovery period and later moved to an outpatient setting for continued therapy. For other women, outpatient treatment was the only therapy they received, but the course of this treatment modality varied from 6 months to several years. Although family and friends were important features of their support systems, personal responsibility was the focus of their success narratives. As one woman explained, "I take responsibility for my behavior now; I have stopped blaming others for what I was doing." Women in this trajectory explicitly acknowledged that the responsibility to not drink was theirs and that the agency for maintaining long-term recovery was internal.

There was one woman in the study who was able to stop drinking without any type of therapy or treatment, and she exemplifies the trajectory of single-handed recovery. For this woman, recovery entailed the decision to stop drinking "cold turkey" and the internal discipline to carry through on intentions. The recognition that her drinking behavior was problematic was an essential component of recovery. Although family and friends provided an external support system, the decision and dedication to change resided within her internal control, "I made a decision to stop drinking. I did not like being out of control. Since that decision was made, I just don't drink. I enjoy being a positive role model for others in my family." The agency in this trajectory was internal.

Connections

Although all the women in this study utilized a variety of recovery trajectories, all the success narratives contained an overarching theme of connections. These connections were an important part of early recovery and had been a missing link prior to sobriety for many of these women. The women often spoke of being inexperienced at making these types of connections, both to others and to themselves. The success narratives demonstrated the powerful role that connections played in their long-term recovery, and the analyses distinguished two unifying concepts labeled (a) beyond self and (b) toward self (see Figure 13.2).

Beyond Self
The unifying concept of beyond self encompassed the connecting relationships that extended to others. However, the therapeutic support provided by these relationships went beyond unilateral emotional connections. The capacity to engage in both giving and receiving was a pivotal aspect of successful long-term recovery for the women in this study. These connections were seen to operate on several levels: transcendental (spirituality), societal (social support), and individual (pets).

The significance of spirituality in successful recovery was described in many ways by the women in this study, but encompassed belief in a higher power, a connection with nature, and finding meaning in life. For some

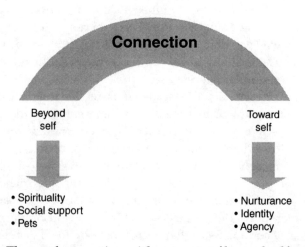

Figure 13.2 *Theme of connection with concepts of beyond self and toward self.*

women, this spiritual connection was found within an organized religion. As one participant said, "My Buddhist religion is very important to me and goes with the AA philosophy of a higher power." For other women, this spiritual connection did not involve organized religion. One participant explained, "Spirituality is important to me, but not organized church." This spiritual connection created a space for personal growth. For some of the women, this was a new belief system, whereas others returned to the spiritual roots of their past.

The importance of social support was seen as another type of connection that extended beyond self. This type of social support was often described as informal helping networks, through which concerns and problems could be addressed. These informal networks encompassed intimate partners, extended family relations, and friendships.

For instance, one participant particularly credited her husband for the support necessary to achieve successful recovery: "My husband is very supportive and also in recovery." Other women referred to their children as either providing support or as the impetus to remain sober. These supportive social networks enhanced the ability for behavioral change and personal growth, and were instrumental in dispelling feelings of isolation. As one participant said, "I feel like I belong to the group, and this is very important to my recovery."

An unanticipated finding of this study was the importance of pets to successful recovery. Of the 21 women interviewed for this study, 19 had at least one pet, one woman had just recently lost her pet, and the one woman who did not have pets was allergic to animal dander. The women were explicit in describing the therapeutic benefits of pet ownership in reducing anxiety, providing comfort, and presenting companionship. As one woman said, "The unconditional affection from my animals makes a difference in my life today." Another woman spoke of her pets as "always being there for me," and of how this emotional connection played an important part in her successful long-term recovery. Other women described the therapeutic benefits of having something that depended on them and of finding healing in the nurturance of others. One woman even said, "I do not trust people who do not have animals in their life."

Toward Self

In contrast to connections that extended beyond the self, there was also a strong unifying concept that described the internal connections made by women in successful long-term recovery. This unifying concept was labeled toward self, and encompassed the reflexive journey that the women experienced. This reflexive journey involved a critical examination of both the feelings and behaviors of the past and present. The three types of connections identified that were directed toward self included nurturance, identity, and agency.

Women in successful long-term recovery explicitly recognized the need for self-nurturance. The ability to honor their personal needs and care for themselves was often described as an important aspect of recovery. As one participant stated, "I had to learn to take care of myself physically and mentally." To do this required a continual process of self-reflection related to both thoughts and emotions. Many women described how they used a technique learned in AA, commonly referred to as HALT (hungry, angry, lonely, or tired). This acronym is used to help AA members more accurately assess their emotional reactions and, thereby, select more appropriate behavioral responses than turning to alcohol as a coping mechanism. Women particularly described these self-nurturance tasks as an ability to maintain balance and focus the correct amount of energy on tasks, based on the corresponding importance given to values and goals. This type of recognition and need for balance often resulted in "saying no when I need to." In addition, these aspects of self-nurturance extended to care of the physical body, as many women spoke of the need to eat right, get enough sleep, and exercise as an essential component in successful long-term recovery.

Another aspect of the reflexive journey toward self-discovery involved aspects of identity. Women in this study described this as a process of awareness of who they were and of what their place was in the world. Some of the women talked of becoming "normal," and of now being able to fulfill legitimized social roles within the confines of the larger society. For some women, this was described as a reclaiming of an identity that had been lost. For instance, one woman said, "I have changed a lot, but the core person of who I am is still the same as before." For others, aspects of identity still revolved around alcohol. As an example, one participant described that she "needed to incorporate the addict but not the bad behavior" into a new identity of who she was.

Finally, the reflexive journey toward self involved a critical examination of agency in the process of successful long-term recovery. Women in successful long-term recovery described having the power to implement and sustain meaningful change, even when this agency invested the power externally. For instance, this was exemplified by the case of the woman who maintained successful recovery by attending daily AA meetings, even after 18 years of sobriety. This example illustrated someone who had identified the self-agency for independent behavior, but placed the power for maintaining successful recovery in an external other. As this woman points out, "I owe my sobriety to attending AA meetings, which is what keeps me from drinking one day at a time." At the other end of the agency continuum were the women who successfully achieved and maintained long-term recovery by placing the power internally. One woman said, "I found the power to make changes in my behaviors . . . I am responsible for my actions." However, no matter where women placed the power for successfully sustaining long-term recovery, each success narrative addressed the individual agency in the healing process that led to a more balanced, productive life.

DISCUSSION

The purpose of this study was to examine and describe the common factors in successful recovery from alcohol abuse among women and to place these factors within the context of both their social networks and the larger social environment. The findings from this ethnographic study suggest that women utilize distinct trajectories to achieve long-term recovery. Recovery typologies were developed, and the three typologies that were identified from the success narratives were AA as ceremony, AA as grounding, and recovery as self-management. In addition, this study found an overarching theme of connections that was a pivotal component of successful long-term recovery from alcohol abuse.

This analysis of the success narratives of women in long-term recovery revealed that although the majority (15 out of 21) of women used AA as a component of their long-term recovery, the meaning and social roles within the context of the organizational structure of AA varied after the early recovery stage. For all these women, the first year or two of early sobriety utilized the traditional, structured 12-step program of AA. However, after this early period, many of the women shifted out of this traditional social neophyte role and into a variety of trajectories that changed the meaning of AA to their well-being. This finding is new to the addiction literature.

Congruent with this study, similar research on women and substance abuse has also found that healing from guilt and shame, social support, and a redefinition of self-identity are all important components of recovery (Bowden, 1998; Ehrmin, 2001; Hall, 2000; Koski-Jannes & Turner, 1999; Millar & Stermac, 2000; Rush 2002). However, most of these studies have focused only on the early years of recovery, sampled only from the AA community, or only attended to special populations of women in recovery (Brudenell, 1996; Chappel, 1993; Hall, 1990; Kearney, 1998).

In addition, previous research has shown that addiction is always a part of a bigger picture that includes history, socioeconomic interactions, and cultural influences, which combine into an individual identity (Brown et al., 2000; Covington, 2002; Kearney, 1997; Rubin et al., 1996). Whereas some of the women in this study talked about a changed identity (from alcoholic to ex-alcoholic), there was an equal number of women who described a redis-covering of a core self. This change in the definition of self is similar to other findings from a sample of substance abusers and people experiencing role changes (Ebaugh, 1988; Marcus, 1998).

An unexpected finding of this study was the importance that animals played in successful long-term recovery. The literature suggests that pets can have a positive impact on one's health (Brenda, 2004; Hooker, Freeman, & Stewart, 2002; Jennings, 1997; Roenke & Mulligan, 1998; Sable, 1995). Whereas some studies found that patients involved in psychotherapy related positively to a pet and demonstrated improved coping and social interactions, other studies have shown that the presence of companion animals reduced auto-nomic reactivity (Baun, Oetting, & Bergstrom, 1991). Some studies involved companion animals and the elderly, and reported decreases in problem-atic behaviors in those with Alzheimer's disease (McCabe, Baun, Speich, & Agrawal, 2002) and an increase in social support for community-dwelling elders (Raina, Waltner-Toews, Bonnett, Woodward, & Abernathy, 1999). One study reported on the use of animals to promote abstinence from addictions and utilized a companion dog during inpatient treatment (Campbell-Begg, 2000). The results of this study showed an improved self-image and enhanced transactions between the patients and nurses in a treatment setting.

Clinical Implications

This study has important practical applications. First, the importance of asking about recovery and recognizing the experiences of women who have achieved successful long-term recovery from alcohol abuse is demonstrated in this research. In this study, the women reported that the telling of their success stories was very helpful to them, and that they had not reflected on their success journey before. Even those active in AA only looked at the "drunkathon" story during meetings, which included the story of hitting bottom and then finding AA, and of where they are now. But it did not focus on what was helping them to stay in recovery. For clinicians, this information can be useful as they interact with women in recovery and ask them to share the strategies that are helping them to maintain success. One of the chance informants reported that telling the success story had moved her patient into productive therapy sessions. On being asked what had made the difference, the participant stated that when she had reflected on the success journey, she felt more empowered to deal with other issues in her life.

The telling of the success story with a focus on the current strategies being used by the women can be referred to as "regrounding in success." Facilitating this "regrounding in success" story for women in recovery assists clinicians in recognizing what is working in the women's lives to maintain long-term recovery. This can be accomplished during clinical interactions by asking clients who are in recovery to share what is helping them stay there, and thus allowing them the opportunity to tell their success story. One way this can happen is by clinicians inquiring about patients' drinking history even after checking that they do not drink; the follow-up questions could be to ask if they ever drank, why they stopped, and when they stopped. Then, if patients are identified as being in recovery, clinicians can ask them to describe what they are doing to maintain their sobriety, thus giving them a chance to share what is working for them and to be recognized for what they have achieved.

Study Limitations

The data generated are limited by the participants' possible inability to articulate all relevant aspects of the recovery experience. One limitation of the study involves the fact that the topic complexity may obscure transferability.

Recommendations for Future Research

More research is needed in the area of long-term recovery from alcohol abuse. Findings from this study show that there are several paths that women use during the journey of long-term recovery. Further exploration of the typology that does not use AA may yield information helpful to clinicians in primary care practices. This information may provide the background for other studies to develop clinical tools to capture the identified components of this recovery process. Future research to investigate the role of companion animals in the recovery process is also needed. This area of research could have implications for both treatment and recovery programs.

REFERENCES

Amaro, H., & Hardy-Fanta, C. (1995). Gender relations in addiction and recovery. *Journal of Psychoactive Drugs, 27*, 325–337.

Anderson, M., Stevens, M., & Post, K. (2001). Sex-role strain in alcoholic women. *Substance Use & Misuse, 36*, 653–662.

Baun, M. M., Oetting, K., & Bergstrom, N. (1991). Health benefits of companion animals in relation to the physiologic indices of relaxation. *Holistic Nursing Practice, 5*(2), 16–23.

Becker, K. & Walton-Moss, B. (2001). Detecting and addressing alcohol abuse in women. *The Nurse Practitioner, 26*(10), 13–22.

Bowden, J. (1998). Recovery from alcoholism: A spiritual journey. *Mental Health Nursing, 19*, 337–352.

Bowser, B. J. (1990). AIDS and "hidden populations." *Multicultural Inquiry and Research on AIDS, 4*, 1–2.

Brady, K., & Randall, C. (1999). Gender differences in substance use disorders. *Addictive Disorders, 22*, 241–251.

Braunstein, M. S. (1993). Sampling a hidden population: Noninstitutionalized drug users. *AIDS Education and Prevention, 5*, 131–140.

Brenda, W. (2004). The therapeutic nature of the human/animal bond: Implications for integrative public health. *Integrative Medicine: A Clinician's Journal, 3*(3), 26–30.

Brown, V., Melchior, L., Panter, A., Slaughter, R., & Huba, G. (2000). Women's steps of change and entry into drug abuse treatment: A multidimensional stages of change model. *Journal of Substance Abuse Treatment, 18*, 231–240.

Brudenell, I. (1996). A grounded theory of balancing alcohol recovery and pregnancy. *Western Journal of Nursing Research, 18*, 429–440.

Callahan, J. (2001). *Alcohol use and abuse*. Boston, MA: Harvard Medical School.

Campbell-Begg, T. (2000). A case study using animal-assisted therapy to promote abstinence in a group of individuals who are recovering from chemical addictions. *Journal of Addictions Nursing, 12*(1), 31–35.

Chappel, J. N. (1993). Long-term recovery from alcoholism. *Psychiatric Clinics of North America, 16*, 177–187.

Chassin, L., & DeLucia, C. (1996). Drinking during adolescence. *Alcohol Health and Research World, 20*, 175–180.

Connors, G., Maisto, S., & Donovan, D. (1996). Conceptualizations of relapse: A summary of psychological and psychobiological models. *Addiction, 91*, S5–S13.

Cook, L. J. (2004). Educating women about the hidden dangers of alcohol. *Journal of Psychosocial Nursing, 42*(6), 24–31.

Copeland, J., & Hall, W. (1995). *Women and drug dependence: An overview for clinicians, policy makers and researchers (Monograph Number 23)*. Sydney: University of New South Wales, National Drug and Alcohol Research Center.

Covington, S. (2000). Helping women recover: A comprehensive integrated treatment model. *Alcoholism Treatment Quarterly, 18*(3), 99–103.

Covington, S. (2002). Helping women recover: Creating gender responsive treatment. In S. L. A. Straussner & S. Brown (Eds.), *The handbook of addiction treatment for women: Theory and practice* (pp. 52–72). San Francisco, CA: Jossey-Bass.

Creswell, J. W. (1998). *Qualitative inquiry and research design.* Thousand Oaks, CA: Sage.

DiClemente, C. C. (2003). *Addiction and change: How addictions develop and addicted people recover.* New York, NY and London, UK: Guilford Press.

Donovan, D., & Chaney, E. F. (1985). *Alcoholic relapse prevention and intervention: Models and methods.* New York, NY: Guilford Press.

Doweiko, H. E. (1990). *Concepts of chemical dependency.* Pacific Grove, CA: Brooks/Cole.

Ebaugh, H. (1988). *Becoming an Ex: The process of role exit.* Chicago, IL: The University of Chicago Press.

Ehrmin, J. (2001). Unresolved feelings of guilt and shame in the maternal role with substance-dependent African American women. *Journal of Nursing Scholarship, 33*(1), 47–52.

Fetterman, D. M. (1998). *Ethnography: Step by step* (2nd ed.). Thousand Oaks, CA: Sage.

Gordis, E. (2001). Improving the old, embracing the new: Implications of alcohol research for future practice. *Social Work in Health Care, 33*(1) 17–41.

Hall, J. (2000). Core issues for female child abuse survivors in recovery from substance misuse. *Qualitative Health Research, 10,* 612–631.

Hall, J. M. (1990). Alcoholism recovery in lesbian women: A theory in development. *Scholarly Inquiry for Nursing Practice: An International Journal, 4*(2), 109–122.

Hammersley, M. & Atkinson, P. (1995). *Ethnography: Principles in practice* (2nd ed.). New York, NY: Routledge.

Helman, C. G. (2001). *Culture, health, and illness* (4th ed.). New York, NY: Arnold.

Hooker, S. D., Freeman, L. H., & Stewart, P. (2002). Pet therapy research: A historic review. *Holistic Nursing Practice, 16*(5), 17–23.

Jennings, L. B. (1997). Potential benefits of pet ownership in health promotion. *Journal of Holistic Nursing, 15,* 358–372.

Kadden, R. (2001). Behavioral and cognitive-behavioral treatments for alcoholism research opportunities. *Addictive Behaviors, 26,* 489–507.

Kearney, M. (1997). Drug treatment for women: Traditional models and new directions. *Journal of Obstetric, Gynecologic, & Neonatal Nursing, 26,* 459–468.

Kearney, M. (1998). Truthful self-nurturing: A grounded formal theory of women's addiction recovery. *Qualitative Health Research, 8,* 495–512.

Kendall, R. E. (1983). Alcohol and suicide. *Substance and Alcohol Actions/Misuse, 4,* 121–127.

Koski-Jannes, A., & Turner, N. (1999). Factors influencing recovery from different addictions. *Addiction Research, 7,* 469–492.

Kvale, S. (1996). *Interviews: An introduction to qualitative research interviewing.* Thousand Oaks, CA: Sage.

Madden, S. K., Montoya, I. D., & Richard, A. J. (1995). Impact of substance abuse on tomorrow's workforce. *Clinical Laboratory Science, 8,* 107–112.

Marcus, M. T. (1998). Changing careers: Becoming clean and sober in a therapeutic community. *Qualitative Health Research, 8*, 466–481.

Marlatt, G. A., & Gordon, J. (Eds.). (1985). *Relapse prevention: Maintenance strategies in the treatment of addictive behaviors.* New York, NY: Guilford Press.

Marlatt, G. A., & Tapert, S. F. (1993). Harm reduction: Reducing the risks of addictive behaviors. In J. S. Baer, G. A. Marlatt, & R. J. McMahon (Eds.), *Addictive behaviors across the life span: Prevention, treatment, and policy issues* (pp. 243–273). Newbury, CA: Sage.

Marlatt, G. A., & VandenBos, G. R. (Eds.). (1997). *Addictive behaviors: Readings on etiology, prevention, and treatment.* Washington, DC: American Psychological Association.

Maxwell, J. A. (1992). Understanding and validity in qualitative research. *Harvard Educational Review, 62*, 279–300.

McCabe, B. W., Baun, M. M., Speich, D., & Agrawal, S. (2002). Resident dog in the Alzheimer's special care unit. *Western Journal of Nursing Research, 24*, 684–696.

McElroy, A., & Jezewski, M. A. (2003). Cultural variation in the experience of health and illness. In G. L. Albrecht, R. Fitzpatrick, & S. C. Scrimshaw (Eds.), *The handbook of social studies in health and medicine* (pp. 191–209). Thousand Oaks, CA: Sage.

Miles, M. B. & Huberman, A. M. (1994). *Qualitative data analysis* (2nd ed.). Thousand Oaks, CA: Sage.

Millar, G. M., & Stermac, L. (2000). Substance abuse and childhood maltreatment: Conceptualizing the recovery process. *Journal of Substance Abuse Treatment, 19*, 175–182.

Morgan, O. (1995). Extended length of sobriety: The missing variable. *Alcoholism Treatment Quarterly, 12*(1), 59–71.

Morse, J. M., & Richards, L. (2002). *Read me first: For a user's guide to qualitative research.* Thousand Oaks, CA: Sage.

Muecke, M. A. (1994). On the evaluation of ethnographies. In J. M. Morse (Ed.), *Critical issues in qualitative research methods* (pp. 187–209). Thousand Oaks, CA: Sage.

National Institute on Alcohol Abuse and Alcoholism (NIAAA). (2000). *Tenth special report to the U.S. Congress on alcohol and health.* Washington, DC: U.S. Department of Health and Human Services.

National Women's Health Information Center. (2000). *Alcohol abuse and treatment.* Retrieved June 18, 2004, from http://www.4woman.org/fag/sa-alcoh.htm

Nelson-Zlupko, L., Dore, M., Kauffman, E., & Kaltenbach, K. (1995). Women in recovery: Their perceptions of treatment effectiveness. *Journal of Substance Abuse Treatment, 13*, 51–59.

New Mexico Department of Health. (2002a). *State of health in New Mexico 2002 report.* Santa Fe, NM: Author.

New Mexico Department of Health. (2002b). *Vision of health in New Mexico.* Santa Fe, NM: Author.

New Mexico Vital Records and Health Statistics Public Health Division. (2002). *New Mexico women's health profile 2001.* Santa Fe, NM: New Mexico Department of Health.

Nixon, S. J. (1994). Alcohol and female sexuality: A look at expectancies and risk. *Alcohol Health and Research World, 18*, 228–231.

O'Connor, L. E., Esherick, M., & Vieten, C. (2002). Drug- and alcohol-abusing women. In S. L. A. Strausner & S. Brown (Eds.), *The handbook of addiction treatment for women* (pp. 75–98). San Francisco, CA: Jossey-Bass.

Raina, P., Waltner-Toews, D., Bonnett, B., Woodward, C., & Abernathy, T. (1999). Influence of companion animals on the physical and psychological health of older people: An analysis of a one-year longitudinal study. *Journal of the American Geriatrics Society, 47*, 323–329.

Rice, D. P., Miller, L. S., & Dunmeyer, S. (1990). *The economic cost of alcohol and drug abuse and mental illness* (DHHS Publication ADM 90-19). Rockville, MD: Alcohol, Drug Abuse, and Mental Health Administration.

Robbins, L. K. (2004). Women's ways of recovery: An ethnography of sustained sobriety. *A focused ethnographic study of women in recovery from alcohol abuse.* (Doctoral dissertation). *Texas Medical Center Dissertations (via ProQuest).* Paper AAI3166187. http://digitalcommons.library.tmc.edu/dissertations/AAI3166187

Roenke, L., & Mulligan, S. (1998). The therapeutic value of the human-animal connection. *Occupational Therapy in Health Care, 11*(2), 27–43.

Rubin, A., Stout, R., & Longabaugh, R. (1996). Gender differences in relapse situations. *Addiction, 91*(Suppl), S111–S120.

Rush, M. (2002). Perceived social support: Dimensions of social interaction among sober female participants in Alcoholics Anonymous. *Journal of the American Psychiatric Nurses Association, 8*, 114–119.

Sable, P. (1995). Pets, attachment, and well-being across the life cycle. *Social Work, 40*, 334–341.

Sandelowski, M. (2000). Whatever happened to qualitative description? *Research in Nursing and Health, 23*, 334–340.

Snow, D., & Anderson, C. (2000). Exploring the factors influencing relapse and recovery among drug- and alcohol-addicted women. *Journal of Psychosocial Nursing, 38*(7), 8–19.

Snow, M., Prochaska, J., & Rossi, J. (1994). Processes of change in Alcoholics Anonymous: Maintenance factors in long-term sobriety. *Journal of Studies on Alcohol, 55*, 362–371.

Suissa, A. J. (2003). Alcoholism as a disease in North America: A critical social analysis. *Journal of Addictions Nursing, 14*, 201–208.

Tomko, M. K. (1988). Recovery: A multidimensional process. *Issues in Mental Health Nursing, 9*, 139–149.

Tonigan, S. J. (2001). Benefits of Alcoholics Anonymous attendance: Replication of findings between clinical research sites in Project MATCH. *Alcoholism Treatment Quarterly, 19*, 67–77.

Tucker, J. A., Donovan, D. M., & Marlatt, G. A. (1999). *Changing addictive behavior: Bridging clinical and public health strategies.* New York, NY: Guilford Press.

U.S. Bureau of the Census. (2000). Retrieved April 14, 2004, from www.census.gov

U.S. Department of Health and Human Services (USDHHS). (2000). *Healthy People 2010: Understanding and improving health.* Washington, DC: U.S. Government Printing Office.

van der Walde, H., Urgenson, F. T., Weltz, S. H., & Hanna, F. J. (2002). Women and alcoholism: A biopsychosocial perspective and treatment approaches. *Journal of Counseling and Development, 80*, 145–153.

Walton, M., Blow, F., & Booth, B. (2001). Diversity in relapse prevention needs: Gender and race among substance abuse treatment patients. *American Journal of Drug and Alcohol Abuse, 27*, 225–240.

Warren, C. (2002). Qualitative interviewing. In J. Gubrium& J. Holstein (Eds.), *Handbook of interview research: Context and method* (pp. 83–102). Thousand Oaks, CA: Sage.

Weaver, G. D., Turner, N. H., & O'Dell, K. J. (2000). Depressive symptoms, stress, and coping among women recovering from addiction. *Journal of Substance Abuse Treatment, 18*, 161–167.

Weiss, S., Kung, H. C., & Pearson, J. L. (2003). Emerging issues in gender and ethnic differences in substance abuse treatment. *Current Women's Health Reports, 3*, 245–253.

Welte, J. W., Abel, E. L., & Wieczorek, W. (1988). The role of alcohol in suicides in Erie County, NY, 1972–1984. *Public Health Reports, 103*, 648–652.

Wilke, D. (1994). Women and alcoholism: How a male-as-norm bias affects research, assessment, and treatment. *Health & Social Work, 19*(1), 29–35.

Wilsnack, R., & Cheloha, R. (1987). Women's roles and problem drinking across the lifespan. *Social Problems, 3*, 231–248.

Wilsnack, R., Vogeltanz, N., Wilsnack, S., & Harris, T. (2000). Gender differences in alcohol consumption and adverse drinking consequences: Cross-cultural patterns. *Addiction, 95*, 251–265.

Wilsnack, S., & Wilsnack, R. (1990). Women and substance abuse: Research directions for the 1990s. *Psychology of Addictive Behaviors, 4*, 46–49.

Zilberman, M., Tavares, H., Blume, S., & el-Guebaly, N. (2002). Toward best practices in the treatment of women with addictive disorders. *Addictive Disorders and Their Treatment, 1*(2), 39–46.

Chapter Fourteen

Personal Privacy and Interactional Patterns in a Nursing Home

Mary Applegate and Janice M. Morse

What a disgrace to be seen crying by that fat Doris. The door of my room has no lock. They say it is because I might be taken ill in the night, and then how could they get in to tend me (*tend*—as though I were a crop, a cash crop). So they may enter my room any time they choose. Privacy is a privilege not granted to the aged or the young (Laurence, 1967, p. 4).

Respect for an individual's privacy is considered a routine part of nursing care, a moral obligation, and, in some situations, a legal requirement of institutional health care. Despite this, the role and responsibilities of providing care dictate that the cultural norm of privacy be violated, and often individuals who are institutionalized feel that privacy norms are not respected (as noted in the *dictum*: "Leave your modesty at the front desk"). In particular, the loss of privacy is significant when elderly persons are admitted to nursing homes, where they are likely to become permanent and often dependent residents.

Loss of privacy may have serious consequences for an individual. The maintenance of privacy allows for a feeling of personal control and the expressing of autonomy, an opportunity for quiet reflection and self-evaluation, and a release from societal expectations and the situational context for sharing personal information (Westin, 1967). Conflict occurs when circumstances inherent to institutional living make the maintenance of privacy difficult, if not impossible. The very nature of the relationship between staff members and residents requires staff members to assume responsibility for caring for residents' intimate personal functions, and many of these care activities are often carried out in areas shared with other residents in the ward (e.g., in a common shower or tub room). The legal implications of supervising residents in self-care activities require staff to have easy access to residents' rooms and communal areas. Deteriorating cognitive and physical functions that accompany old age include the often accurate assumption that the elderly may no longer be able to make informed and responsible decisions or to perform daily tasks without assistance; therefore, although actions to protect residents' privacy are viewed as important, staff members may passively accept the premise that privacy as a right and as a norm is not feasible with the roles and responsibilities of staff for "getting the work done." Hence, privacy norms defined by the dominant culture are redefined in the professional caregiving relationship between the nurse and the patient. Therefore, in this chapter, we define *respect for an individual's right to privacy* as valuing and respecting the individual as a *person*, and respecting individual rights and property within the confines of institutional life.

Despite the suggested importance of privacy for the well-being of all individuals and particularly the well-being of nursing home residents, the literature describing the phenomenon is largely descriptive. Only a few concrete suggestions are offered for improving the maintenance of privacy for residents of nursing homes, for example, protecting the patient's modesty or possessions. This research has been largely conducted from the perspective of the investigator using a proscriptive inventory or checklist of acts or incidents that may constitute a violation of privacy, but this approach has contributed little to our understanding of the causes underlying the problem. Clearly, there was a need to investigate the problem differently, using research methods that consider the context and behavioral norms of the setting, so that a new perspective of the concept of privacy and privacy maintenance could be obtained.

REVIEW OF THE LITERATURE

There is a lack of agreement regarding the essential nature of the concept of privacy. The word privacy is derived from the Latin word *privatus,* meaning withdrawn or apart from public, peculiar to oneself, or belonging to an individual (Hoad, 1986). Theoretically, it has been described as a feeling (Bates, 1964), as a right (Westin, 1967), as a state (Boone, 1983; Kelvin, 1973), or as a freedom (Halmos, 1953). Other writers have suggested that privacy can be conceptualized as a process of control, but they disagree on whether the control is over personal transactions (Margulis, 1977), access to self (Altman, 1975), or personal information related to one's identity. These control definitions have been criticized because they define the process of attaining privacy rather than the meaning of privacy (Garrett, 1974). However, these definitions are useful in establishing moral or legalistic claims to privacy (Greenawalt, 1974) as well as in providing a conceptual basis for identifying culturally normative behaviors in North American culture associated with privacy maintenance.

The discussion of privacy has revolved around two important questions: Is privacy attainment an individual's right, or is privacy derived from other interests? (Benn, 1971; Blple, 1984; Gross, 1971; Prosser, 1984; Simmel, 1971; Warren & Brandeis, 1980). The concept of human dignity and the autonomous nature of humans are inherent in many of these discussions. Privacy has been considered an important component of the development and maintenance of a sense of self (Reiman, 1976). The ability to selectively disclose information that reveals the real self is instrumental in the development of relationships (Beardsley, 1971; Henderson, 1975).

Westin (1967) identifies four main states of privacy: solitude (or the ability to withdraw or be alone), anonymity (when there is a separation of the social identity and the action), intimacy (relaxed and frank relationships are developed with some by exercising corporate seclusion of others), and reserve (when psychological withdrawal or nonparticipation creates a psychological barrier against unwanted intrusion; Henderson, 1975; Schuster, 1972, 1976a, 1976b; Schwartz, 1968; Westin, 1967).

Although important, these four states of privacy add little to our knowledge about the context of privacy maintenance or our understanding of privacy violation. It is clear that privacy is a culturally defined concept that is dependent on context and situation. As an abstract concept, privacy cannot be observed per se; one may observe *violations of the privacy norm*, but only if one first learns what that norm *is* in a given context. While the dominant culture may adhere to certain cultural rules or patterns for respecting the privacy of others, exceptions to these rules may be condoned, accepted, and expected in designated settings or situations. Thus, privacy is a culturally defined and abstract concept that is situation-dependent.

The nursing home setting is one such "exception" to the norm of the dominant culture. For example, while it is accepted that a young female in the role of a nurse may ask an elderly male resident if his bowels have moved that day or assist him with toileting, such actions would be accepted with shock or horror outside of the nursing home setting. Yet, despite the culturally condoned (and essential) reformulation of boundaries in the professional caretaking nurse–patient relationship, many researchers have noted that even these reformulated privacy norms are often not respected and frequently violated in nursing home settings. In addition, despite the culturally condoned and necessary reformulation of boundaries in the caretaking nurse–patient relationship, norms in the nursing home subculture are not described; hence, violations of these norms are poorly understood.

One contributing factor is undoubtedly related to the architectural structure of the building. Roosa (1981) notes that nursing home residents unanimously select solitude or aloneness as the definition of privacy, and he speculates that this is because of the residents' loss of private space. As illustrated in Laurence's (1967) quotation at the beginning of this chapter, the structure of providing care, although essential for physical well-being, may be considered a psychological violation. Thus, there is a need for further investigation and development of this important concept.

METHODS

Investigation into the nature and rationale of privacy *as a concept* must be conducted inductively. Although indicators of privacy violations or respect may be observed in a checklist fashion, these checklists add little to our theoretical understanding of privacy *as a concept.* Furthermore, because of its conceptual nature, the *a priori* development of an observational schedule, a checklist, or set of interview questions necessarily leads to a deductive approach, which in qualitative inquiry threatens validity. Therefore, the concept of privacy was "bracketed" or put aside and the basic premise of participant observation held, and the setting was entered without a preconceived framework. However, once the observational phase of the research was completed and some interviews had been conducted, data were analyzed to ascertain the antecedents, causes, and conditions involved in respect for or violation of an individual's privacy.

How then is an abstract concept investigated? We suggest that the most valid way is to observe it in the setting until normative behaviors are understood *in context.* By becoming a part of the setting as a nonparticipant observer (i.e., an observer who does not blend into the setting by using a work or participant role), the investigator may be able to record normal behaviors as they occur in the day-to-day setting. Analysis of these behaviors within the framework of an abstract concept adds insights that would be obtained through interviews or by using checklists.[1]

Setting

Data were collected in a 75-bed unit of a veteran's home in a large Canadian city, over a 6-month period. The residence was a spacious single story brick building, with large windows reaching to the floor. The unit contained several day areas with chairs around the periphery, and these areas had a television that was usually turned on. Residents' rooms were mostly shared, with two residents per room; there were only two single-bed and two four-bed rooms. The facility had a large "activities" room and a dining room, but there was a lack of space where a resident could be alone, if desired. Although the unit was connected to another unit of similar size, there was infrequent mingling of the residents, and the residents from each unit had their meals in the dining room separately.

The residents were all male, had been members of the Canadian Armed Forces, and had served in active duty overseas, primarily in the Second World War or the Korean War.[2] The ages of the men ranged from 64 to 102 years. Five men were 64 years of age, 35 men were between 65 and 74 years of age, 14 men were between 75 and 85 years of age, and 17 men were over 85 years of age. The residents had a variety of physical and mental conditions that resulted in their institutionalization. Written consent for participation was obtained from the institution, the staff, and most of the residents. If a resident was considered impaired and unable to give consent, permission was obtained from that resident and consent obtained from his legal guardian. If a resident did not wish to participate in the study, then the researcher left the area whenever the resident made an appearance.

Approximately one half of the men were considered mentally competent, and two thirds of the residents required wheelchairs for mobility. Many of the men had a history of alcohol abuse prior to their admission. The level of care required by the residents ranged from minimal to total care, and their length of stay at the facility ranged from newly admitted to 24 years. In addition to ethical clearance obtained from the university and hospital Human Subjects' Committees, permission was obtained from the Residents' Committee and individually from all residents, and the staff knew of the nature and purpose of the study. Only one resident refused to participate, and observations were not conducted when he was present.

Data Collection

The primary method of data collection, nonparticipant observation, allowed the observation of the setting and resident activity from the perspective of those within the setting and without the work role interfering with the process of data collection. The researcher was not a staff member and was not involved in the actual care activity, with the exception of providing minimal assistance with bed-making and meals. On the unit, short periods of observation were conducted, after which the researcher left the setting to record brief handwritten notes about observations and informal interactions.

These notes were expanded into field notes at the end of the day. Personal feelings, impressions, and hunches were recorded in a separate diary. Observations were made from a variety of settings within the facility, including the sunroom, coffee shop, arts and crafts room, desk area, front hallway, dining room, corridors, and residents' rooms. During these periods of observation, information conversations with residents and staff members often took place. These conversations allowed the researcher to confirm observations with participants and to verify tentative patterns or themes. The researcher participated as an observer in regularly scheduled occupational and physical therapy sessions, recreational activities, and special events. Staff members also included the researcher in their organized events.

Most of the information was collected through observations and informal conversations with the informants. Formal interviews were conducted with the primary informants *later* in the study, and they were guided by the use of broad, descriptive, open-ended questions to obtain the residents' perspective of normal life at the facility. The focus of the interviews was on the daily lives and activities of the residents. Prompts such as asking for descriptions of routines or changes in the lifestyles and care activities of residents were often required, and these descriptions were later analyzed to determine the circumstances under which privacy violations occurred. Interviews were conducted either in the resident's room or in an office adjacent to the unit. Formal interviews were taperecorded and transcribed for coding and analysis. The interview tapes were numerically coded to ensure anonymity.

Once analysis commenced, other residents and staff were interviewed on an ongoing basis to confirm the findings and to ensure validity. A model that best fit the concept of privacy was developed, and this model was verified with the other staff.

RESULTS

The most striking feature of the unit was the absence of conversation among the residents. Although mentally competent residents sat together within a comfortable conversational distance, they normally sat in silence. Many of the men appeared to ignore others in the unit, passing them in the corridor without verbal or even nonverbal acknowledgment. Only two or three of the residents did not consistently conform to this pattern, and every day, they circulated around all the residents, conversing and exchanging small talk. The response of the less communicative residents to those who made the effort to chat with them was varied. Some responded with enthusiasm, some were more reticent, and others acknowledged the greeting with a wave or a nod. The overall "tone of the unit was cordial, with reserved cooperation among residents."

Types of Interactions in Relation to Privacy

Analysis of the residents' interrelationships revealed three kinds of interactions, and the respect for the individuals' right to privacy was consistent with the way they perceived each other. The first type of interaction was labeled *as a friend* relationship; there was recognition of the person as a unique individual with specific qualities or characteristics. The second type of interaction was labeled *as a stranger* and reflected a relationship that was depersonalized and in which no attempt was made to acknowledge the uniqueness of the person. In the *as a stranger* interaction, the interaction was rote, infrequent, and lacked warmth. The third type of interaction was labeled *as an object* and reflected a relationship where the resident was dehumanized and interactions were impersonal, where individuals were spoken *at* rather than spoken *to*. In the *as an object* interaction, it was as though the person who was the object of the interaction was not present. In the interaction *as a friend,* there was an acknowledgment of the individuality of each person and a recognition of his right to self-determination. This characteristic was less apparent in the *as a stranger* mode of interaction, and it appeared to be absent in the *as an object* mode of interaction.

Four routes of interaction were identified that directly or indirectly involved residents. They were resident to resident, resident to staff, staff to resident, and staff to staff. The descriptions of each of the three interaction *patterns* (i.e., as a friend, as a stranger, or as an object) are discussed for each communication route. As patterns of interaction become increasingly dehumanized, respect for the person as an individual is lost, and privacy norms are disregarded (see Table 14.1). Therefore, we suggest that privacy is best understood within the context of understanding the nature of interaction patterns and relationships between residents and caregivers.

Interacting "As a Friend"

Resident to Resident
Despite the lack of communication, some residents appeared to demonstrate a genuine interest in other residents and recognized their individuality. These residents would observe what was going on, anticipate the needs of other residents, and offer help. In the coffee shop, these men would notice when a resident got out a cigarette and required assistance to light it. They would get up from their seat and go over and automatically light the cigarette. At meal

Table 14.1 *Patterns of Interaction in a Long-Term Care Setting: Relationship to Privacy*

Communication Route	Patterns of Interaction		
	As a Friend	**As a Stranger**	**As an Object**
Resident to resident	**Caring behaviors** • anticipated needs of others • offered assistance or advocacy **Relationship** • friendship –warmth, sharing humor, reciprocal	• lacked involvement • formal –superficial, cordial conversations trite	• ignored each other • no relationship –courtesies ignored no acknowledgement of frailties
Resident to staff	**Appreciation of the person** • acknowledged in the total social context • mutual respect • sharing of personal information	• acknowledged in caregiving role • care rewarded or punished • employee–employer relationship	• acknowledged in task context • manipulation • master/servant relationship
Staff to resident	**Appreciation of the social context of the resident** • "care of the person" • bends rules/routines to allow for individual preferences • care is past, present, and future oriented	**Interaction context is role-based** • "care of the resident" • bends rules/routines to accomplish care activities • care is present and future oriented • distant, professional	**Interaction context is task-based** • "completion of the task" • unit routine is enforced • care is present-oriented • invisible

	Interactions about residents aimed at a personalized plan of care	Interactions about residents aimed at staff control over the plan of care	Interactions aimed at organizing and completing tasks efficiently/ expediently
Staff-to-staff	• mutual goal setting between resident and staff • residents' confidences are respected • shared stories reveal the personhood of the resident	• resident input into the plan of care controlled • residents' confidences are shared by the staff • stories told for interest	• shared stories criticize, demean, or ridicule the resident
Relationship to privacy	**Privacy is respected** • personal respect is conveyed naturally (inherent in relationship) • function of relationship	**Social norms of privacy are acknowledged** • compliance with ascribed rules of privacy	**Privacy is violated** • privacy not considered necessary or important

Source: Applegate and Morse (1994, p. 418). Reprinted with permission.

times, some residents could be slowly wheeling their chairs to the dining area. One resident in particular would approach a wheelchair-bound resident to offer a "free" push to or from the dining room; the wheelchair-bound resident reported: "He says, 'Going down or going home.' He treats me like a person who has the choice to receive his help." Another resident reported that he liked it when he was able to sit by one particular elderly resident to keep his "eye on him" and to assist him with activities that might prove difficult because of his physical impairments.

The men also demonstrated normal expressions of friendship. They would greet the less mentally competent residents in the corridor with an enthusiastic "Hello there, old timer!" or "Hello, young fella!" and the other resident would immediately brighten with a wave. Other expressions of friendship included good-natured "kidding" that accompanied watching televised sporting events. They included teasing those who supported the losing team or rehashing victories.

Courtesies were extended to both the mentally competent and the mentally incompetent residents. Competent residents seldom interrupted conversations between the researcher and the informants. Once, when the researcher was walking up to a competent resident, a mentally incompetent resident joined them at the table. The competent resident politely acknowledged the comments of the mentally incompetent man each time he spoke, even though the content was irrelevant to the ongoing conversation.

Residents also acted as advocates for other residents by "watching out" for them and complaining to the staff if they felt their care was inappropriate or substandard. Sometimes this assistance was merely ringing the bell to call a staff member or attempting to ensure that all were included in the exercise class by deliberately hitting the ball toward those who were less involved, with an encouraging "Atta, boy!" These residents behaved in a protective manner toward other residents. For instance, one morning an elderly resident fell. He was not injured, but he was shaken and returned to bed for a few hours. His roommate stayed with him just to keep "an eye on him" and to make sure that the staff members allowed him to rest.

Resident to Staff

When interactions were personalized, residents appreciated the staff and perceived them more as individuals responsible for their care. Staff members' personal lives outside the workplace were acknowledged and were of interest to residents. Although the residents may have been dependent on the staff members for specific assistance, they appreciated that staff members also had lives beyond the nursing home.

Despite the fact that these residents were not always able to identify particular staff members by name, it was obvious from the expressions on their faces when they received care from staff members with whom they felt comfortable. Spontaneous smiles and warm greetings were evidence of this recognition, and, in turn, this recognition was appreciated by the staff. Such acknowledgments were facilitated when residents knew their assigned caregiver for the day and were able to distinguish individual caregivers.

A common interest would often provide the grounds for a special relationship between staff members and residents. Residents could identify staff members who shared an interest in a hobby, a language, a sports event, or gardening. Such points of interest would be the basis for regular conversations, and the sharing of a mutual interest gave residents an opportunity to relate to the staff members outside of care activities.

Residents were sensitive to the problems caregivers may have had when caring for residents. If there were unexpected delays, they were philosophical about it. One man said about his back, "It would be nice to be done early, but what the heck do I need to rush for?" These residents realized that the staff was human too:

> Here you can ask them [the staff] to do anything for you with reason, and they'll do it. I've seen some of these guys yell and bellyache. They [the staff] are the only people trying to do a job, too, and some of these guys expect too darn much. We have a wonderful staff here.

In a friendly interaction, the resident approached the staff member as an individual. Residents would express an interest in the staff member's health and safety. They worried about winter road conditions when the staff member left work and inquired about his or her other family members' health. Residents would demonstrate an appreciation of a particular staff member's uniqueness. This was demonstrated by simply knowing the staff person's name or by discussing a common interest. The residents also appreciated those activities that were care-related, and selected staff members were rewarded with gifts such as candy bars, chocolate, pop, coffee, or compliments.

Staff to Resident

In *"as a friend"* relationships, the staff to resident interaction was based on the question "who is this *person* I care for?" There was an attempt to view the resident in a broader social context beyond his role as a resident in the institution.

Many of the residents were anxious to share their lives and to tell their stories, and the staff realized that the resident had a past, a present, and a future. On the corridor walls, there were photographs reflecting the military experience of the residents. In addition, in the residents' rooms, photographs of family gave staff members something to discuss with the resident. They would sit with the residents and go through photograph albums that told the story of the residents' life beyond the facility. The staff would then reciprocate by bringing their own photographs of family and special events. Celebrating milestones in the residents' life, such as birthdays or anniversaries, required the staff to plan ahead to make sure residents had appropriate clothes or that their clothing was cleaned and pressed so that such occasions would indeed be special. In many ways, resident–staff and staff–resident interactions were reciprocal. When a staff member treated a resident with dignity and attempted to acknowledge his individuality, the resident was more likely to feel comfortable and reciprocate.

Staff to Staff
One way to discern how the staff perceived a resident was to analyze how that resident was referred to during staff conversations. When the pattern of interaction was personalized, staff-to-staff communication resulted in the development of a personalized plan of care for a resident that accommodated the need of the resident within the restrictions of institutionalized life. Specifically, these interactions demonstrated respect for the confidences of the resident, included the resident in decision making, and supported the uniqueness of the resident. Objective reporting of factual information that affected the care plan was communicated between shifts. Information such as the development of reddened areas that required special skin care, the need to alter a medication, or a change in the resident's condition that required staff members to adjust the resident's normal routine were most frequently reported.

Informally, nurses told stories to each other about the residents. Even if these anecdotes were humorous, they were told with warmth and respect, often revealing, for example, an appreciation of the staff member for the resident's patience and occasionally showing errors in the staff's own judgment. For example, one resident (who was cognitively impaired) complained that he was unable to find his room since the ducks had left. At first, the aide assumed the resident was confused, until she remembered that the lawn ornaments, just outside the window, had been put away for the winter. Outside the resident's window was a family of ducks.

Staff who recognized the resident as an individual reported difficult or unusual behavior in the context of the situation. There was an attempt to understand the occurrence and to offer an explanation for the behavior. For example, one resident was particularly uncooperative and unpleasant, once even refusing his dinner and all care. His behavior was reported to a staff member who volunteered the information that the resident had been out with his family for the afternoon and was unhappy about returning to the facility. The staff member also acknowledged that the resident was quite tired from the excursion. This explanation was accepted, and the resident was allowed to rest. When the resident was treated as a person, confidences were respected. Personnel were often involved in letter writing or banking for residents, and residents said it was important that this information not be communicated to anyone. Thus, when interacting *as a friend*, normal courtesies are observed, care is considerate, and privacy norms are respected.

In summary, when staff and residents treated each other as friends, then each person was acknowledged as a unique individual. Persons acknowledged and respected the other individual as a person, and caring behaviors were evident. Within such a relationship, the respect for personal privacy was conveyed naturally, as a part of the interaction.

Interacting "As a Stranger"

Resident to Resident

When a relationship becomes depersonalized, there is no attempt to consider the individual outside of the patient's role or beyond the context of the required interaction. Many of the men seemed to be indifferent to those who shared the facility with them. Residents would walk along the corridor with their eyes straight ahead and not acknowledge those near them. They would enter and leave the sunroom without even glancing at the other residents. If they did interact, they were cordial but superficial and trite. For example, one man explained that he greeted another resident at every meal with the same expression "I see you made it," to which the second man replied, "Yes, and I see you did, too." Other than this exchange, no words were spoken during the meal.

Despite the fact that approximately half the men were mentally competent, only four residents actually knew the name of all the men in the unit. Other residents were able to identify their roommates, but when asked with whom they shared a room, several competent men replied, "Oh, I know them to see them." The same response was obtained from men who shared tables in the dining room, despite the fact that the men sat at the same tables for many months or even years. The absence of a resident would go unnoticed. One resident was transferred to a hospital with cardiac arrhythmia one Friday evening. When the researcher inquired about him on Monday morning, several of the residents were surprised that he was not in the facility. Although this man spent much of his time outside his room, his absence was unnoticed by several of the men. Thus, when resident-to-resident interaction was depersonalized and "as a stranger," the main characteristic of the interaction was the residents' lack of involvement with each other. Communication was superficial, with no real attempt to acknowledge any familiarity. Although there were no negative feelings, there were also no feelings of warmth between residents. Residents were not interested in learning about each other, and because of this disinterest in each other, privacy concerns were respected.

Resident to Staff
Incidents of resident–staff interaction were predominantly associated with care activities. The depersonalized resident-to-staff relationship was characterized by residents appreciating the staff only as long as their own care needs were met. The resident would approach a staff member if he had a request or question concerning his care. Residents offered rewards, such as sweets, based on their satisfaction with the nurses' care. It appeared to be an employee–employer relationship, with the residents serving as the bosses. Many residents did not attempt to learn the names of individual staff members or to distinguish one staff member from another even though many of the staff members had been employed in the unit for more than a year:

Researcher: What about the staff—do you know the staff very well?

Resident: Well, it's pretty hard to know them because they come and go all the time.

Researcher: Do you know them by name?

Resident: Well, I know _____; she works Sunday afternoons. She has been here since I came. And there's _____. She's on the other end. The rest, they are changing all the time, I don't know why either.

Researcher: Do you know the ward clerk or the health nurse?

Resident: No, she's gone.

Researcher: What about the assistant?

Resident: No, not very much.

In the *as a stranger* mode of interaction, if some aspect of the care was unsatisfactory, then the staff *in general* would suffer the brunt of the resident's displeasure. Little effort was made to identify the staff person responsible. Staff members could identify residents who would "punish" them when they were unhappy with their care. One resident would refuse to speak to any staff member, even to the point of refusing to say "Good morning." The staff felt that this man saw them only as his employees and therefore put them in a subservient position. For example, this employee–employer relationship would be emphasized when a resident threatened to report a staff member for not carrying out his wishes, and sometimes residents would refuse to cooperate with care, delay staff, or become very demanding. In addition, conflicts often developed over the extent to which residents were expected to be independent in caring for themselves. Thus, residents who interacted with the staff "as a stranger" saw them only in their roles as caregivers and not as individuals; their relationship was one of employee–employer.

Staff to Resident

When interacting as strangers, staff members defined their relationship with residents only in the context of their roles as caregivers. They defined their role as one of caring for the *resident* as opposed to caring for the *person*, a distinction one would find in a personalized relationship. One resident noticed this distinction when he received his nightly prescription of brandy. He reported that one of the nurses would hold the glass up at eye level and measure his "medication" to the precise drop. Another nurse would just pour his shot of brandy with the salutation "Cheers." Although a simple example, the resident perceived the first nurse as treating him like a resident and the second as treating him like a person.

The *as a stranger* relationship was cordial, but distant. Often, decisions were made for the residents, and they were denied the autonomy normally afforded competent adults. One resident said that the staff "too often are doing service to a *thing*—to a person of no account." Another man recognized this and said, "You see, I've reverted back to an infant, if you get what I mean. Maybe I don't squawk—and I guess I squawk more than a baby does." Thus, such residents felt they were treated as if they were less than men.

Residents were labeled as *demanding* if they refused to accept decisions made for them by others or they were particularly specific about how care activities should be performed. Residents were also labeled manipulative or dependent if they attempted to get assistance beyond the level that staff considered necessary.

In the *as a stranger* interaction, the staff ignored residents' complaints and observations and challenged the residents' abilities to make reasonable judgments. One resident reported the following:

> The toilet was plugged up. I went and told the nurse, "I need a plumber." Well, they looked down at me like the bunch they've got tied down—you know, they have men tied down? One of the nurses came down and flushed the toilet and water went all over the place. It wasn't good enough, my word wasn't good enough to tell them. And I said to the nurse, the same nurse I reported it to: "Why—is not my word good? You run down and flush the toilet." I don't see good, but I can see when a toilet's flushed. If I'm good enough to go and tell them about it, they should be good enough to listen.

Broken promises and broken time schedules that were not followed also irritated the men:

> So they give you a promise, and you know the most used words in here by the staff are "just a minute, I'll be right with you." They forget to come back, and the minutes turn into hours. They are heavily used words.

The use of such expressions to simply put off any further discussion of the delay seems to deny the residents' right to an adequate discussion. On the other hand, routines were often adhered to even when it was detrimental to the residents. One morning, a resident was excessively short of breath. He returned to bed to rest before his weekly tub bath. A staff member insisted that he get up again as she was making the beds and "wanted to get his room done." Thus, when the staff treated residents *as strangers*, the residents were not treated as persons, only as residents requiring care. Residents were often treated as less than men by the staff, and instead of encouraging residents to share meaningful information in an atmosphere of trust, their interactions were frequently rote and often directive.

Staff to Staff

In the *as a stranger* mode of interaction, staff-to-staff interactions related to residents were aimed at staff control over the plan of care. Change of shift reports would focus on care activities that had occurred in the previous shift, but there would be little attempt to describe the situation or the context of the behaviors. Interactions in team conferences would center on the discussion of care that had been completed or on the identification of difficulties. Often, the need to involve the resident in the planning of care was acknowledged; *however*, the resident would become involved at the point of changing the actions and not at the point of establishing goals for care. For example, during one report, the staff decided that one resident should have his bath day changed, and it was scheduled for the same day as his "bowel day" and his physiotherapy day. He was given the choice of two other days, but he was not asked if he wanted the actual change.

The staff often made the decision as to what information should be shared with other staff members, and this often included information that the resident had shared with the staff on a personal level. Although residents seldom identified information as confidential, notice that such information would be shared and used for planning care could have given residents more control over such information. Thus, staff-to-staff communication at the *stranger*, depersonalized level did reflect the special concerns of the resident, but the staff viewed the resident from a caretaker's perspective. Although physical needs would be acknowledged, the individual's specific input would be limited. Because *respect* for the individual was limited, privacy norms were violated to some extent.

In summary, when residents and staff treated each other *as a stranger*, interactions were cordial and polite, but lacked involvement and concern for the other. However, as shown in Table 14.1, the social norms of privacy were acknowledged and followed.

Interacting "As an Object"

Resident to Resident

As one resident in a wheelchair moved into the dining room, he referred to some of the slower residents as "the unavoidable and unfortunate obstacles that needed to be dealt with." This comment demonstrated the tendency of some residents to regard other residents without consideration for their humanness and frailties, to treat them as if they were objects or life forms with no redeeming qualities. Some residents would either ignore any attempt by other residents to address them or else respond aggressively. They did not use common courtesies such as "Please" or "Excuse me." Residents who adopted this pattern of communication would deliberately attempt to interfere with other residents by impeding the flow of traffic with their wheelchairs.

Some of the equally competent residents did not show compassion for those who were mentally incompetent and would even physically threaten them. One resident developed a great hostility toward a man he discovered going through his possessions. Also, sometimes the intrusion was a deliberate search for cigarette or candy; often it was done by an incompetent resident, unaware of what he was doing. After this incident, he would threaten the residents with his cane for any minor irritation. Some of the residents would react to other residents in ways that showed no compassion or understanding, and this was most noticeable in their behavior toward the mentally incompetent residents. When interactions were *as an object*, privacy norms were violated. Such behavior was in contrast to the behavior of other residents who recognized the humanness of the mentally impaired men and treated them with respect even if it was not reciprocated.

Resident to Staff

In the *as an object* interaction between residents and staff, residents referred to staff members as a means of "getting something done." Thus, staff members were viewed in a more subservient way than in an employer–employee relationship; this relationship resembled a master–servant relationship. In these situations, the residents expected staff members not just to provide care, but also to wait on them. Some staff members believed that residents saw it as a woman's duty to look after men. These residents, who were veterans, believed that they had earned the right to be cared for and to be waited on as well.

At times, residents attempted to manipulate staff members so that they could achieve their individual objectives. Residents would test new or relief staff members in these situations, often seeking assistance more frequently than required for establishing a more stringent schedule.

Staff to Resident

When staff members treated a resident as a nonperson, their interactions did not demonstrate the simple human attributes of compassion, understanding, and kindness. In the dehumanized interaction pattern, the resident was reduced to an object, a task, or even to a nonhuman life form. In this situation, the staff saw the day's assignments as tasks to be completed, and these tasks were organized so that they could be accomplished as quickly and as expediently as possible. The individual needs of residents and the appropriate norms for care were not considered. Because the resident was viewed as an object, little attempt was made to maintain privacy during physical care. For example, curtains and doors were not closed when assisting the resident with personal tasks, thus physically exposing him.

Residents would be treated as if they did not exist. For example, although a resident was directly in the line of vision of staff members, he would be ignored. He would wait patiently to be addressed, often unsure whether he was noticed or not. Sometimes staff members would initiate an activity with a resident, doing something to him without any explanation or warning. A resident in a wheelchair would suddenly be moved to an alternative location. Decisions would be made without attempting to inform the resident. On other occasions, the staff would approach the resident with a rhetorical question, and even if the resident answered appropriately, his response would be ignored. For example, a staff member approached a resident in a wheelchair and began pushing the man to his room, asking if he wanted to go to bed. This man responded, "Why did you give me a choice? I have no choice." The staff member did not even acknowledge that she had heard.

At meal times, residents would be fed quickly, given food in amounts and at a rate that made chewing difficult. Also, the television or radio would be played loudly for the distraction of the staff rather than for the enjoyment of the residents. Thus, the interaction was strictly dehumanized and task-oriented, without caring. The routine of the unit directed all interactions, rather than the needs of the residents. Many times, residents were ignored as if they were invisible. Things were done to residents without consideration for their feelings, including respect for their privacy. When patients were viewed as an object, the staff made no attempt to knock when they entered the bathroom. One nurse was observed changing an incontinent patient's pants in the corridor. The staff showed no consideration for the patient; for example, the staff did not request permission to enter their lockers. They merely went ahead as if the patient was not present and the contents were common property.

Staff to Staff

In the *as an object* mode of interaction, the resident was dehumanized when the staff members geared the plan of care to task completion without consideration for individual differences. The need to finish the work overrode any particular need of a resident. Things such as bath lists were inflexible even when circumstances made following the schedule difficult or impossible. Formal reports were rote, with the staff reporting on the tasks completed. Even if they mentioned individual residents, they communicated little that would help the plan of care.

When a resident was treated as an object, there was no attempt to understand the resident's perspective; instead, the staff would create a situational context that reflected their biases and values. Stereotypical expectations were expressed about residents, with little evidence to support such expectations. For example, a large percentage of the residents had abused alcohol in the past. Stories told by the staff members reflected the residents' continued abuse of alcohol and were told in a derogatory manner. Although some of these stories were confirmed by the staff and residents, on other occasions, the stories were not verified and were used to ridicule or discredit the residents, and were unrelated to any plan of care. In the *as an object* mode of interaction, the residents' privacy was not respected; personal information was not treated confidentially.

In summary, when interactions between residents and the staff were *as an object interaction*, there was little concern for the other person's feelings, rights, or welfare (see Table 14.1). Residents were unaware of the needs of others and treated as if they were servants or handmaidens. Residents selfishly manipulated situations for tasks to be completed at their own convenience.

The staff provided routinized task-oriented care, and the work routine was completed without any consideration for the residents' needs. During reports, the staff spoke of the residents in stereotypical terms, often criticizing, demeaning, or ridiculing them.

Changing Relationships, Contexts, and Interactions

When the context was changed, the normative patterns of silence were not maintained. It was observed, and residents and staff members confirmed, that increased interactions occurred between residents and staff members during informal or recreational situations. Social events within the facility, such as the "happy hour" and pub nights, would foster resident-to-resident communication that resembled the chatter of pub talk. During happy hour, residents would deliberately sit with each other and initiate conversation. Similarly, recreational events broke the normative behavioral patterns and permitted the staff to see the residents in a context outside the caregiving role, making them respond by interacting with the residents as friends. These special situations seemed to help the caregivers view the residents differently, and they shared their observations about residents with one another. As one nurse explained to the researcher, "This is 'a *natural* experience'—something that they might have done before they were admitted to the unit. I think it helps them remember those times." Beyond their therapeutic value, these recreational events provided staff members with the opportunity to share an experience with the residents and to see residents as people, and thus, they provided common experiences outside the normal caregiving role. However, as soon as the social event ended, the patterns of interactions resumed the normal, nonverbal state. This norm was illustrated when, one weekend, the residents travelled to a scenic national park. Two residents, who normally shared a room, continued to be partners and continued to share a room on the trip. They both appeared to enjoy the trip immensely, chatting as old friends—yet, on their return, they resumed their nonverbal patterns. One of the residents wrote a note to his roommate in the next bed expressing how much he had enjoyed his company on the trip.

Types of Interactions in Relation to Privacy

From the preceding data, it was evident that a staff member's relationship with the resident determined how the staff member was treated and whether or not the resident's privacy was respected. Privacy was naturally respected when residents and staff acknowledged each other's personhood and inter-actions. Respect for privacy *was* respecting the individuality of the other and thus acknowledging the value of each person. Activities related to maintaining privacy were activities that generally demonstrated respect for the individual. The dignity, self-esteem, and autonomous nature of the person was promoted, and thus, the personhood of the resident was reaffirmed.

In the study, it was important to note that the staff members' respect for the patients' right to privacy varied from one resident to the next despite the fact that all residents were theoretically exposed to the same *potential* for dehumanization. For example, Gubrium (1997) has noted that the "bed and body work" is a "leveler" with the staff's priority of completing tasks taking precedence over the individual resident's needs. In this particular study, there appeared to be a greater mix of patients requiring different levels of nursing care than in Gubrium's study. Nevertheless, cognitive intactness did not appear to be an adequate condition to ensure respect from the staff or from other patients. As reported in other nursing home settings (such as Kayser-Jones, 1981), residents engaged in reciprocal relationships with the staff, thus inhibiting the dehumanization process (see e.g., Morse, 1991).

In "Murray Manor" (Gubrium, 1997), staff behavioral norms appeared to inherently respect some aspects of privacy in the *residents'* areas. For example, before entering a room, the staff knocked and waited for permission to enter (p. 31). On the floors where patients were more confused (and the staff believed these patients were mostly disoriented to time and place), doors were left open and patients' privacy was less respected (pp. 33–34). As in this study, some patients in "Murray Manor" vigorously protected their territory and their possessions from wandering disoriented patients.

In 1966, Vail suggested a very useful framework for understanding dehumanization. This involved treating the person (a) *as trivium,* or as a child; (b) as an inanimate object or the product of another's work; (c) as an animal or a lower life form; and (d) as the other, as a non-person. Although they are distinct, Vail (1966) notes that these types may be attributed to a single person simultaneously.

In this study, there was evidence for all four types of dehumanization. For instance, the action of exposing a resident while he was being changed or bathed may be considered one aspect of treating a person *as trivium*. If the resident was considered to lack self-awareness, to be asexual, and to have feelings resembling a childlike innocence, caregivers may unconsciously not have considered it necessary to conform to adult modesty norms. In situations in which the resident was not viewed as an individual and was acknowledged *only* as a resident in the facility (i.e., as an inanimate object), the right to privacy was defined solely within the context of the resident's role as a resident. Respect for privacy was demonstrated as respect for the resident/stranger in the facility. Privacy was viewed from the perspective of the institution. Rules for privacy are normally incorporated in the policies and procedures of the institution. From the staff's perspective, the objectives of the caregiver took precedence, and privacy was invaded if care requirements for the resident or the needs of the institution were seen as more important. As a result, the autonomy of the resident may be jeopardized, and ultimately, the loss of self-worth and dignity may occur.

Finally, if the personhood of the resident was totally ignored and the resident was dehumanized (i.e., as a nonperson), then the right to privacy was not considered. In these situations, there was no respect for the person, and the resident was treated as an object. Because an object has no feelings, normal considerations that maintain a person's dignity were not observed. Thus, personal privacy was not a consideration and was violated. An important extension of this research would be to continue this inquiry, linking the privacy violation with the type of dehumanization manifested.

The lack of communication between residents in the nursing home was important. Residents who sat at the same dinner table for years but did not communicate showed little interest in the other residents as persons. Residents who were not interested in others, or who were unwilling to communicate, sat within conversational range of another resident; it appeared culturally acceptable in the subculture of the nursing home to isolate oneself in silence from the others. This normative mode of interacting was also evident behaviorally when these residents made no effort to care for, or to watch out for, residents who were less aware, to the extent that they would even knock them down in the corridor or with a remarkable lack of empathy, chase them away from their belongings with a cane. As a few residents did not subscribe to these behaviors and did engage in daily caring communication with all residents, greeting others and assisting them with their needs, the normative pattern of communication revealed in this study in Saville-Troike's (1985) framework may be considered "individually determined/negotiated silence." Another function that may have contributed to the lack of communication was the physical limitations of the residents themselves. As with all elderly, conversation with some residents with hearing loss was difficult. However, the dramatically changed levels of conversation that occurred with the change of scene (as on "pub night") revealed that changing the "rules" by changing the social context permitted—and even fostered—interaction. "Pubs" are typically noisy, friendly conversational places, in which the gender-related reserve is relaxed and strangers may converse.

IMPLICATIONS

Genuine respect for privacy was demonstrated through actions that confirmed a respect for the resident as a person of worth and dignity rather than through actions that merely conformed to designated rules. Closing the curtains around the resident may create the impression of privacy for the staff member, but if the resident was not treated with respect for his personhood, little advantage was gained from the action. Protecting residents' privacy became a function of the caregiver when residents were totally dependent on others and were unable to rely on their own resources to maintain privacy. For the staff member who did not view residents as individuals, the need to protect residents' privacy involved a narrow range of behaviors. A broader perspective of privacy maintenance was revealed when respect for privacy was defined in the wider context of respect for the individuality of the person. By identifying depersonalization as an antecedent to privacy invasion, actions that would ultimately lead to the respect of privacy were identified. These actions should establish opportunities for both staff members and residents to view each other as individuals. For instance, if the staff observes that having a pub night facilitates "pub talk," then serious consideration should be given to making the "happy hour" a daily event.

To genuinely respect the individuality of other people, both staff members and residents must appreciate each other beyond the immediate interaction of the care activity. This may require some staff members and residents to reformulate the role expectations of the staff to include activities outside of "bed and body" work—a term used by the staff that reveals an attitude that dehumanizes the residents. Staff members need to help residents in getting to know them as individuals. This includes introducing themselves daily to their assigned residents, wearing name tags that clearly display their names, sharing personal information, and providing care that accommodates individual habits and preferences of residents. In turn, residents also need to recognize staff members as individuals. In this study, some residents mistakenly identified staff turnover as the reason why they were unable to learn staff names. This mistaken perception could be eliminated by having smaller units that would reduce the number of staff in contact with each resident, thus facilitating recognition and fostering relationships. It is also possible that uniforms interfere with the recognition of staff and the necessity, purpose, and functions of the uniform dress code should be re-examined.

Previous studies have noted the lack of interaction between residents in nursing homes and have tried to foster communication with strategies such as remotivation therapy or reorganization of seating arrangements (Tate, 1980). This lack of communication has been attributed to distancing or withdrawal by residents as a response to the lack of privacy (Berdes, 1987). From the study, it appears that the most fruitful way to facilitate communication is to periodically change the social context by providing opportunities for residents and staff to interact outside the roles of residents and caregivers. Outings, special events, and celebrations allow the staff and residents to participate in informal situations. Such activities create new normative patterns of interaction and allow both residents and staff members to see each other from different perspectives.

Similarly, relationships between residents need to be fostered. Admission to a nursing home facility disrupts established friendship patterns, and formulating new relationships and institutions often proves difficult (Noelker & Poulshock, 1984). Despite the fact that aggressive behavior has been attributed to overcrowding and lack of privacy, residents have been found to prefer open wards over any other type of institutional accommodation (Kayser-Jones, 1986). This has been interpreted as the need for companionship being greater than the need for privacy. Yet this selective approach to the problem appears too simplistic: Residents, like all persons, need both companionship *and* privacy, and the need for privacy or for aloneness varies from day to day. Just as residents sometimes need to be alone, so do they need to interact with others to maintain their sense of identity. It is a matter of individual preference. Further, it must be recognized that there is a difference between being left alone and being left out. When a resident chooses to be alone and can do so, then the resident has some semblance of privacy. However, an individual who has been shipwrecked and is alone on a deserted island has no privacy because an alternative does not exist. Just so, the resident who is alone in his room has no privacy if he has no opportunity to interact with others in ways that establish his identity among others. The presence of others provides a milieu against which one can test the authenticity of one's personal identity.

Avoiding interaction with others has been identified as privacy-maintenance behavior (Schuster, 1976a, 1976b; Tate, 1980). In this nursing home, *reserve* (Westin, 1967) became the main strategy to maintain privacy in an environment that was constantly public. Paradoxically, in some situations, this technique appeared to actually work against obtaining privacy: by continuing noninvolvement with others, some residents did not achieve reciprocal respect as a person either from the other residents or from the staff. Thus, others' respect for a resident's privacy seems to be inherent in the relationship that the resident was able to establish with others. Interestingly, increasing his interaction with others ultimately increases the resident's privacy. Providing situations that could allow staff and residents permission to move out of their established roles selectively breaks the norm of silence that is often seen in nursing home facilities.

Many residents were unable to actively protect their privacy because of their physical or cognitive impairments. The caregiver was then responsible for giving respectful care—not just to the person now known, but to the person of the past. As Knepfer and Johns (1989) observe, "They [the elderly] need a nurse to guard and preserve their personalities, their memorabilia and person rituals, the symbols of their lives that remind them of who they were and are" (p. 163). Thus, respect for privacy goes beyond the realm of purely physical or bodily domains and captures the personal element that reflects the individual. The pictures on the corridor walls of the institution where this study was conducted show residents as they once were—strong and independent. As the residents recognized themselves in their pictures on the wall, so their past became a part of the present that they could recognize, to *know again* (Vesperi, 1985, p. 75). The residents' stories told of life events that were unique or commonplace, but those stories revealed aspects of these men who were now dependent on others. Respect for privacy was respect for the person revealed in those pictures and stories.

Finally, we cannot agree that dehumanization was an essential condition for every instance of privacy violation. Rather, we suggest that when one person violates another's privacy, and the relationship between the two is not one of indifference, then the person violating the other's rights will experience guilt. The greater the process of dehumanization, the less a person experiences guilt when invading another's privacy.

The nebulous, dynamic, and abstract nature of the context of privacy has been difficult to define, describe, and delineate. Descriptions of the essence of privacy have eluded social scientists, philosophers, and legal writers. Yet it is an important concept, for violating an individual's right to privacy "threatens our liberty as individuals to do as we will, just as an assault, battery or imprisonment of our person does" (Bloustein, 1984, p. 187). From the study, it was evident that an individual's expectation and experience of privacy was influenced by both personal and environmental factors. Because privacy was context-bound, the experience of privacy for an individual living outside a nursing home facility was both quantitatively and qualitatively different from that of an individual who is institutionalized and dependent on others for some aspect of care. Conceptualizing privacy as respect for the individuality of a person acknowledges these variations and enables facilities providing care to ultimately enhance the protection of privacy.

ACKNOWLEDGMENTS

The authors wish to thank the staff and the residents of the host institution. The authors also acknowledge the assistance of Dr. D. Forrest and Dr. J. Storch. This research was conducted as a part of the MN degree requirements for the first author. Financial support was provided by the Alberta Foundation for Nursing Research, the Alberta Association of Registered Nurses, and by an NHRDP/MRC Research Scholar Award to Dr. Morse.

NOTES

1. The concept of health provides a sample of the problems related to using deductive methods for concept development. Researchers using interviews to obtain information on health practices, invariably, obtain information that resembles a grade school health class post-test—such as information on vitamins, sleep, and exercise—yet this information bears little resemblance to the researchers' observations of actual behavior. From this perspective, it is odd that researchers are still puzzled about the discrepancy in reported and observed behavior in studies on health. Therefore, in this study, the inductive method of nonparticipant observation was used, with the researcher entering the setting as a stranger (to both the staff and the residents) and as a researcher rather than a nurse.
2. As Canada did not enter into the war in Vietnam, unlike the United States, veterans are now elderly and male. This is reflected in the patient regulations and veterans' hospitals

REFERENCES

Applegate, M., & Morse, J. M. (1994). Personal privacy and interactional patterns in a nursing home. *J Aging Studies, 8,* 413–434.
Altman, I. (1975). *The environment and social behavior: Privacy, personal space, territory, and crowding.* Monterey, CA: Brooks/Cole.

Bates, A. P. (1964). Privacy—a useful concept? *Social Forces, 42*(4), 429–434.

Beardsley, E. (1971). Privacy: Autonomy and selective disclosure. In J. Pennick & J. Chapman (Eds.), *Privacy* (pp. 56–70). New York, NY: Atherton.

Benn, S. (1971). Privacy, freedom, and respect for persons. In J. Pennick & J. Chapman (Eds.), *Privacy* (pp. 1–26), New York, NY: Atherton.

Berdes, C. (1987). The modest proposal nursing home: Dehumanizing characteristics of nursing homes and of nursing home residents. *Journal of Applied Gerontology, 6*(4), 372–388.

Bloustein, E. J. (1984). Privacy as an aspect of human dignity. Privacy as an aspect of human dignity. In F. Schoeman (Ed.), *Philosophical dimensions of privacy: An anthology* (pp. 156–197), New York, NY: Cambridge. (Reprinted from *NYUL Rev.,* 1964, *39*, 962–1007.)

Boone, C. K. (1983). Privacy and community. *Social Theory and Practice, 9*(1), 1–30.

Garrett, R. (1974). The nature of privacy. *Philosophy Today, 18*(19741), 264–284.

Greenawalt, K. (1974). Privacy and its legal protections. *Hastings Center Studies, 2,* 45–68.

Gross, H. (1971). Privacy and autonomy. In J. Pennick & J. Chapman (Eds.), *Privacy* (pp. 169–181). New York, NY: Atherton.

Gubrium, J. F. (1997). *Living and dying at Murray Manor.* Charlottesville, VA: University of Virginia Press.

Halmos, P. (1953). *Solitude and privacy.* London, UK: Routledge & Kegan Paul.

Henderson, M. R. (1975). Acquiring privacy in public. *Journal of Contemporary Ethnography, 3*(4), 446–455.

Hoad, T. (1986). *The concise Oxford dictionary of English etymology.* Oxford: Clarendon Press.

Kayser-Jones, J. S. (1981). *Old, alone, and neglected: Care of the aged in the United States and Scotland.* Berkley, CA: University of California Press.

Kayser-Jones, J. S. (1986). Open-ward accommodations in a long-term-care facility: The elderly's point of view. *The Gerontologist, 26*(1), 63–69.

Kelvin, P. (1973). A social-psychological examination of privacy. *British Journal of Social and Clinical Psychology, 12*(3), 248–261.

Knepfer, G., & Johns, C. (1989). *Nursing for life.* Sydney: Pan Books.

Laurence, M. (1967). *The stone angel.* Toronto, CA: McClelland & Stewart.

Margulis, S. T. (1977). Conceptions of privacy: Current status and next steps. *Journal of Social Issues, 33*(3), 5–21.

Morse, J. M. (1991). Negotiating commitment and involvement in the nurse–patient relationship. *Journal of Advanced Nursing, 16*(4), 455–468.

Noelker, L. S., & Poulshock, S. W. (1984). Intimacy: Factors affecting its development among members of a home for the aged. *The International Journal of Aging and Human Development, 19*(3), 177–190.

Prosser, W. (1984). Privacy: A legal analysis. In F. Schoeman (Eds.), *Philosophical dimensions of privacy: An anthology* (pp. 104–141). New York, NY: Cambridge.

Reiman, J. H. (1976). Privacy, intimacy, and personhood. *Philosophy & Public Affairs, 6*(1), 26–44.

Roosa, W. (1981). Privacy and congregated living as viewed by nursing home residents. *Dissertation Abstracts International, 41*(9–13), 3389.

Saville-Troike, M. (1985). The place of silence in an integrated theory of communication. In D. Tannen & M. Saville-Troike (Eds.), *Perspectives on silence* (pp. 3–18). Norwood, NJ: Ablex.

Schuster, E. A. (1976a). Privacy and the hospitalization experience. *Communicating Nursing Research, 7,* 153.

Schuster, E. A. (1976b). Privacy, the patient, and hospitalization. *Social Science & Medicine, 10,* 245–248.

Schwartz, B. (1968). The social psychology of privacy. *American Journal of Sociology, 73,* 741–752.

Simmel, A. (1971). Privacy is not an isolated freedom. In J. R. Pennock & J. W. Chapman (Eds.), *Privacy: Nomos XIII* (pp. 77–87). New York, NY: Atherton Press.

Tate, J. W. (1980). The need for personal space in institutions for the elderly. *Journal of Gerontological Nursing, 6*(8), 439–449.

Vail, D. J. (1966). *Dehumanization and the institutional career.* Springfield, IL: CC Thomas.

Vesperi, M. D. (1985). *City of green benches: Growing old in a new downtown.* Ithaca, NY: Cornell University Press.

Warren, S. D., & Brandeis, L. D. (1980). The right to privacy. *Harvard Law Review, 4*(5), 193–220.

Westin, A. F. (1967). *Privacy and freedom.* New York, NY: Atheneum.

CHAPTER FIFTEEN

CULTURAL VARIATION IN BEHAVIORAL RESPONSE TO PARTURITION: CHILDBIRTH IN FIJI

Janice M. Morse

Due to the pain and suffering of labor and the possibility of life-threatening complications, childbirth is considered a time of acute physiological stress for both the mother and the infant and a time of psychological stress for the mother, family, and community. As the timing of the birth event is relatively predictable, all cultures have responded to the risk of birth by developing methods of caring for the pregnant and parturient woman. All cultures have allocated the specialist role of the management of labor to the traditional birth attendant (TBA). Many practices have developed to minimize the risks to the mother and the infant. Similarly, perinatal explanatory beliefs have developed to reduce the psychological stress of childbirth. These beliefs are congruent with the broader cultural context (Mead & Newton, 1967; Wellin, 1978).

In spite of the interest in traditional birth practices over the past decade, the majority of existing research consists of descriptive ethnographic accounts of the birthing process (e.g., Kay, 1982; MacCormack, 1982). Few researchers have conducted comparative studies and attempted theoretical explanations for birthing practices. This study, examining childbirth in Fiji, compares and contrasts the culturally specific methods used during childbirth to control pain and to reduce the risk of injury to the mother and the infant and examines the maternal response to pain.

Reprinted from Janice M. Morse (1989). Cultural variation in behavioral response to parturition: Childbirth in Fiji. *Medical Anthropology*, 12(1), 35–54. Reprinted by permission of the publisher, Taylor & Francis Ltd. (www.tandf.co.uk/journals; www .informaworld.com). Original from dissertation Morse (1981).

FIJI

Fiji was selected for the site of this research because the country has several unique characteristics. The population consists of two distinct cultural groups: the Fijian and the Fiji-Indian. Although these two cultures have coexisted in one country for more than a century, there has been limited interaction between the two cultural groups. There has been little cultural borrowing, and intermarriage is rare. Both groups have retained their own cultural heritage and have maintained dualism within a limited geographical area. As the Fiji Government provides one health care system for both cultural groups, Fiji is a unique environment for comparative health studies: Two distinct cultural groups exist in a similar ecological environment using the same health care system.

In spite of the universal health care system in Fiji, the morbidity and mortality rates of the two groups differ significantly. The 1976 census reported the infant mortality rate as 37 per 1,000 for Fijians and 54 per 1,000 for Fiji-Indians. The early neonatal mortality rate (i.e., the number of infant deaths within 7 days of birth) is 32.8 per 1,000 for Fiji-Indians and 15.2 per 1,000 for Fijians (Ministry of Health n.d.a, n.d.b). The maternal mortality rate for 1976 was 125.7 per 100,000 live births, with the Fiji-Indian maternal mortality rate 26% higher than the Fijian (Ministry of Health, n.d.b, p. 2). In 1975, the rate of anemia in Fiji-Indian pregnant women was 89% higher than in Fijian pregnant women and 172% higher than other racial groups. The Fiji-Indian government noted that anemia was cited as the cause of maternal mortality in 12% of the deaths and possibly a contributing factor in an additional 37% of deaths attributed to hemorrhage and hypovolemic shock (Ministry of Health, n.d.a., p. 5). Similarly, the rate of preeclampsia per 100,000 live births was 186% higher in the Fiji-Indian than in the Fijian pregnant women. Preeclampsia was present in 7% of Fiji-Indian women at delivery, as compared to 2.4% of Fijian women (Ministry of Health, n.d.a, p. 8).

The Fijians

Although the pressures of modernization are resulting in the breakdown of traditional village life, kinship, extended to social units forming a village community, still plays a vital role in the identity of the Fijian. Even if the Fijian migrates to the city for educational purposes or for occupational reasons, he continues to make a financial contribution to the village general fund and frequently returns to the village. The Fijian social organization is based on kinship, rank, and sex (see Quain, 1948). Patrilineal descent and patrilocal residence (with less consideration to the matriline) establishes connections between members of the social unit. The rank structure divides the people into two groups: the chiefs and the commoners. The chief has authority over all members of the village and is entitled to special privileges and tokens of respect. Seniority, based on age and sex, orders social interaction among individuals. Within the family, the senior male member has authority over all members; males over females and the older over the younger. The villages show many indications of a society in transition (Frazer, 1973). The traditional *bure* (i.e., house) is being replaced by single room structures of wood or corrugated iron. An intensive public health campaign is attempting to replace latrines (situated on the periphery of the village) by supplying each village with water seal privies and piped water. Most villages own a commercial vehicle, such as a small truck, to take supplies to the nearest market.

The concept of "community" and "sharing" are highly integrated into the Fijian life, and its importance cannot be overestimated. The society is based on mutual service rather than individual effort (Lester, 1946). This concept is essential for the economic structure, continuity, and interpersonal relations within the group. Satisfactory interpersonal relations are highly desired. An informant stated that:

> We share things, we are willing to sacrifice anything for our friends. In this way we get confidence in our people. [By giving?] By giving—not so much in receiving—it's what you give that counts.

This thought is so pervasive that when asked to define health, a 26-year-old replied:

> Good health, in my own Fiji interpretation—is plenty of food in the garden—ripe, ready to pick—and everybody in the village loves you. [Health is] when you are on good terms with everybody in the village.

Conversely, ill health and death are caused by enemies, assisted by spirits or the devil (Spenser, 1966), through sorcery (*vu-ni-duvu*). Disease is also caused by these evil spirits as a punishment for wrongdoing, or even one's ancestor's wrongdoing, so that numerous rituals and taboos are observed to stay healthy. Spirits linger, waiting for an opportunity to observe a transgression and then to enter the body of an offender. Life, I was told repeatedly, was a *"fight"* between good and evil. All natural disasters, such as hurricanes, were caused by the devil, and illness and deaths were explained within this framework. The Fijian response to childbearing is not an exception to this pattern.

The Fiji-Indians

At the end of the 19th century, the need for labor to assist in the growing of sugarcane led to the adoption of the indenture system and the importation of East Indian labor into Fiji. The utilization of Indian labor was not unique to Fiji. The indenture system had been established in 1833 in the British Colonies and laborers had been recruited for more than 50 years to work in Natal, Trinidad, British Guiana, Mauritius, and Dutch Guinea (Kerr & Donnelly, 1976). Unfortunately, the indenture system had been in operation long enough for its abuses to be refined, and the Indian recruiter, or *arkati*, often used unscrupulous methods to enlist laborers for Fiji (Naidu, 1980). In addition, push factors existed in India at that time. Several years of crop failures made the recruiters' exaggerated descriptions of Fiji resemble paradise. Although regulations regarding recruitment existed to protect the emigrants, these were often disregarded and not enforced. The indenture system was in operation in Fiji between 1878 and 1920, during which time 60,500 Indians were indentured into Fiji (Kerr & Donnelly, 1976). Workers were recruited from throughout India, but the majority originated from South India.

The cramped conditions in the boats bringing the workers to Fiji resulted in the breakdown of the caste system, but religious barriers remained. On their arrival in Fiji, the new immigrants were quarantined and then assigned to a grower for working in the sugarcane fields or the sugar mills on the "dry" (i.e., western) side of Viti Levu. Cramped housing in coolie lines further facilitated the merging of Indian cultures. Linguistic changes occurred, and today, Hindustani (i.e., Hindi, with Urdu and English words occurring within the vocabulary) is most commonly spoken.

Following the absolution of the indenture system, the Indian became upwardly mobile in Fiji using education and economic enterprise. Although many Fiji-Indians still reside in hamlets farming sugarcane, a large percentage also reside in the city. Much of the control of government and industry is by the Fiji-Indian. Many Indian customs and traditions have survived intact. Although some younger women now wear western clothing, most wear the traditional *sari* or the Moslem tunic. Food is prepared according to Indian customs with spices imported from India. Patrilineal descent and patrilocal residence dictate the female role. A common practice is for the adolescent to help her mother at home until marriage is arranged at the age of 17 or 18 years. Only in the cities is the Fiji-Indian woman employed. At the present time, Fiji-Indians comprise 52% of the total population (Parliament of Fiji, 1977). The main religious groups for this population are Hindu (80%), Moslem (15%), and Christian (4%; Parliament of Fiji, 1977).

CROSS-CULTURAL STUDIES OF CHILDBIRTH

In spite of significant maternal physiological variation and differences in infant birth weight, investigation into racial variation in the course of labor has revealed no major differences. Duignan, Studd, and Hughes (1975) found no significant differences in the duration of pregnancy, the duration of the first stage of labor, or the progress of labor or cervical dilation rate when examining 1,306 parturients from the three racial groups: Caucasian (West European), Asian (immigrants from India, Pakistan, and Bangladesh), and Black (immigrants from Africa and the West Indies). In Israel, Melmed and Evans (1972) compared Arab patients with foreign-born Jews and found no differences in cervical dilation rate, gestational age, the position of the head at the onset of labor, and the type of delivery (spontaneous, assisted delivery, or cesarean section). A third study (Lim, Wong, & Sinnathuray, 1977), examining Malay, Chinese, and Indian parturients, found no difference between groups for mean maturity in weeks, the fetal presenting part, or the duration of the second stage of labor. Rates of cervical dilation were the same for all groups, except that Indian women experienced a slight delay at 5 cm. Therefore, for the purposes of this study, it was assumed that the physiological birth process and the pain stimulus of birth would be similar for both the Fijians and the Fiji-Indians.

CULTURAL PATTERNING OF CHILDBIRTH

Mead and Newton (1967) noted the regularity of the societies' care and concern for the pregnant women and the variation of these caring patterns between cultures. They also noted that the assessment of childbirth within a culture cannot be separated from the cultural context and presented a framework suggesting factors that affect the cultural attitude and caring patterns regarding childbirth. The first aspect to be considered in this assessment is the amount of importance that the culture places on the birth event. This includes consideration of the amount of social support the mother receives, the amount of preparation for the birth event, and the changes in routine necessitated by other members of the community. Some indication of the importance may also be evidenced by the amount of knowledge (such as the physiological understanding and the treatment of abnormalities) existing in the culture. The second aspect, whether birth is viewed as an illness or as normal physiology, also determines the attitudes toward the parturient woman and the care that she receives. Third, the amount of secrecy and privacy of the birth event varies interculturally. Some members do not give information regarding reproduction to members until the marriage ceremony, with stories explaining "where babies come from." On the other hand, other cultures, accepting birth as normal and natural, do not exclude anyone who wishes to participate in the birth event. The fourth consideration is the sexual implications of birth. Some cultures do not associate sexual intercourse with birth, whereas many others react with extreme modesty and do not permit men to participate in the birth. Childbirth may also be considered as "dirty or defiling," with the woman secluded in a special area until cleansed and able to resume her normal role. The last factor is the consideration of birth as a supernatural event, out of the control of man. In this context, an extraordinary event, such as the death of the mother or the infant, is particularly horrifying. All of these aspects have implications for the analysis of child birthing systems—the roles, attitudes, and ecology of childbirth. To some extent, these factors have resulted in different practices being utilized in birthing systems and in varying patterns of behavior. Their study provides insights into the underlying rationale for the cultural context of childbirth.

In 1978, Jordan published an extensive cross-cultural study of childbirth of four cultural groups from the Yucatan, Holland, Sweden, and the United States. She noted major differences between each culture in the birth environment, the birth attendants and support systems, the available technology, medications used, and locus of decision making, which were reflected in the women's behavior during labor and delivery. She observed that pain becomes a different "object" in different systems. The system determines "whether it is highlighted or discounted, what kinds of occasions its occurrence provides for displaying the nature of systems . . . [and] what role it plays in making birth visible as a medical or natural 'kind of event'." In a system, for example, where pain is in control of the medical attendant, it is the role of the patient to convince and negotiate with the attendant by "producing the appropriate display of pain experienced" to obtain analgesics (Jordan, 1978, p. 36). This and the pathological panic behaviors frequently exhibited in the American obstetrical ward result in comparatively high levels of noise and hysteria. This contrasts with Sweden, where informed patients maintain self-control and make their own decisions regarding analgesics, and with the Dutch and Yucatan cultural systems in which birth is considered a natural event and is accepted with patience while "nature takes its course" (Jordan, 1978).

The ethnographic literature is replete with examples of preparations used to reduce maternal anxiety and pain associated with childbirth and to maximize the chances of a successful outcome (i.e., a healthy mother and infant). Expectant mothers are protected from malevolent spirits through community actions, social support, and restrictions on her behavior (e.g., Chen, 1973; McCain, 1975) or from strong emotions (e.g., Cosminsky, 1977). Dietary restrictions are usual but sometimes inappropriate, reducing, rather than increasing, protein levels (Cosminsky, 1977; Mead & Newton, 1967; Paul, 1967). Physiological preparation for labor is common and takes the form of changes in the work role (Gillam, 1973), massage, including external version of the fetus (Cosminsky, 1977; Jordan, 1978), and preparation of the perineum by stretching and massaging the vulva (Mead & Newton, 1967). Body mechanics, or the position the mother uses during labor, also affects the length of labor. Most common positions are squatting (DeVidas, 1947), semi-prone with a support person behind (Cosminsky, 1977), right lateral, or with the mother lying on her back. Support systems play an important role in comforting and encouraging the laboring women. Jordan (1978) gives an excellent example of "birthing talk" in the Yucatan. Herbal medicines are frequently used as analgesics or to strengthen contractions (e.g., Cosminsky, 1977), and the application of heat to the abdomen or back is also used to reduce pain (Cosminsky, 1977; Mead & Newton, 1967).

METHODS

Both qualitative and quantitative methods were used in this study. Initially, the research was conducted using the ethnographic approach. Interviews and participant observation were conducted in the hospital, the community, and the surrounding villages. These beginning observations and findings were evaluated, and this initial analysis directed the subsequent research process. Hypotheses were developed and tested until an explanatory theory was derived. Such an approach is the method of choice when literature is sparse and the basic information for deductive research is not available or appropriate. Thus, as the research progressed, relevant events were compiled, compared, and continuously evaluated, and quantitative research methods were used to confirm, refute, or explore new research questions as they evolved.

The research was conducted between October 1980 and March 1981. The researcher's background as a nurse facilitated entry into the setting and the health care system. Multiple methods of data collection were used. First, unstructured interviews were used to elicit the context of birth in each culture from TBAs. Four Fijian "wise ladies" (*yalewa vuku*), one from the upper

Sigatoka River, one from a small village between Sigatoka and Nadi, one from the Ba District, and the fourth from a mountain village behind Tavua, served as informants. Also, four Indian *dai*, three from villages near Ravi-ravi and the fourth from Ba township, served as the main informants for the Fiji-Indian group. These informants supplied information about the context of birth in each culture, which included a description of the traditional and present-day practices for the management of pregnancy, labor and delivery, and the immediate postpartum period and also the beliefs and expectations of behavior for the parturient women. This information was verified with multiparous women in the community, with elderly women, by a lesser number of men, and by observations in the pre- and postnatal clinics and the local hospital. Second, participant observation was conducted in the delivery room, and parturient women were interviewed about their birth experience and beliefs and practices about childbirth. Thirty-two mothers were observed during labor with observations being coded every 30 minutes from the time of admission until contractions were 2 to 3 minutes apart and then every 10 minutes until the second stage, when observations were continuous. Blood pressure and pulse were recorded every 10 minutes to obtain an assessment of maternal distress and a tape recorder was used continuously.

Hypotheses arising from the interviews and observations of women were tested by surveying hospital records. Finally, the cultural perceptions of the painfulness of childbirth, as compared to other painful stimuli, were measured by administering the *Morse Pain Scale* to Fijian and Fiji-Indian mothers in the postpartum period, to mothers who had given birth sometime previously, to nulliparous women (i.e., women who have not experienced childbirth), to nurses (who had indirect experience with childbirth by observation), and to men from both cultural groups, which gave a total sample of 140.

The Morse Pain Stimulus Scale

The Morse Pain Scale was developed using Thurstone's method of paired comparisons (Green, 1954/1974; Nunnally, 1978). This technique permits the ordering and scaling of stimuli that are close together so that the individual would normally have difficulty choosing between them. As there is variation in the selection of paired stimuli, the distribution of judgments of each stimuli are normally distributed on a continuum, and these distributions overlap. The painfulness of certain conditions, including childbirth, can be measured this way. As Zborowski (1952, 1969) and others have shown, the pain experience is culturally shared and transmitted by behavioral cues and verbal descriptors. To ensure cultural relevance of the questionnaire, the pain stimuli included on the scale were obtained by asking Fijian and Fiji-Indian nurses and community members to list the ten most painful conditions they could imagine. The nine most frequently mentioned conditions were heart attack, childbirth, broken leg, a migraine, a stomach cramp, a bad burn, toothache, a kidney stone, and a crushed thumbnail. These were combined in all possible paired combinations resulting in 36 questions. The respondents were asked to answer all the items by circling the more painful condition in each pair. The scale was analyzed by assessing the proportion of subjects responding to each choice in every item. Z-scores were obtained, and the results were reported on a line graph after multiplying each result by ten (see Nunnally, 1978). Results were obtained for both the Fijian and the Fiji-Indian sample.

RESULTS

The Fijians

The Fijian Context of Childbirth

The communal nature of the Fijian life does not exclude children from the knowledge of the physiology of conception, pregnancy, and birth. Small children know and understand "how babies are made" and "where babies come from" and understand the similarity between their own bodies and the bodies of animals they have seen giving birth. Children, as a part of their everyday lives, will have observed pregnant women in the early stage of labor, but not seen a birth. They will have observed nursing women and assisted with the care of her child as a part of their everyday life, and when menarche occurs in adolescence, the girls will have been prepared for the event.

"Love and marriages" are becoming increasingly common, and the traditional customs surrounding the arranged marriage are mostly observed in remote areas. At the time of marriage, Fijian women know what to expect on their wedding night and understand the procreative functions of intercourse.

When pregnancy occurs, the care of the pregnant woman is the responsibility of the whole community with the final responsibility for care allocated to the *yalewa yuku*. However, there was some role differentiation between the four TBAs interviewed. Two provided complete prenatal care, prescribed herbal medicines, supervised the delivery of the infant, and provided postnatal care. The other two did not prescribe herbs, but rather left this to the village women to administer. One described herself as the *nasi ni koro* or village nurse. She reported that she often sought assistance of the *yalewa yuku* when complications arose. The men also had a role in the caring, with the husband relieving the wife of her cooking and gardening responsibilities and other males supporting the husband during delivery. Even the children were sent to find delicacies, such as sea slugs, so the pregnant woman was "spoilt like a baby." Consequently, the care of pregnant women appears to be the responsibility of the entire community. This responsibility manifests itself as a hierarchy that consists of the *yalewa yuku*, the *nasi ni koro*, the women, the men, and lastly the children.

For this caring network to be activated, it is essential that the woman disclose her pregnancy as soon as possible, and many beliefs exist to ensure that this occurs. The Fijians believe in the "power of the unborn embryo" and in the evil power that the newly conceived embryo can exert on other pregnant women, women who have just delivered, and other babies. These embryos have the ability to cause a miscarriage, to make another infant sick, or to cause his hair to fall out. They also believe that an unborn embryo may cause other disasters, such as storms that can upset the canoes and drown men fishing in the ocean. The power of the embryo is removed when the pregnancy is disclosed. Therefore, the fear of causing harm to others forces mothers, especially those in the shameful position of conceiving out of wedlock, to reveal their pregnancy. Several other beliefs also pressure the mother to reveal her pregnancy. In two regions, the Yasawa Islands and the upper Sigatoka River, there are caves with very narrow entrances. If a mother has not disclosed her pregnancy, then her abdomen will enlarge while she is in these caves and she will not be able to get out. Another belief is that if a woman is pregnant, a hooting owl will fly over her house every night. A third belief is that pregnancy cannot be hidden, as changes on the back of the woman's heel are obvious. As the pregnancy progresses, so does the shape and size of the heel until it resembles a pregnant abdomen.

As soon as a woman realizes she is pregnant, she tells her husband who informs the village councilman who, in turn, informs the chief. The pregnancy is then announced at the next village meeting, and multiple caring and support systems are initiated. The woman is never left alone lest *tauriliyalone*, stealing of the embryo (from breaking away or stealing the soul) should occur; *tauriliyalone* can be prevented if another person is in attendance at all times. Fijians also believe in maternal impression. The Fijian mother must watch for someone walking behind her back because this is an attempt to "put his face on the baby." She must think happy and kind thoughts so that the baby will be happy and because "bad" thoughts will cause the infant's face to be distorted and ugly. Expectant mothers are urged to sit for short periods of time and to continue to work on light tasks. A daily walk is essential because it is believed that a lazy mother will have a long and difficult labor. It is also dangerous to sit with one's legs facing the door because a spirit will enter the vagina; in later pregnancy, it is desirable to sit on one's heels to stretch the perineum in preparation for delivery. Pregnant women are given the choicest foods and are encouraged to eat large portions. Traditionally, the husband, or nowadays frequently a young relative, will remain home to care for the expectant mother, to wash clothes in the river, to carry water and firewood, and to do other chores. The *yalewa yuku* performs a bimanual examination (*sili*) early in pregnancy to confirm the pregnancy and assess the position of the uterus and the width of the pelvic outlet. Coconut oil is used as a lubricant, or the women sit in a bowl of warm water for the examination. Herbs[1] may be prescribed (see Table 15.1) because these have the common characteristic of producing a slimy substance (to help the baby slip out easily) when prepared by the shred method.[2] During pregnancy, the *yalewa yuku* performs massage (*bobo*) and may perform external version if the position of the fetus is breech or transverse. The *yalewa yuku* also manually stretches the perineum in preparation for delivery.

At the onset of labor, the woman is encouraged to walk slowly until "one leg is shorter than the other." She gives birth in a specially prepared *bure*, usually her mother's house. A *tapa* cloth divides the room and fresh mats are placed on the ground. Men wait around a *yagona* bowl on one side—where they can hear, but not see, the delivery. Women assist with the delivery

Table 15.1 *Common Herbs Used During Pregnancy and Parturition by Fijian Women*

Herb	Stage of Pregnancy	Purpose
Bele (*A. manihot*)	From the 6th month	To help the baby slip out easily
Verevere (*Clerodendrum inerme* Linn.)	From the 6th month	To help the baby slip out easily
Red hibiscus (*Hibiscus rosasinensis*)	Early pregnancy	To relieve morning sickness
	Mid and late pregnancy	To help the baby slip out easily
Red hibiscus and bele	During labor	To hasten delivery
Vuvudi (*Polyalthia laddiana*)	During labor	To hasten delivery; to stop pain; to clean out the afterbirth
Botebotekoro (*A. Conizoides* Linn.)	During labor and postpartum	To increase contractions; to "make the stomach hard"
Vativati (*Acrostichum aureum* Linn.)	During labor	To stop pain
	Postpartum	To "make the stomach hard"; to cleanse the insides

using soothing phrases roughly translated as "this is the pain you have to bear" and "it will soon be over." Although pain is expected, it is also tolerated. It is not culturally acceptable to cry out. One mother reported that:

Other women laugh at you when you cry. They say "you should not be crying, it [having a baby] is a part of your duty," and, "if you know it hurts, why did you go around doing this to yourself?" They gossip—it's degrading if you cry. Old ladies always admire quiet ladies.

During labor, massage is continued for the relief of pain. The legs and thighs are rubbed to prevent cramping, the abdomen to assist with contractions, and the small of the back to relieve pain. The woman is physically supported by female relatives, and a rope for the woman to pull on may be tied to the rafters. If the labor is difficult, the woman's husband may be admitted to support his wife. When the infant's head appears at the perineum, the *yalewa yuku* lets the birth occur naturally only "pulling the baby out" if the shoulders become impacted. She then smokes a cigarette and relaxes before cutting the cord with a slither of bamboo, a sharp shell, or scissors. The center vein of a coconut palm leaf, which was traditionally used to tie the cord, has been replaced with string, with the cord stump being swabbed with methylated spirits or Dettol® antiseptic. The female relatives then take the infant while the placenta is delivered, and the husband buries the placenta. Nothing is planted on the placenta, nor are there any beliefs concerning the disposal of the placenta. The infant is not placed on the ground, and if it is a chiefly infant, the baby is constantly carried.

The woman rests for 4 days. During this time she will be shown the baby, but since there is a belief that colostrum is poisonous for the infant, the mother will not breastfeed. The infant is fed by the nearest lactating relative, or it is fed *lolo* or coconut milk. The mother is given herbs to cleanse the uterus and does not comb her hair for fear of draining her strength.[3] On the 4th day, there is a feast of thanks for the *yalewa yuku*, and she is presented with mats, cloth, and kerosene as payment. She then returns to her own home but continues to visit the mother daily to administer a massage. When the infant's cord separates, the infant's grandmother or grandfather keeps the cord in a bag and gives a feast to honor the child. Afterwards, the dried cord stump is buried and a coconut palm planted on top. If this is not done, the child will be "flighty" or hyperactive, always searching for his or her cord. The pattern of community caring continues. The infant is carried constantly, passed from one older woman to another. One mother, whose home was half a mile from the village, said that the old women came to fetch her baby at dawn each day because it is believed that early morning rays are especially beneficial for the infant. They cared for the infant to the extent that frequently she did not know where her baby was. Fijian fathers are especially caring toward their infant and display affection openly.

Hospital Delivery

The labor and delivery of three Fijian women[4] (two primigravida and one multigravida) were observed. All women had prepared for labor by taking herbs regularly during the pregnancy. One mother labored for 23 hours, and at one stage she became distressed and whimpered. Valium® 10 mgm IM was given at 3 to 4 cm dilation, and a mixture of nitrous oxide and oxygen was used at the end of the second stage. The other two mothers labored quietly without any signs of distress, lying very quietly and still.

Perception of Childbirth Pain

Analysis of the results of the Morse Pain Scale ($n = 67$) showed that the pain of childbirth was perceived as most severe by the Fijian population (Figure 15.1). Childbirth pain was ranked high (15.51), much higher than a kidney stone (11.36) or a broken leg (10.02) (see Figure 15.1). A comparison of Fijian males and females showed that males (with a score of 18.65) perceive this event to be considerably more painful than females (with a score of 13.17).

Assessment of the Cultural Context

Using the framework presented by Mead and Newton (1969), birth in the Fijian culture is considered an important, natural event that is prepared for extensively. The health of the pregnant mother and the safe birth of the infant are considered the responsibility of the entire community and are shared by the entire community. However, to activate the extensive community support systems that have developed to ensure the safety of the mother and the infant, a system of beliefs exists that coerce the mother to disclose her pregnancy in the first trimester.

The Fiji-Indians

Fiji-Indian Context of Childbirth

In the Fiji-Indian culture, female purity, innocence, and virginity are highly valued. Therefore, sex and topics that are associated with sex (including childbirth) are not discussed. Thus, when a small child asks, "where do babies come from?" he is told, "from New Zealand," "from the store," or "from the

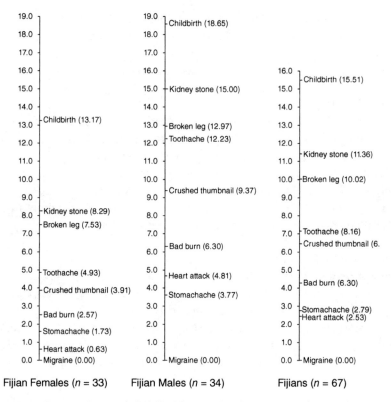

Figure 15.1 *Preceptions of childbirth pain in the Fijian culture: Total group, males and females.*

hospital." Should he realize that an infant is developing within his mother and asks, "how does the child get out?" he is given incorrect information:

> Indian people, they don't want their children to know these things. So they will not tell their children—they just don't answer. My son—he is 5 years—asked how it (the baby) will get out from the stomach and I say, "by the mouth."

To maintain purity in young girls, it is especially important that they remain ignorant of "the facts of life." When they reach adolescence, they know nothing of menstruation until the bleeding begins. Even then, some informants reported that they were too shy to tell their mothers, and instead they sought help from an older sister or sister-in-law. Only a few informants reported knowing about such developmental changes. This information is now a part of the school curriculum (at the fourth form or 8th year), but many girls do not attend school at this age, or menarche has already occurred.

The stress, community suspicion, gossip, and danger of pregnancy that accompanies the loss of purity are controlled by careful cloistering of the females. There is no system of courtship and virtually no interaction between the sexes, even in late adolescence. Consistent with these cultural norms, the student nurses at the local hospital were not permitted to leave the hospital compound alone. In the daylight they left in pairs. If students wished to go to an evening movie they had to be accompanied by a staff nurse. If their parents permitted them to speak to a boy or receive phone calls, they had to bring a parental letter of consent to the hospital matron.

Arranged marriages were the norm. These were contracted several weeks before the wedding ceremony with the bride and groom usually seeing each other only once. At the time of marriage, the Fiji-Indian woman did not know about intercourse, but she is usually informed about this by her husband. Because this information shocked many new brides, it was not uncommon for brides to run away on their wedding night. It is interesting that this knowledge was not withheld from the males and that adolescent boys discussed sexual matters freely among themselves. Adolescent males shared these things in secret, but if one of them "tried something with a girl," the story was repeated and exaggerated. Boys got pictures of women from magazines and shared them, but they were beaten if a teacher caught them. Elderly women were also free to discuss these things among themselves, but they reported that they were "too shy" or "too embarrassed" to give this information to their daughters and daughters-in-law. The person most likely to give assistance, support, and information to the new bride was a sister-in-law, provided she was senior to the bride and a good relationship existed between the two.

When conception occurred, many women did not realize that they were expecting, as they were ignorant of the symptoms of pregnancy. Several informants reported that when they missed their periods and experienced morning sickness, it was the husbands who informed them that they were pregnant. Others were unaware of their condition until quickening occurred. The knowledge of the new pregnancy is kept a close secret by the husband and wife, and even the mother-in-law often does not know about the pregnancy until the fifth or sixth month when the increasing abdominal size can no longer be concealed. Thus prenatal care for the pregnant women is delayed until mid or late pregnancy. One female physician reported that "it is almost impossible to examine them [Indian women]. You cannot see what you are doing, juggling all that *sari*." Even if vaginal examination is performed to assess pelvic adequacy, the women are frequently too tense for examination to provide any meaningful information.

Once the pregnancy is known, no special concessions are made regarding the pregnant woman's work role. If she is married to a cane farmer, she continues her work in the fields. She receives no nutritional supplementation, and because she has the lowest status in the household, she is served food last. Although it is not required that pregnant women observe a fast, a Muslim woman explained that "one got more care from God if this was observed—and the baby would be safer." There are no preparations made for the infant. It is considered "bad luck" to purchase anything for the infant or to choose a name prior to birth.

In spite of this suppression and denial of pregnancy, a few beliefs exist to reduce the mother's anxiety. Most Hindu parents go to a temple and obtain a cord, or *tabeez*, that is tied around the pregnant woman's abdomen to protect the infant. Temple ash is frequently mixed with water and drunk. A penknife may be tied to the woman's undergarment to provide protection from evil eye, and if an eclipse occurs, a pregnant woman must remain indoors with her eyes open. If she sleeps she will miscarry. Many believe that it is dangerous to cut things, especially pumpkin, because this causes a part of the baby to be missing, and the infant will be born with a hare lip, without a finger, or the sex of the infant will be changed from male to female with the severing of the penis. Also, care is taken not to step over a rope that is tethering a cow because this would cause a difficult labor.

In addition, the midwife, or *dai*, did not provide care until the labor began. She would conduct the labor in the mother-in-law's house alone unless the labor was long and difficult at which point the mother-in-law would be admitted. The birth would take place on the floor often with the woman's head and shoulders propped against the wall. The *dai's* role was mostly one of passive nonintervention, watching and waiting. Comfort was provided verbally, rather than by touch. They instructed the mothers to keep pushing ("*gatero, gatero, gatero*") and not to make noise. The *dai* believes that the birth can take place by itself and only sometimes supports the infant's head. After the birth, the cord is cut with a new razor blade soaked in hot water, and the cord is tied with string. Warm charcoal is mixed with *ghee* and rubbed on the cord. The third stage of labor is accelerated by rubbing or "jiggling'" the fundus. Once, when a delay in the delivery of the placenta occurred, one *dai* reported that she stuffed the woman's unbraided hair into her mouth to make her vomit. The resulting Valsalva (or gag reflect) expelled the placenta. Traditionally, the placenta is burned with cow's milk being poured on top of it and the hole is filled and some flowers planted to mark the place. After the birth, the mother and the infant are massaged with coconut oil, and a hot, spiced milk drink called *sont*[5] is given to the mother to restore her strength and to enhance lactation. Colostrum is not given to the infant because it is believed that the "breasts are empty." Until the third day, the infant is fed glucose and water from an enamel bowl or a feeding bottle. The mother is permitted to rest until the 10th day. During this time, a perineal toilet is given by placing warm charcoal in a pan and adding *ghee* or *jarwine* (for warmth). This produces smoke to which the perineum is exposed and then washed. Daily care of the child, and decisions regarding his care, are the privilege of the mother-in-law rather than the new mother.[6] Male infants are especially valued.

Childbirth in a Nontraditional Setting: The Fiji-Indian

Twenty-nine Fiji-Indian women were observed during labor and delivery in the hospital setting. The sample consisted of 22 Hindus, six Muslims, and one Gujarati. Of this group, 13 were primigravida, and 16 were multiparous (gravida ranging from 2 to 9). Three did not deliver normally; one had an epidural anesthetic and forceps delivery, and two others had a lower uterine cesarean section. Subjects age ranged from 18 to 40 years (mean 24.4 years). Three subjects had no education, and all but one had an arranged marriage. None of the women were employed, nor had they ever been employed outside the home. Their husbands, with the exception of one teacher and two clerks, were in nonprofessional positions.

Interviews in the delivery room revealed that the primigravida did not have basic knowledge regarding the birth process, nor did they know what to expect. Women asked questions such as:

Why is it paining [sic] and then stop?

Sometimes my stomach gets very hard and then it pains me.

One woman cried when she was told that the birth process—and the pain—would continue for a number of hours. Some women did not know how the baby would get out. Others told me that they guessed that it "would come from there, as that's where the doctor examines, eh?"

Crowded conditions at the hospital and other responsibilities of the nurse resulted in the patient often laboring alone for long periods of time. This, combined with ignorance on the part of the patient, resulted in a panicked patient. Patients called out constantly in labor, wailing and praying to *Allah* or calling for *uma* (mother) and openly crying. The vocalizations continued between contractions, and as the labor progressed they became more intense during contractions. Patients were considered to be uncooperative by the staff. Some multigravida pushed too early in the labor (before the cervix was fully dilated), and other patients continued to push between contractions. Other patients tried to touch the perineum (considered, by the nurses, as a contaminating action) and frequently would not lie still. Many patients begged for the doctor to "cut the baby out." Most patients were left in the care of the staff in the hospital. Only occasionally did the patient's mother or mother-in-law remain in the ward or on the hospital grounds. If a

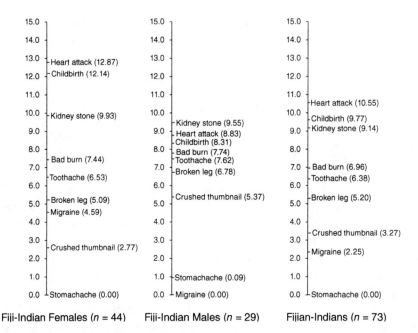

Figure 15.2 *Preconceptions of childbirth pain in the Fiji-Indian total group, males and females.*
Source: Morse (1982). Reprinted with permission by the Transcultural Nursing Society.

husband brought his wife to the hospital, he left quickly and did not return until the infant was born. The nurses were astounded when told that their patients did not know what was happening to their bodies during the birthing process, and the nurses continued to confirm this observation with all Fiji-Indian patients admitted. Because the nurses had learned the anatomy and physiology of reproduction as a part of their nursing education, and as the taboo against discussing such matters worked both ways, they had not previously recognized the patients' innocence and ignorance.

Perception of Childbirth Pain

The Pain Stimulus scale was administered to 29 Fiji-Indian males and 44 females (Figure 15.2). The results showed that the pain of childbirth was ranked lower than that caused by a heart attack by the females, and ranked third, which is much lower, by the males.

Assessment of the Context of Childbirth

Again using Mead and Newton's (1967) framework, childbirth in the Fiji-Indian culture is suppressed, ignored, and denied. When women were asked questions concerning what they did to care for themselves during pregnancy, they replied "nothing." When asked how their lives changed when they became pregnant, they replied that "nothing was changed." The sexual implications of pregnancy and the intimate examinations and exposure associated with the delivery are very stressful and shameful to the Fiji-Indian. This culture copes with this stress by concealing the pregnancy as long as possible, which jeopardizes the health of the mother and the infant by limiting dietary supplements, not permitting adjustments in the work role, inhibiting a supportive environment, and denying information on how to cope with labor and delivery. This pattern of denial includes cultural devaluing of the parturition pain, especially by the males, who are not associated with the delivery at all. Although pleased with the new infant, especially a son, the integration of the mother and the infant proceeds only after purification rituals. For the mother, the postpartum period is one of uncleanliness, and she is excluded from the temple for 30 days. In the first week of life, the Hindu infant must have his head shaved because the dirty hair (i.e., that which has been inside his mother) must be removed. New, strong, clean hair grows to replace the first hair. It is during this time, however, that the mother is cared for, massaged, and given a high-protein ginger drink, *sont*, to enhance lactation.

DISCUSSION

As shown, the child birthing systems in the Fijian and Fiji-Indian cultures are divergent. Whereas childbirth in the Fijian culture is natural and the pregnancy is revealed as early as possible, in the Fiji-Indian culture the pregnancy is concealed as long as possible. In the Fijian culture, there is a system to care for the mother in the form of massage, herbal medicines, dietary supplements, changes in the work role, and protective beliefs, whereas in the Fiji-Indian culture there are only a few protective religious and folk beliefs to help the women cope. It is possible that these beliefs, such as it being "bad luck" to purchase anything or to choose a name for the infant before the birth, exist to reduce maternal attachment. This, however, needs to be investigated further. The lack of relief in the work role for the pregnant Fiji-Indian women is a serious health risk, and it is recognized by the nurses. When the nurses were giving prenatal care they routinely inspected the women's hand for calluses (as a sign of working in the cane fields), and to ensure rest they frequently admitted mothers with signs of early toxemia into hospital. On the other hand, the Fijians care for the pregnant mother by using both the traditional therapies prescribed by the *yalewa yuku* and the hospital clinic. Even in labor, the Fijians continued to take herbal remedies for pain and to speed labor. When asked how they got the medicines, they told the investigator that they "sneaked them in—unless the doctor is Fijian or broad-minded!"

At the onset of labor, the time that the women report to the hospital is statistically significant between the two groups.[7] The Fijians arrived at the hospital late in labor, frequently fully dilated with "head on view." Mothers explained that they would rather give birth in the village "where they felt loved" than in the hospital, so they stayed home as long as possible. On the other hand, the Fiji-Indian mothers reported very early, frequently with false labor, or late with the cervix fully dilated. These problems were caused because the Fiji-Indian mother did not know the signs and symptoms of labor or was "too shy" to report to the family that the contractions had started.

The importance of privacy regarding topics with a sexual connotation impeded the research process and required changes in the research plan. Initially the researcher attempted to conduct interviews in the ward with mothers in early labor and following birth, combined with observations in the labor room. This plan was quickly discarded when the lack of privacy in the ward resulted in a virtual nonresponse from the mothers. It was from the interviews in the labor or delivery room, where the researcher acted as a support person and privacy was ensured, that significant information was obtained.

The difference was also apparent when interviewing the TBAs. Interviews with the *yalewa yuku* were public events, with all interested villagers, including children and males, serving as interested spectators. Interviews were uninhibited, and included detailed discussions and simulated demonstrations of positions used for delivery. Information was frequently sought from the researcher as to "how things were done in America"—a topic that provoked much laughter. On the other hand, interviews with the Indian *dai* commenced only when the *dai* could be assured that no one would overhear the interview. The *dai* took care to send their daughters and daughters-in-law on an errand so that they would not overhear the conversation. Interviews with elderly Fiji-Indian women were sometimes conducted in small groups, provided the women were age peers and related and if privacy was ensured. The researcher was privy to such information only after she had established her status as a married woman with children.

In the labor room, there were striking differences in the behavioral expression of pain between the two groups. The Fijians tended to labor silently, lying still and quietly, whereas the Fiji-Indians were restless and noisy patients. In spite of the evidence that the Fiji-Indians appeared to suffer more, the amount of pain associated with childbirth was rated higher by the Fijians. It is important to note that the scale measures the amount of pain *thought* to be associated with childbirth. In the Fijian culture, in which the risk of childbirth is acknowledged and prepared for, there are herbs, psychological support, and other physiological comfort measures to reduce the pain. The Fijian males indirectly learn about the painfulness of childbirth by listening to, but not seeing, a birth. This secondary role, helping only with minor tasks and assisting with only the most difficult labors, projects the severity of the pain to the males, yet denies them full participation in the birth process and the opportunity to relieve anxieties through direct caring tasks. Thus, childbirth pain is rated highest by this group. The listening and the waiting of the males are probably also associated with the Fijian value on silent labor and the urging of women not to cry out. Conversely, Fiji-Indian males are excluded from participation in the birth event and are not required to assist the mother in the postpartum period. Because childbirth is suppressed and denied, the associated pain is rated low.

These differences in cultural beliefs and practices of mothers in both cultures are reflected in the different rates of maternal and infant mortality within the two groups. As previously mentioned, Fiji-Indian maternal mortality is 26% higher than the Fijian rate (Ministry of Health, n.d.b). Although the number of births conducted by TBAs is declining, these births totalled 6.5% of the 88% of total births registered (Parliament of Fiji, 1977, p. 232). The ethnographic data in this study provides insights into the reasons for the greater utilization of the TBA by the Fijians than by the Fiji-Indians, even in areas where both groups have equal access to services. In Fiji, it does not appear that the TBAs contribute to the inequity in maternal morbidity rates between the two groups. Rather, the comparison of cultural beliefs and practices between the two groups provides insights into the problem. There is evidence that it is the poor diet, intestinal parasites, and the work role of the Fiji-Indian women that contribute to the high rate of anemia and preeclampsia in that population.

Although labor and delivery are the periods of greatest risk to the mother and the infant, the government policy of increasing health care to women throughout pregnancy will reduce the maternal mortality rate. However, the government's task appears difficult because the work role, diet, and cultural attitudes toward the pregnant women in the Fiji-Indian culture are an integral part of the entire social system. Therefore, the primary target group to achieve change is not the pregnant women, but rather, considering the sociocultural construction of pregnancy in this patriarchal society, the primary target group is the mothers-in-law. Change will be slow, and it will probably accompany trends of increased health status in the total group.

CONCLUSION

Examining the effects of culturally patterned behavior provides important insights into the health of each group. The Fijians viewed the extensive traditional caring patterns as a valid and preferable replacement for hospital care, whereas modesty *and* the wish to conceal pregnancy delayed antenatal care for the Fiji-Indian. The support and the caring that the Fijian women received in the village resulted in the reluctance to abandon this setting and to travel to the hospital at labor onset. Fiji-Indians, on the other hand, not knowing the mechanics of labor and delivery, transferred to the hospital either at the first twinges of labor or very late in labor and displayed very panicked behaviors during delivery and were unable to cooperate with the nurses. The Fijians' natural perspective of birth, support systems, and prenatal care prepared them for delivery and for the expected pain of childbirth. On the other hand, there was little support or traditional care for the Fiji-Indian until after the delivery. Pregnancy was denied and suppressed. These differences in the cultural caring systems are reflected in the governmental statistics for maternal–infant morbidity and mortality.

NOTES

Janice M. Morse is professor of nursing and National Health Research Scholar in the Faculty of Nursing, University of Alberta, Edmonton, Alberta, Canada T6G 2G3. Her research interests are in the cultural aspects of health care.

1. Identified using Parham (1972).
2. The leaves (or, in the case of the hibiscus, the outer layer of the stem) are torn into small pieces in a bowl and cold water is added. The leaves are squeezed with the finger, and the resulting shiny, foamy infusion (rather like egg-white) is immediately drunk.
3. This explanation differs from Lester's (1946). He attributes this custom to the wish for postnatal women to appear unattractive to their husbands to assist maintaining the postnatal sexual taboo.
4. The number of Fiji women observed in labor was less than expected because the Fijians were "boycotting" the hospital. Although the hospital served both Fijians and Fiji-Indians, it was originally built to serve the Indians. Consequently, most of the staff were Fiji-Indian, and Indian food was usually served.

5. See Morse (1984).
6. Johnston (1977) noted that this also occurred in Trinidad. She noted that this practice affirms the lowly status of the new mother by separating her from her achievement.
7. Chi square comparison of the degrees of cervical dilation of Fijian (n = 35) and Fiji-Indian (n = 38) mothers at the time of admission to the labor ward was statistically significant (χ^2 = 9.58, df = 4, $p \leq .05$). Cervical dilation was measured as: 0 (false labor); 1–3 cm; 4–7 cm; 8–9 cm; and fully dilated.

REFERENCES

Chen, P. C. Y. (1973). An analysis of customs related to childbirth in rural Malay culture. *Tropical and Geographic Medicine, 25*, 197–204.

Cosminsky, S. (1977). Childbirth and midwifery on a Guatemalan Finca. *Medical Anthropology, 1*(3), 69–101.

De Vidas, J. (1947). Childbirth among the aranda, Central Australia. *Oceania, 18*, 117–119.

Duignan, N. M., Studd, J. W. W., & Hughes, A. O. (1975). Characteristics of normal labor in different racial groups. *British Journal of Obstetrics and Psychiatry, 82*, 593–601.

Frazer, R. (1973). The Fijian village and the independent farmer. In H. Brookfield (Ed.), *The Pacific in transition: Geographical perspectives on adaptation and change* (pp. 75–96). London, UK: Edwards Arnold.

Gillam, B. (1973). Beliefs of the Wapei people about conception, childbirth and early childcare. *Tropical Doctor, 3*, 85–87.

Green, B. (1954/1974). Paired comparison scaling procedure. In G. M. Maraneli (Ed.), *Scaling: A sourcebook for behavioral scientists* (pp. 93–97). New York, NY: Aldine.

Johnston, J. (1977, December). *The household context of infant feeding practices in South Trinidad.* Paper presented at the Annual Meeting of the American Anthropological Association. Houston.

Jordan, B. (1978). *Birth in four cultures: A cross-cultural Investigation of childbirth in Yucatan, Holland, Sweden and the United States.* Montreal: Eden Press Women's.

Kay, M. A. (1982). *Anthropology of human birth.* Philadelphia, PA: F.A. Davis.

Kerr, G. J. A., & Donnelly, T. A. (1976). *Fiji in the Pacific* (3rd ed.). Hong Kong: The Jacaronda Press.

Lester, R. H. (1946). A few customs observed by Fijians in connections with birth, betrothal, marriage and death. *Fiji Society of Science and Industry, 2*, 113–129.

Lim, M. A., Wong, W. P., & Sinnathuray, T. A. (1977). Characteristics of normal labor among different racial groups of Malaysia. *British Journal of Obstetrics and Gynaecology, 84*, 600–604.

MacCormack, C. P. (Ed.). (1982). *Ethnography of fertility and birth.* London, UK: Academic Press.

McCain, C. (1975). Ethno-obstetrics in Ajijic. *Anthropological Quarterly, 48,* 38–56.

Mead, M., & Newton, N. (1967). Cultural patterning of perinatal behavior. In S. Richardson & A. E. Guttnaler (Eds.), *Childbearing—Its social and psychological aspects.* Baltimore, MD: Williams and Wilkins.

Melmed, H., & Evans, M. I. (1976). Patterns of labor in native and immigrant populations in Israel. *Israel Journal of Medical Science, 12*(2), 1404–1409.

Ministry of Health. (n.d.a). *Complications of childbearing in Fiji, 1973–1975.* Unpublished Report, Suva: Government of Fiji.

Ministry of Health. (n.d.b). *Maternal mortality in Fiji, 1976–1979.* Unpublished Report, Suva: Government of Fiji.

Morse, J. M. (1981). Descriptive analysis of cultural coping mechanisms utilized for the reduction of parturition pain and anxiety in Fiji. Unpublished doctoral dissertation, University of Utah. University microfilms No. DA8208935.

Morse, J. M. (1982). "Does it Hurt?" Cultural variation in the perception of painful events. In C. N. Uhl & J. Uhl (Eds.), *Transcultural nursing. Proceedings from the seventh transcultural nursing conference* (pp. 45–53). Salt Lake City, Utah: University of Utah and the Transcultural Nursing Society.

Morse, J. M. (1984). The cultural context of infant feeding in Fiji. *Ecology of Food and Nutrition, 14,* 287–296.

Naidu, V. (1980). *The violence of the indenture of Fiji.* Fiji Monograph Series, No. 3. Suva: The World University Science.

Nunnally, J. C. (1978). *Psychometric theory.* New York, NY: McGraw-Hill.

Parham, J. W. (1972). *Plants of the Fiji Islands.* Suva: Government Printer.

Parliament of Fiji. (1977). *Report on the census of the population.* 1976, Vol. 1, Part 4. Parliamentary Paper 13 of 1977. Suva: Government Printing Department.

Paul, J. P. (1967). Childbirth among the lawa people of northern thailand. *Obstetrics and Gynecology, 30,* 756–757.

Quain, B. (1948). *Fijian village.* Chicago, IL: University of Chicago Press.

Spenser, D. M. (1966). *Disease, religion and society in the Fiji islands.* Seattle: University of Washington.

Wellin, E. (1978). Theoretical orientations in medical anthropology: Change and continuity over the past half-century. In M. H. Logan & E. E. Hunt, Jr. (Eds.), *Health and the human condition* (pp. 23–39). North Scituate, MA: Duxbury Press.

Zborowski, M. (1952). Cultural components in response to pain. *Journal of Social Issues, 8,* 16–30.

Zborowski, M. (1969). *People in pain.* San Francisco, CA: Jossey-Bass.

COMMENTARY TO "CULTURAL RESPONSES TO PARTURITION: CHILDBIRTH IN FIJI"

Backstage Ethnography

Once, in the middle of writing my dissertation (Morse, 1981), a professor gave me some advice: "In a few years you will not even want to use it as a doorstop!" I mulled this over and kept on writing.

This professor was both right and wrong. Let's start with *wrong*: It did take a few years for the full-length dissertation to be published as an article (Morse, 1989)—almost a decade, to be exact, before the articles were in print. Meanwhile, the dissertation findings spurred a few more studies on the cultural assessment of the painfulness of painful events (Morse & Morse, 1988; Morse & Park, 1988a, 1988b)—but no one seems to have noticed, so I am grateful to Mary de Chesnay for giving this research a second chance. And in the field, I learned how to do ethnography— the hard way, the traditional way, on my feet. I now believe we owe to the new ethnographers (and to the literature) a glimpse into the backstage, bringing it forward. Doing ethnography is not easy—in fact, it is grueling—and again, I appreciate the opportunity to tell the story of foreign fieldwork.

But this cynical professor was also *right*—some parts belong in the doorstop. I realized the potential of the study but did not write about the potential as specifically as I should have, believing in graduating without sticking out my neck. I realize now that this was a mistake, and I should have taken the research the full theoretical nine yards. Again, I thank Mary for this space. The second realization was that descriptive, ethnographic fieldwork cannot be given justice in a 20-page article, and the research should have been published as a monograph. Of course, complete dissertation copies were presented to the Minister of Health, Government of Fiji, to the University of South Pacific Library, and to the Hospital where the study was done, as well as University of Michigan, but that is not *true* dissemination. And now I worry about students who are forced into writing ethnographies as three or more articles for publication. This practice breaks the cohesiveness of the ethnography and destroys its wholeness.

Backstage

As a doctoral student, I was fascinated by the differences in the cultural responses to pain. Zborowski's (1952, 1969) study showed that the painfulness of painful events were culturally learned, and these differences were behaviorally manifest. But in doing a pain study, did I have to *measure* pain? June Abbey, our professor in physiology, came to my rescue and told me all about pulse transit time (PTT) machines, which measured the transit time for the R-wave to the finger. In theory, the faster the pulse, the greater is the pain being experienced. I ordered one of these machines with my meager doctoral stipend and was very impressed. It was battery powered, had leads and electrodes, dials and flashing lights. Indeed, this machine may be credited for getting me into a hospital as a researcher—as a *scientist*—but it failed almost as soon as I started data collection. Apparently, the golden rule for anthropology fieldwork is that all equipment should be taken upto the roof and dropped. Then, if it still works, take it with you. Failure of essential equipment is formula for panic: Did I still have a research project?

Other technical difficulties with my "protocol" involved documenting the sounds of distress during labor. My protocol instructed me to place a tape recorder on the patient's locker, but all I recorded was the roar of the air conditioner when the sun shone or the roar of rain on the title roof when it did not.

Critical in my proposal were interviews with women in early labor to find out their expectations of the birthing experience. Everyone, it seemed, stayed in bed in the ward, even those in early labor. The entire ward it seemed—20 other postpartum mothers—listened intently to my interview questions. Beds in the mission hospital were very close together, and the ward was silent, with no TV or radios. All they heard was my voice, for none of the mothers being interviewed answered my questions. The only response of the interviewees was an occasional nod. I had examples of the world's worst interviews. And I am embarrassed to tell you how many interviews I conducted before I realized that it was a fruitless way to collect data, especially in a culture where no one discussed such matters. Fortunately, I kept these tapes, and once I understood why these mothers were silent, they proved to be excellent examples of the power of the modesty taboo.

My excellent proposal also recommended that my role during delivery would be that of an *observer*. I coded behaviors and recorded the course of labor, physiological signs, and caregiver actions on a spreadsheet. But I did not feel I was learning anything and had no idea how these marks would be interpreted—statistical tallying seemed inadequate to capture what I was seeing, and I was very aware that my sample size would be too small at the end of data collection to be meaningful. As the staff became accustomed to me, they increasingly left me alone in the delivery room, knowing I would call them once the delivery was imminent. They found my meticulous recording of blood pressure, the timing of contractions, and so forth, very handy to copy onto the patient's charts to ensure their records were complete, but then I had little data about nurse–patient interactions.

It was in such a situation, alone in the delivery room, that one of Agar's (1982) rich points occurred: A young primigravida asked: "Doctor, what is happening? How is the baby going to get out?" Oh. I sat on her bed and became a midwife, rubbing her back and giving her sips of water. "Now," I said, "Here's the bargain: You tell me what you know, and I'll tell you what I know."

It was at this point that I became an ethnographer. I had conducted interviews with TBAs in the villages for several months, and all that they had told me then clicked into place. The traditional practices of childbirth of both Fijian and Fiji-Indian cultures were reflected in their present attitudes and behaviors. I stopped collecting physiological data and stopped doing the ridiculous, silent pre- and postnatal interviews. Instead, I interviewed women in the delivery room, sitting on their beds, rubbing their backs. Suddenly, I understood the role and strength—no, the amazing force—of the modesty taboo in the Fiji-Indian culture. I immediately saw how it impacted on the behavior of the parturient women, how it interfered with care, and I also saw its ramification on the maternal and infant morbidity rate. I understood that the vocalizations of Fiji-Indian women and the silence of the Fijian during delivery were because of cultural patterning and not the intensity of pain being experienced. And the question, "How is the baby going to get out?"—the cultural concealing of the mechanics of birth from the Fiji-Indian first-time pregnant mothers—was also because of the essential maintenance of the cultural purity of females (Mead & Newton, 1967). The silence during birth may be attributed to the communal approach to birth in the Fijian culture, with the males sitting and listening outside the hut. I was astonished to see these micro–macro linkages . . . but realized that I was not finished yet.

I asked the nurses, "How do you know who has pain, and who does not?" They all said: "I don't know—I have never had a baby!" But I knew they knew, because I had watched them make decisions about who was to be given analgesia and when, and I had observed nurses and listened to the way they spoke about "naughty patients" (those who were vocalizing, screaming, and did not follow instructions) and "good patients" (those who were obedient and silent). I recalled from my psychometrics class how to measure and rank close stimuli using Thurstone's technique of paired comparisons (Nunnally, 1967). And importantly, this time I knew my way around—back to the stationery shop for stencils; type the questionnaire, one manual key at a time; beg favors for it to be translated into Fijian and Hindi; and run back to the church basement to run off mimeographed copies. Now I had lots of assistants—nurses and even the hospital chaplain took my questionnaires out to their villages and into the town to be completed. Once fieldwork makes sense, it's great fun.

Afterward

Then back home, with the dissertation defended and settled into a position, I realized I was not quite finished. I needed some additional data about the "cultural response to pain." I realized the implications: that caregivers viewed the painfulness of pain events from their cultural perspective, and if the patients' behavior did not match the caregivers' cultural frame, proper pain control was not given.

I needed more data and used Thurstone's technique again, comparing perceptions of pain between mothers who had home births with mothers who had hospital births (Morse & Park, 1988a), the cultural differences in pain expectations between East Indian, Hutterite, Ukrainian, and Anglophone Canadians (Morse & Morse, 1988), and even an encyclopedia entry (Morse & Park, 1988b).

Implications

By this stage, I recognized the full implications and how this work extended Zborowski's (1969) study showing that pain behaviors were culturally learned and culturally transmitted. I recognized that *how painful* something was perceived to be determined whether or not the person in pain received compassion, kindness, analgesics, or care. Even today, we have several illnesses that are not culturally recognized, and those suffering from such conditions as fibromyalgia or females with symptoms of a heart attack have not received care in the past, although this is now changing. And I learned painfully how nonmainstream my thinking was by submitting an article to *Pain*. The reviewer wrote: *This is a peculiar paper. The authors are measuring pain, based on people's guesses according to folklore.* I recognized that this was true, but also that the physician reviewing the article did not know anthropology, nor understand culture, nor appreciate the power of human interaction. When presenting the study, many people asked me, "how could people who had not experienced the pain, evaluate the painfulness of the pain—for instance, men evaluate childbirth?" I would reply that we are taught how painful these conditions are; we observe people in pain with these conditions; and, of course, we care for them, evaluate their pain, and do decide when it should or should not be treated. Knowing the perceived painfulness of painful conditions is a part of our cultural understanding of ourselves, something that is used in interaction, in caregiving, and medical care. Perhaps we do not yet fully understand it nor put it in the equation when providing care.

Are some questions too large for a dissertation? Perhaps; but they are worth tackling, and fun to do so. If they do become a doorstop, at least they become interesting ones.

REFERENCES

Agar, M. (1982). *The professional stranger*. New York, NY: Wiley.

Mead, M., & Newton, N. (1967). Cultural patterning of perinatal behavior. In S. Richardson & A. F. Guttnaler (Eds.), *Childbearing: Its social and psychological aspects*. Baltimore, MD: Williams & Wilkins.

Morse, J. M. (1981). *Descriptive analysis of cultural coping mechanisms utilized for the reduction of parturition pain and anxiety in Fiji*. (Unpublished doctoral dissertation). University of Utah. University microfilms No. DA8208935.

Morse, J. M. (1989). Cultural variation in behavioral response to parturition: Chilbirth in Fiji. *Medical Anthropology, 12*(1), 35–54.

Morse, J. M., & Morse, R. M. (1988). Evaluation of the pain experience of others: Cultural variation in the perception of painful events. *Journal of Cross-Cultural Psychology, 19*(2), 232–242.

Morse, J. M., & Park, C. (1988a). Hospital births and home deliveries: Comparison of the perceived painfulness of parturition. *Research in Nursing and Health, 11*, 175–181.

Morse, J. M., & Park, C. (1988b). Differences in cultural expectations of the perceived painfulness of parturition. In K. Michaelson (Ed.), *Childbirth in America: Anthropological perspectives* (pp. 121–129). South Hadley, MA: Bergin & Garvey.

Nunnally, J. C. (1967). *Psychometic theory*. New York, NY: McGraw Hill.

Zborowski, M. (1952). Cultural components in response to pain. *Journal of Social Issues, 8*, 16–30.

Zborowski, M. (1969). *People in pain*. San Francisco, CA: Jossey-Bass.

LIST OF JOURNALS THAT PUBLISH QUALITATIVE RESEARCH

Mary de Chesnay

Conducting excellent research and not publishing the results negates the study and prohibits anyone from learning from the work. Therefore, it is critical that qualitative researchers disseminate their work widely, and the best way to do so is through publication in refereed journals. The peer review process, although seemingly brutal at times, is designed to improve knowledge by enhancing the quality of literature in a discipline. Fortunately, the publishing climate has evolved to the point where qualitative research is valued by editors and readers alike, and many journals now seek out, or even specialize in publishing, qualitative research.

The following table was compiled partially from the synopsis of previous work identifying qualitative journals by the St. Louis University Qualitative Research Committee (2013), with a multidisciplinary faculty, who are proponents of qualitative research. Many of these journals would be considered multidisciplinary, though marketed to nurses. All are peer reviewed. Other journals were identified by the author of this series and by McKibbon and Gadd (2004) in their quantitative analysis of qualitative research. It is not meant to be exhaustive, and we would welcome any suggestions for inclusion.

An additional resource is the nursing literature mapping project conducted by Sherwill-Navarro and Allen (Allen, Jacobs, & Levy, 2006). The 217 journals were listed as a resource for libraries to accrue relevant journals, and many of them publish qualitative research. Readers are encouraged to view the websites for specific journals that might be interested in publishing their studies. Readers are also encouraged to look outside the traditional nursing journals, especially if their topics more closely match the journal mission of related disciplines.

NURSING JOURNALS

Journal	Website
Advances in Nursing Science	www.journals.lww.com/advancesinnursingscience/pages/default.aspx
Africa Journal of Nursing and Midwifery	www.journals.co.za/ej/ejour_ajnm.html
Annual Review of Nursing Research	www.springerpub.com/product/07396686#.UeaXbjvvv6U
British Journal of Nursing	www.britishjournalofnursing.com
Canadian Journal of Nursing Research	www.cjnr.mcgill.ca
Hispanic Health Care International	www.springerpub.com/product/15404153#.UeaX7jvvv6U
Holistic Nursing Practice	www.journals.lww.com/hnpjournal/pages/default.aspx
International Journal of Mental Health Nursing	www.onlinelibrary.wiley.com/journal/10.1111/(ISSN)1447-0349
International Journal of Nursing Practice	www.onlinelibrary.wiley.com/journal/10.1111/(ISSN)1440-172X
International Journal of Nursing Studies	www.journals.elsevier.com/international-journal-of-nursing-studies
Journal of Advanced Nursing	www.onlinelibrary.wiley.com/journal/10.1111/(ISSN)1365-2648
Journal of Clinical Nursing	www.onlinelibrary.wiley.com/journal/10.1111/(ISSN)1365-2702
Journal of Family Nursing	www.jfn.sagepub.com
Journal of Nursing Education	www.healio.com/journals/JNE
Journal of Nursing Scholarship	www.onlinelibrary.wiley.com/journal/10.1111/(ISSN)1547-5069
Nurse Researcher	www.nurseresearcher.rcnpublishing.co.uk
Nursing History Review	www.aahn.org/nhr.html
Nursing Inquiry	www.onlinelibrary.wiley.com/journal/10.1111/(ISSN)1440-1800
Nursing Research	www.ninr.nih.gov
Nursing Science Quarterly	www.nsq.sagepub.com
Online Brazilian Journal of Nursing	www.objnursing.uff.br/index.php/nursing

(continued)

Journal	Website
The Online Journal of Cultural Competence in Nursing and Healthcare	www.ojccnh.org
Public Health Nursing	www.onlinelibrary.wiley.com/journal/10.1111 /(ISSN)1525-1446
Qualitative Health Research	www.qhr.sagepub.com
Qualitative Research in Nursing and Healthcare	www.wiley.com/WileyCDA/WileyTitle/product Cd-1405161221.html
Research and Theory for Nursing Practice	www.springerpub.com/product/15416577#.Ueab lTvvv6U
Scandinavian Journal of Caring Sciences	www.onlinelibrary.wiley.com/journal/10.1111 /(ISSN)1471-6712
Western Journal of Nursing Research	http://wjn.sagepub.com

REFERENCES

Allen, M., Jacobs, S. K., & Levy, J. R. (2006). Mapping the literature of nursing: 1996–2000. *Journal of the Medical Library Association, 94*(2), 206–220. Retrieved from http://nahrs.mlanet.org/home/images/activity/nahrs2012selectedlist nursing.pdf

McKibbon, K., & Gadd, C. (2004). A quantitative analysis of qualitative studies in clinical journals for the publishing year 2000. *BMC Med Inform Decision Making, 4*, 11. Retrieved from http://www.ncbi.nlm.nih.gov/pmc/articles/PMC503397

St. Louis University Qualitative Research Committee. Retrieved July 14, 2013, from http://www.slu.edu/organizations/qrc/QRjournals.html

ESSENTIAL ELEMENTS FOR A QUALITATIVE PROPOSAL

Tommie Nelms

1. Introduction: Aim of the study
   a. Phenomenon of interest, and focus of inquiry
   b. Justification for studying the phenomenon (how big an issue/problem?)
   c. Phenomenon discussed within a specific context (lived experience, culture, human response)
   d. Theoretical framework(s)
   e. Assumptions, biases, experiences, intuitions, and perceptions related to the belief that inquiry into a phenomenon is important (researcher's relationship to the topic)
   f. Qualitative methodology chosen, with rationale
   g. Significance to nursing (How will the new knowledge gained benefit patients, nursing practice, nurses, society, etc.?)
   Note: The focus of interest/inquiry and statement of purpose of the study should appear at the top of page 3 of the proposal
2. Literature review: What is known about the topic? How has it been studied in the past?
   Include background of the theoretical framework and how it has been used in the past.
3. Methodology
   a. Introduction of methodology (philosophical underpinnings of the method)
   b. Rationale for choosing the methodology
   c. Background of methodology
   d. Outcome of methodology
   e. Methods: general sources, and steps and procedures
   f. Translation of concepts and terms

4. Methods
    a. Aim
    b. Participants
    c. Setting
    d. Gaining access, and recruitment of participants
    e. General steps in conduct of study (data gathering tool(s), procedures, etc.)
    f. Human subjects' considerations
    g. Expected timetable
    h. Framework for rigor, and specific strategies to ensure rigor
    i. Plans and procedures for data analysis

WRITING QUALITATIVE RESEARCH PROPOSALS

Joan L. Bottorff

PURPOSE OF A RESEARCH PROPOSAL

- Communicates research plan to others (e.g., funding agencies)
- Serves as a detailed plan of action
- Serves as a contract between investigator and funding bodies when proposal is approved

QUALITATIVE RESEARCH: BASIC ASSUMPTIONS

- Reality is complex, constructed, and, ultimately, subjective.
- Research is an interpretative process.
- Knowledge is best achieved by conducting research in the natural setting.

QUALITATIVE RESEARCH

- Qualitative research is unstructured.
- Qualitative designs are "emergent" rather than fixed.
- The results of qualitative research are unpredictable. (Morse, 1994)

KINDS OF QUALITATIVE RESEARCH

- Grounded theory
- Ethnography (critical ethnography, institutional ethnography, ethno-methodology, ethnoscience, etc.)
- Phenomenology
- Narrative inquiry
- Others

CHALLENGES FOR QUALITATIVE RESEARCHERS

- Developing a solid, convincing argument that the study contributes to theory, research, practice, and/or policy (the "so what?" question)
- Planning a study that is systematic, manageable, and flexible (to reassure skeptics):
  - Justification of the selected qualitative method
  - Explicit details about design and methods, without limiting the project's evolution
  - Attention to criteria for the overall soundness or rigor of the project

QUESTIONS A PROPOSAL MUST ANSWER

- Why should anyone be interested in my research?
- Is the research design credible, achievable, and carefully explained?
- Is the researcher capable of conducting the research? (Marshall & Rossman, 1999)

TIPS TO ANSWER THESE QUESTIONS

- Be practical (practical problems cannot be easily brushed off)
- Be persuasive ("sell" your proposal)
- Make broad links (hint at the wider context)
- Aim for crystal clarity (avoid jargon, assume nothing, explain everything) (Silverman, 2000)

SECTIONS OF A TYPICAL QUALITATIVE PROPOSAL

- Introduction
  - Introduction of topic and its significance
  - Statement of purpose, research questions/objectives
- Review of literature
  - Related literature and theoretical traditions
- Design and methods
  - Overall approach and rationale
  - Sampling, data gathering methods, data analysis
  - Trustworthiness (soundness of the research)
  - Ethical considerations
- Dissemination and knowledge translation
  - Timeline
  - Budget
  - Appendices

INTRODUCING THE STUDY—FIRST PARA

- Goal: Capture interest in the study
  - Focus on the importance of the study (Why bother with the question?)
  - Be clear and concise (details will follow)
  - Provide a synopsis of the primary target of the study
  - Present persuasive logic backed up with factual evidence

THE PROBLEM/RESEARCH QUESTION

- The problem can be broad, but it must be specific enough to convince others that it is worth focusing on.
- Research questions must be clearly delineated.
- The research questions must sometimes be delineated with sub-questions.
- The scope of the research question(s) needs to be manageable within the time frame and context of the study.

PURPOSE OF THE QUALITATIVE STUDY

- Discovery?
- Description?
- Conceptualization (theory building)?
- Sensitization?
- Emancipation?
- Other?

LITERATURE REVIEW

- The literature review should be selective and persuasive, building a case for what is known or believed, what is missing, and how the study fits in.
- The literature is used to demonstrate openness to the complexity of the phenomenon, rather than funneling toward an a priori conceptualization.

METHODS—CHALLENGES HERE

- Quantitative designs are often more familiar to reviewers.
- Qualitative researchers have a different language.

METHODS SECTION

- Orientation to the Method:
  - Description of the particular method that will be used and its creators/interpreters
  - Rationale for qualitative research generally and for the specific method to be used.

QUALITATIVE STUDIES ARE VALUABLE FOR RESEARCH

- It delves deeply into complexities and processes.
- It focuses on little-known phenomena or innovative systems.

- It explores informal and unstructured processes in organizations.
- It seeks to explore where and why policy and local knowledge and practice are at odds.
- It is based on real, as opposed to stated, organizational goals.
- It cannot be done experimentally for practical or ethical reasons.
- It requires identification of relevant variables. (Marshall & Rossman, 1999)

SAMPLE

- Purposive or theoretical sampling
  - The purpose of the sampling
  - Characteristics of potential types of persons, events, or processes to be sampled
  - Methods of making decisions about sampling
- Sample size
  - Estimates provided based on previous experience, pilot work, etc.
- Access and recruitment

DATA COLLECTION AND ANALYSIS

- Types: Individual interviews, participant observation, focus groups, personal and public documents, Internet-based data, videos, and so on, all of which vary with different traditions.
- Analysis methods vary depending on the qualitative approach.
- Add DETAILS and MORE DETAILS about how data will be gathered and processed (procedures should be made public).

QUESTIONS FOR DATA MANAGEMENT AND ANALYSIS

- How will data be kept organized and retrievable?
- How will data be "broken up" to see something new?
- How will the researchers engage in reflexivity (e.g., be self-analytical)?
- How will the reader be convinced that the researcher is sufficiently knowledgeable about qualitative analysis and has the necessary skills?

TRUSTWORTHINESS (SOUNDNESS OF THE RESEARCH)

- Should be reflected throughout the proposal
- Should be addressed specifically, with the relevant criteria for the qualitative approach used
- Should provide examples of the strategies used:
  - Triangulation
  - Prolonged contact with informants, including continuous validation of data
  - Continuous checking for representativeness of data and fit between coding categories and data
  - Use of expert consultants

EXAMPLES OF STRATEGIES FOR LIMITING BIAS IN INTERPRETATIONS

- Planning to search for negative cases
- Describing how analysis will include a purposeful examination of alternative explanations
- Using members of the research team to critically question the analysis
- Planning to conduct an audit of data collection and analytic strategies

OTHER COMPONENTS

- Ethical considerations
  - Consent forms
  - Dealing with sensitive issues
- Dissemination and knowledge translation
- Timeline
- Budget justification

LAST BITS OF ADVICE

- Seek assistance and pre-review from others with experience in grant writing. (plan time for rewriting)
- Highlight match between your proposal and purpose of competition.
- Follow the rules of the competition.
- Write for a multidisciplinary audience.

REFERENCES

Marshall, C., & Rossman, G. B. (1999). *Designing qualitative research.* Thousand Oaks, CA: Sage.

Morse, J. M. (1994). Designing funded qualitative research. In N. Denzin & Y. Lincoln (Eds.), *Handbook of qualitative research* (pp. 220–235). Thousand Oaks, CA: Sage.

Silverman, D. (2000). *Doing qualitative research.* Thousand Oaks, CA: Sage.

OUTLINE FOR A RESEARCH PROPOSAL

Mary de Chesnay

*T*he following guidelines are meant as a general set of suggestions that supplement the instructions for the student's program. In all cases where there is conflicting advice, the student should be guided by the dissertation chair's instructions. The outlined plan includes five chapters: the first three constitute the proposal and the remaining two the results and conclusions, but the number may vary depending on the nature of the topic or the style of the committee chair (e.g., I do not favor repeating the research questions at the beginning of every chapter, but some faculty do. I like to use this outline but some faculty prefer a different order. Some studies lend themselves to four instead of five chapters.).

Chapter I: Overview of the Study (or Preview of Coming Attractions) is a few pages that tell the reader:

- What he or she is going to investigate (purpose or statement of the problem and research questions or hypotheses)
- What theoretical support the idea has (conceptual framework or theoretical support). In qualitative research, this section may include only a rationale for conducting the study, with the conceptual framework or typology emerging from the data.
- What assumptions underlie the problem
- What definitions of terms are important to state (typically, these definitions in quantitative research are called *operational definitions* because they describe how one will know the item when one sees it. An operational definition usually starts with the phrase: "a score of … or above on the [name of instrument]"). One may also want to include a conceptual definition, which is the usual meaning of the concept of interest or a definition according to a specific author. In contrast, qualitative research usually does not include measurements, so operational definitions are not appropriate, but conceptual definitions may be important to state.

- What limitations to the design are expected (not delimitations, which are intentional decisions about how to narrow the scope of one's population or focus)
- What the importance of the study (significance) is to the discipline

Chapter II: The Review of Research Literature (or Why You Are Not Reinventing the Wheel)

For Quantitative Research:
Organize this chapter according to the concepts in the conceptual framework in Chapter I and describe the literature review thoroughly first, followed by the state of the art of the literature and how the study fills the gaps in the existing literature. Do not include non-research literature in this section—place it in Chapter I as introductory material if the citation is necessary to the description.

- Concept 1: a brief description of each study reviewed that supports concept 1 with appropriate transitional statements between paragraphs
- Concept 2: a brief description of each study reviewed that supports concept 2 with appropriate transitional statements between paragraphs
- Concept 3: a brief description of each study reviewed that supports concept 3 with appropriate transitional statements between paragraphs
- And so on, for as many concepts as there are in the conceptual framework (I advise limiting the number of concepts for a master's degree thesis owing to time and cost constraints.)
- Areas of agreement in the literature—a paragraph, or two, that summarizes the main points on which authors agree
- Areas of disagreement—where the main issues on which authors disagree are summarized
- State of the art on the topic—a few paragraphs in which the areas where the literature is strong and where the gaps are, are clearly articulated
- A brief statement of how the study fills the gaps or why the study needs to be conducted to replicate what someone else has done

For Qualitative Research:
The literature review is usually conducted after the results are analyzed and the emergent concepts are known. The literature may then be placed in Chapter II of the proposal as shown earlier or incorporated into the results and discussion.

Chapter III: Methodology (or Exactly What You Are Going to Do Anyway)

- Design (name the design—e.g., ethnographic, experimental, survey, cross-sectional, phenomenological, grounded theory, etc.)
- Sample—describe the number of people who will serve as the sample and the sampling method: Where and how will the sample be recruited? Provide the rationale for sample selection and methods. Include the institutional review board (IRB) statement and say how the rights of subjects (Ss) will be protected, including how informed consent will be obtained and the data coded and stored.
- Setting—where will data collection take place? In quantitative research, this might be a laboratory or, if a questionnaire, a home. If qualitative, there are special considerations of privacy and comfortable surroundings for the interviews.
- Instruments and data analysis—how will the variables of interest be measured and how will sense be made of the data, if quantitative, and if qualitative, how will the data be coded and interpreted—that is, for both, this involves how the data will be analyzed.
- Validity and reliability—how will it be known if the data are good (in qualitative research, these terms are "accuracy" and "replicability").
- Procedures for data collection and analysis: a 1-2-3 step-by-step plan for what will be done
- Timeline—a chart that lists the plan month by month—use Month 1, 2, 3 instead of January, February, March.

The above three-chapter plan constitutes an acceptable proposal for a research project. The following is an outline for the final two chapters.

Chapter IV: Results (What I Discovered)

- Some researchers like to describe the sample in this section as a way to lead off talking about the findings.
- In the order of each hypothesis or research question, describe the data that addressed that question. Use raw data only; do not conclude anything about the data and make no interpretations.

Chapter V: Discussion (or How I Can Make Sense of All This)

- Conclusions—a concise statement of the answer to each research question or hypothesis. Some people like to interpret here—that is, to say how confident they can be about each conclusion.

- Implications—how each conclusion can be used to help address the needs of vulnerable populations or nursing practice, education, or administration.
- Recommendations for further research—that is, what will be done for an encore?

Index